Louis Gifford
Aches and Pains

Book Two

Aches and Pains 15-20

Nerve Root 1-5

CNS Press, Aches and Pains Ltd., Kestrel, Swanpool,
Falmouth, Cornwall, TR11 5BD, UK

Email:info@achesandpainsonline.com
www.giffordsachesandpains.com

A CIP catalogue record for the book is available from the British Library.

First published 2014
Reprinted 2015, 2016 (thrice), 2017 (twice), 2018 (thrice), 2019 (twice), 2020 (thrice), 2021 (twice)

ISBN 978 1 7399486 1 0

Louis Gifford Aches and Pains

Book 1 Aches and Pains Sections 1-14. Book 2 Aches and Pains Sections 15-20. Nerve Root 1-5. Book 3 Graded Exposure 1-4. Case Histories 1-4.

Louis Gifford MApplSc FCSP

Editing — Philippa Tindle, Mick Thacker and Paula Ross

Typesetting and
Figures redrawn by — Harriet Gendall and Julian Tredinnick

Printed and bound by — TJ Books Limited, Padstow, Cornwall, UK.

Contents

ACHES AND PAINS

NERVE ROOT

Section 15

FASCINATING STRESS

Chapter 15.1
Neuroendocrine stress systems, brains and healing

Windmills of your mind

Round, like a circle in a spiral
Like a wheel within a wheel.
Never ending or beginning,
On an ever spinning wheel
Like a snowball down a mountain
Or a carnival balloon
Like a carousel that's turning
Running rings around the moon

Like a clock whose hands are sweeping
Past the minutes on its face
And the world is like an apple
Whirling silently in space
Like the circles that you find
In the windmills of your mind

Part of the soundtrack from the film: 'The Thomas Crown Affair.' The song made the top ten in the UK charts in 1968, sung by Noel Harrison. Written by Alan and Marilyn Bergman and Michael Legrand (the original French composer).

I've already been discussing the notion that high levels of mental stress can mess with and stall the physiological efficiency of healing. We've used the phrase 'stress puts healing on hold', or perhaps more accurately, 'dampens its efficiency', for a long time now. We particularly use it when explaining things to patients and there is now plenty of evidence to support this, some of which you can easily make patient palatable.

Let's go back to some basic physiology and anatomy of the classic stress response and briefly turn our attention to two of the four major systems involved: namely, the neuroendocrine and the sympathetic systems; both of which are activated by any sort of threat or stressor, both are associated with having the capability of producing not only immediate effects, but also vast and far- reaching longer term ones too. The neuroimmune and the motor systems are the third and fourth big players respectively.

The sympathetic (autonomic), neuroendocrine and neuroimmune systems are common to a major swathe of the animal kingdom in one form or other. Their ultimate role being to 'act' or 'respond' in order to restore homeostasis, as well as 'prepare' the body's physiology for any physical action, via the motor system – that may be required. Simply, all four respond to threat and excitement in all its guises.

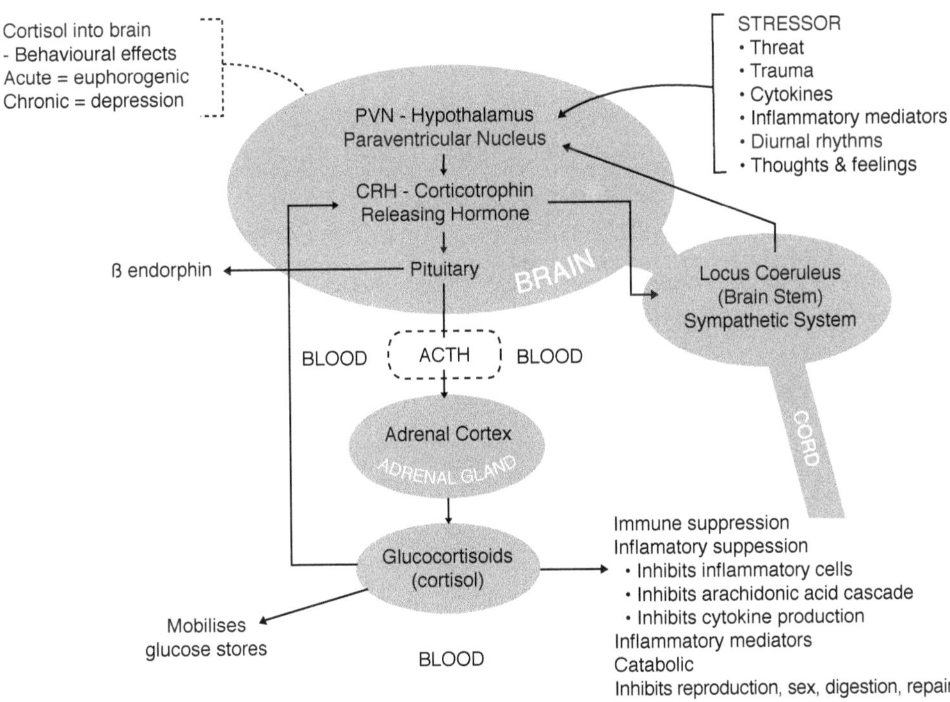

Figure 15.1 Stress System involving 'Cortisol' – the Hypothalamic-Pituitary-Adrenal (HPA) Axis.

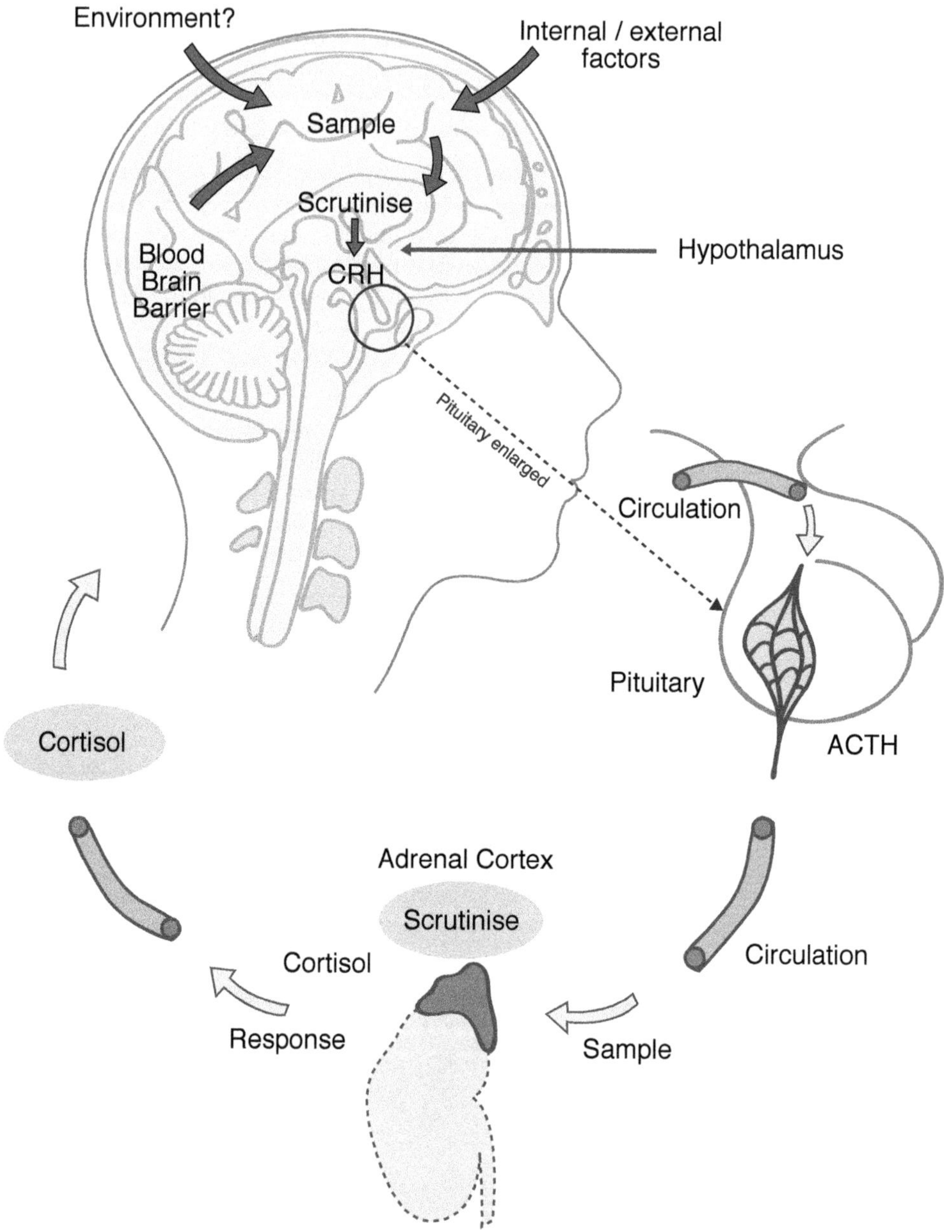

Figure 15.2a More detail of the HPA axis.

I have summarised the anatomy and function of these systems in four diagrams (figures 15.1, 15.2a & b here and in 15.8 and 15.9 later on). I'll come back to these figures very soon.

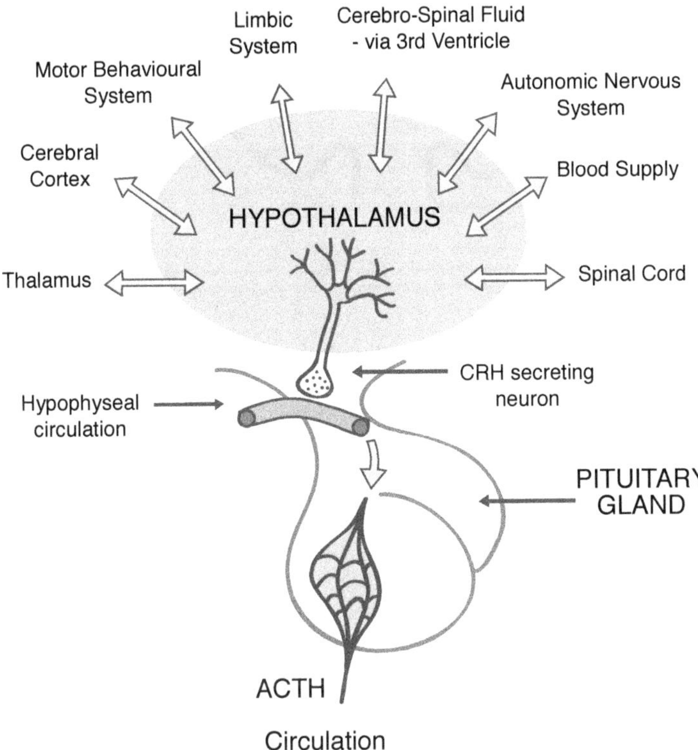

Figure 15.2b Highlighting the role of the hypothalamus and the pituitary in the HPA axis.

The neuroendocrine system was really brought into the spotlight by the work and writings of Hans Selye all those years ago. It is classically referred to as the HPA axis, the 'Hypothalamic-Pituitary- Adrenal axis.

I am no brain anatomist but there are a quite a few bits about it we should all know. It's quite hard I think, but hey, since it has been described as 'probably the most complex thing in the universe', we are excused. No we're not. If you're going to be good at understanding pain—and I think all clinicians dealing with pain should—you have to have a good grounding in the brain and how it works. The following few chapters are how I've managed to make it interesting and easy for myself as well as relevant to the patients I see. I'm hoping it will help you too?

Zoologists always look at the brain as being divided into three basic parts that moved in evolutionary terms from primitive and lowly up the scale to more advanced and more complex (check figure 15.3, it'll help you follow this):

1. There's the lowly hindbrain, termed the Rhombencephalon. Well known parts of it are, medulla oblongata, pons and cerebellum. The pons houses the locus coeruleus (ceruleus in American English), which is often viewed as the brain's centre in relation to sympathetic output. I shall return to it shortly. We've already come across the RVM – the rostroventral medulla that's involved in the

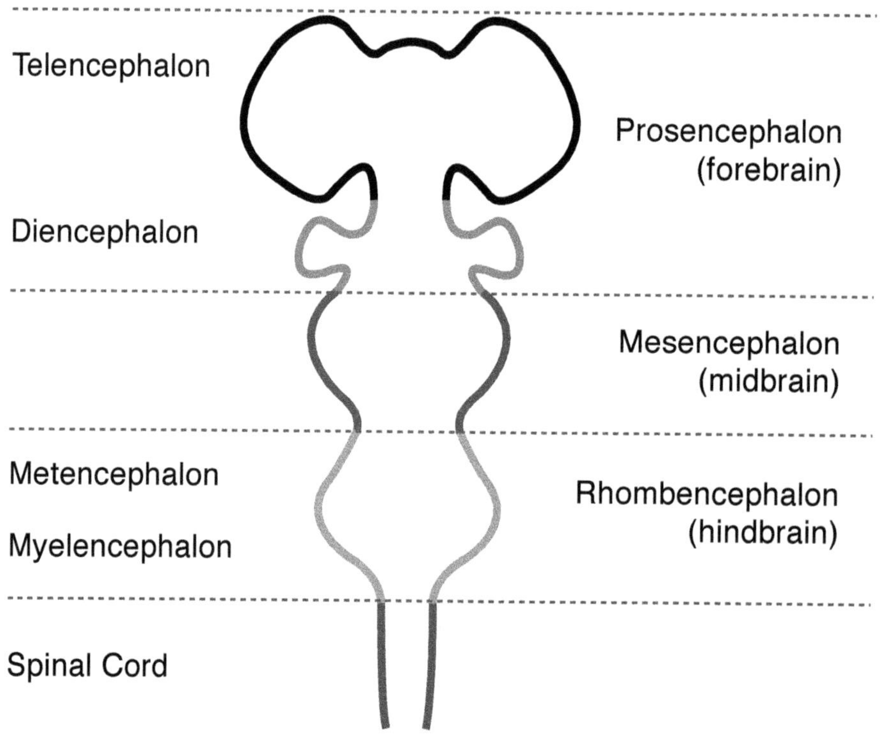

Figure 15.3 Highlighting the three basic parts of the brain and their subdivisions.

processing of nociception, it's found here too. Note also that this is where most of the fourth ventricle resides and several of the cranial nerves emerge – the vagus (10th), glossopharyngeal (9th), facial (7th) and trigeminal (5th) being well known ones.

2. The midbrain is called the Mesencephalon. The substantia nigra is probably the most well known zone for most physiotherapists as it is concerned with motor control and dopamine production.

3. The lofty forebrain, or the Prosencephalon, is further divided into: the more primitive diencephalon and the more 'advanced' telencephalon. It's the telencephalon that contains the cerebral hemispheres, those important and so massive areas of the human brain, that are said to make us who we are. For the basic stress response interest is mainly focused on the thalamus and hypothalamus – both of which are major parts of the diencephalon.

All three parts can be thought of as a simple continuum, with the hindbrain merging out of the spinal cord and then the mid and forebrains following – often depicted as a straight line with swellings at each division. Comparing embryos of all vertebrates reveals a remarkable similarity, so much so that, it is virtually impossible to tell them apart, by simple observation, in the early stages of development. The same applies to the early nervous systems of these embryos because they all conform to the same 'primitive' layout. In the more complex and bigger brained vertebrates, the massive development of the forebrain and its requirement of fitting into a limited cranial space, overwhelm the basic linear appearance and oblige it to fold, twist and turn to accommodate. Compare our brains to that of a goldfish (figure 15.4) for example! Goldfish's brains have got everything we've got; it's just that ours is a great deal larger and we've got proportionately a great deal more of the highly complex bit at the front – the telencephalon!

The hypothalamus is about the size of an almond and sits just under the thalamus and just above the pituitary (figure 15.2). With the larger thalamus it forms the major tissues of the more primitive part of the forebrain, the diencephalon. The hypothalamus sits very close to the pituitary gland and together they are famous for their role in connecting the brain to the body, via hormonal messenger release into the blood stream. In a romantic kind of way they can be seen as orchestrators of the body, dictated to by the yet higher conductor that is the thinking and perceiving brain. Well, not entirely!

Let's follow things via the figure (15.1 and 15.2):

In the stress literature the most famous part of the hypothalamus is the PVN – the paraventricular nucleus. It is this hot spot that receives inputs from the threat processing and scrutinising brain and from where it gets stimulated into action. What is fascinating is the great variety of inputs into the PVN that are able to activate it (to right in figure 15.1). Threat comes in many guises. Think: that which may come from the environment, or from the body, or from our thinking and imagination. Note how 'threat' is so open to huge individual differences in interpretation. Coming across a snake like an Adder may be of great interest to one person, yet to another, a massive source of anxiety. Modern human brains seem particularly good at coming up with 'stressors' that would be ridiculed by our wild animal cousins if only we could talk to them. 'You're worried about your finger nails cracking and you can't go out tonight because you've got split-ends? You want to come and spend a day with me...' (from a recently recorded conversation with a Polar Bear!).

Here we're obviously talking 'top-down' stressors', but there are 'bottom-up' stressors as well and they're best seen in terms of any 'threat' to homeostasis. I discuss this in detail in section 18. Trauma, injury and musculoskeletal 'disease', like osteo and rheumatoid arthritis, can all be viewed as 'threats' or 'stressors' to homeostasis.

If we look deeper and further down the microscope of 'bottom-up', we find messengers of bad tidings arriving in the brain, coming up from the stressed areas of the body – like inflammatory mediators and cytokines (interleukins). These are the chemicals that are released from injured, inflamed and healing tissues of the body into the blood, which can get their scripts heard, registered and acted upon by the brain. Remember the tuber cinereum of the hypothalamus from the 'MOM' chapter earlier (section 10). It's one of the areas of the hypothalamus where neurones can sample and 'sniff' the blood for all these messenger chemicals (see next chapter 15.2). The PVN is also notable in having 'bottom-up' type inputs from an area in the brain-stem called the locus coeruleus, mentioned just now (figs 15.1, 15.8 and 15.9). It is the sympathetic nervous system's hot spot! Put simply, it's one of the brain's

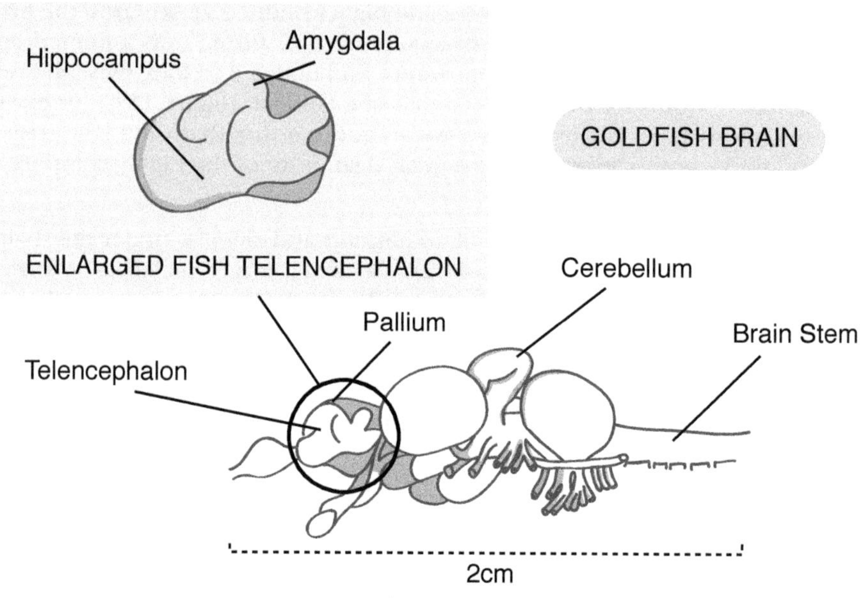

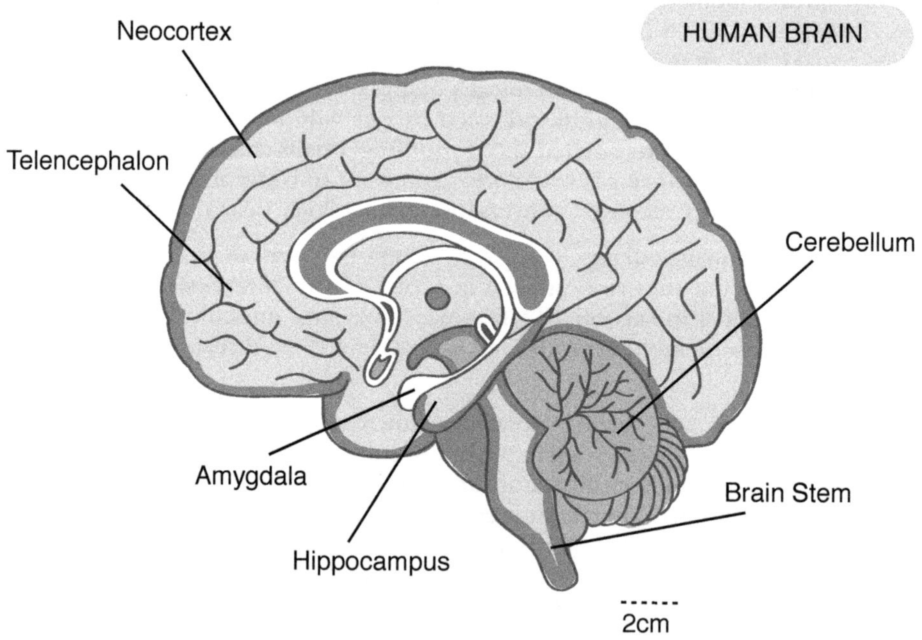

Figure 15.4 A comparison of a goldfish brain to a humans. Redrawn from: Braithwaite, V. (2010) Do fish feel pain? Oxford University Press, Oxford.

major neural 'panic-buttons'! If you're interested, locus coeruleus means 'dark blue spot' in Latin, so named because it actually does appear blue!

The PVN receives all the incoming scary and threatening stuff; so it could be viewed that it is from here that 'stress response action' gets going. Or, could it be from that ridiculous thought you had just now about finger nails! Perhaps, but what caused the thought in the first place? Remember the MOM – things always come in circular circuits: i.e. on-going 'sample-scrutinise-respond-sample again' circuits... so you can really *start* from anywhere on the circle... remember the song... *'Like a wheel within a wheel, never ending or beginning, on an ever spinning wheel, as the images unwind, like the circles that you find, in the windmills of your mind.'* Apologies, it's a song from the 1968 film 'The Thomas Crown Affair' that made the hit parade back then! I'm very fond of it. And the point of this little madness is that, if you can bring yourself to think in circles, then you can give an explanation for something beginning anywhere on that circle's circumference. Further, as you progress around it so you can pick-up more support for the issue you're observing.

So the PVN gathers all the incoming scary, threatening and exciting stuff (which includes sexual opportunity – definitely a risk taking strategy!) and off fire its neurons, that then relay to the nearby pituitary gland (figures 15.1 and 15.2b). These specialised neuro-secretory fibres are stacked with one particular neuro-hormone, 'corticotrophin releasing hormone' (CRH), which kicks off a series of events via the craziest route.

CRH gets released from these fibres at the stalk of the 'neural' part of pituitary (the 'posterior' pituitary); then it diffuses into the 'hypophyseal' circulation; gets whisked downstream for a only a very few millimetres, before being dragged out on the opposite bank of the circulation to enter the 'endocrine' or 'anterior' part of the pituitary; where it now stimulates the release of 'adreno-corticotrophic-stimulating-hormone, (ACTH for short), as well as β endorphins back into the circulation (see figures 15.1, 15.2). Robert Salposky reckons this takes about fifteen seconds and that is SLOW!

For those of you who want to get more comfy with the notion of evolution, this zany 'neural- chemical-circulatory-glandular-chemical-circulatory-and-off-it-goes' pathway, is a good example of something that is definitely not 'intelligent-design'! It's a wonderful example of evolution bodging what it's already got! (Another 'crazy-route' example is coming up when we look at the Sympathetic system!).

It's pretty obvious to state that **adreno-cortico**trophin-stimulating hormone's target – is the adrenal cortex (adreno-cortico). This is where the vast majority of ACTH receptors are found and it's where the famous stress chemical 'cortisol' is produced in the body – in the outer or 'cortical' layers of the little adrenal gland, that sits on top of the kidneys (figure 15.2a). Thus, when ACTH finally arrives at the adrenal cortex, that's several minutes by the way, it stimulates it to dump cortisol into the general circulation, which then goes off to find its target receptors and produce its effects. You'll note from the figure (15.1) that the term 'glucocorticoid' is used. It basically means steroid hormone and cortisol is just one form of glucocorticoid. 'Cortisol' is invariably reserved for human glucocorticoid. Break the word down and it explains its major function, where it's from and what it is! Hence: 'gluco' –

involved in glucose metabolism, 'corti' – from the adrenal cortex and 'coid' referring to steroid! Simple!

In figure 15.1, I've listed several effects of cortisol and you can quite happily look up the vast array of effects of it in any good textbook or online. What you find is rather dependent on the type of textbook you read, try comparing what you find in texts devoted to endocrine systems, to pain and to immunology for example. What frustrates me is that the majority of these sources never seriously look at it in terms of the 'evolutionary' 'WHY' question. Why does cortisol suppress; inflammation, the immune system, reproduction and digestion? And yet at the same time mobilise stores of glucose and stimulate glucose production? Think about it and you realise you're dealing with one hellishly powerful and far reaching chemical!

The answer to the 'WHY' question is simply that it's useful for survival!

In stressful situations what do you need?

You need vast amounts of energy – glucocorticoids stimulate 'gluconeogenesis' – the 'new' or 'neo'- genesis, or 'generation', of glucose. For example, in the liver it promotes glucose production from stores of amino acids, glycerol and lactate and/ or propionate. Also in the liver, but in muscle cells too (right where it's needed), it promotes the breakdown of the energy storing molecule glycogen (which consists of long chains of glucose molecules) into glucose. So here it's 'glycogenolysis'! ('Lysis' means breakdown). It can also stimulate the breakdown of fat – yet another source of energy should it be needed. (Starvation is clearly a form of stress/threat).

In contrast, but still basically supporting the same useful thing, cortisol halts energy 'storage', for example, it blocks the uptake of glucose and other nutrients into cells involved in storage. It effectively blocks the action of insulin, whose major role is in facilitating the uptake and storage of 'energy' molecules for use in the future. The sum total of this aspect of its action is therefore to make sure there is an adequate supply of energy (glucose) when and where it is needed.

Cortisol is often branded as a 'catabolic' steroid meaning 'breakdown' (as opposed to the opposing 'build-up' or 'anabolic' steroids so well known for their misuse by athletes and body-builders).

Think about patients on long term steroid treatments, but also think of those TV pictures of the stress of surviving in places like Eritrea, Somalia and Ethiopia, or even the disastrous and seemingly unnecessary results of 'modern stress' like anorexia. If you leave cortisol to its own devices it ultimately slowly eats you – or the bits of you that don't matter too much and can easily be replaced later on when times improve. Thus, it allows you to keep going while you wait for better times to come, or maybe to go in search of them. Long term stress, thanks to cortisol, can produce muscle weakness and wasting and loss of bone (hence bone thinning in long term stress situations). 'Slowly eat yourself' is a clever strategy to adopt when resources are very scarce and where a constant supply of energy is required! Start with the glycogen and fat stores, then when they're finished, move on to muscle. Don't waste energy on keeping bones stronger than necessary.

Tucking into one-self, though difficult to contemplate, is quite an amazing adaptation to the stress of hard times. It also helps us to see how on-going mental stress (where we think we're in dire straits, but in reality, compared to a polar bear's existence, we're being a bit pathetic), when viewed from a 'catabolic' perspective, can be physically and physiologically harmful. Remember Selye's rats – many died!

Think of the stress of long term pain and relate to, muscle wasting and not that uncommonly, loss of bone density too. The discussion here relates to one aspect, the effect of stress and cortisol on muscle and bone, the other of course, is simple 'lack of use' and deconditioning.

Time for a little aside about restricting the amount you eat and longevity (see Weindruch 1996) (This might help ease the torment caused by naming and explaining little bits of the brain!).

It was highly likely that our ancestors, in quite regular cycles, lived through times of plenty and times of hardship. All organisms do of course, but modern human ingenuity has seen to it that a few of us lucky ones, in the middle class western world, have never even contemplated the notion of hard times, particularly starvation. With not even a nod of appreciation, we blithely live in times of constant plenty – yup, most of us are over-weight and boozed-up, yielding to the ancient wisdom of evolutionary success that demands that when times are good – make the best of it, fill up, get fat and store up, so that when times get bad we'll be ready. Some of you may have noticed how easy it is to turn the calories into storage – we're fat in a jif, but also how long it takes for the fat to disappear. It is weeks, or even months to lose a modest pound or two. I recall the evolutionary biologist Steven Jones noting that if the average American stopped eating on the 1st January they'd still be fit and well on the 1st May! Think about it in evolutionary terms and you realise we're endowed with a very smart system, that kicks in when we're exposed to the fluctuating resources of nature. The two pronged rule is: 'Turn any excess calories into fat storage as quickly as possible, but only use sparingly when needed.' No wonder losing weight quickly is so difficult; we're just not supposed to do it! And, we are supposed to yo-yo!

What's even smarter, but quite startling really, is that modest starvation seems to increase length of life. For example, a white rat on a normal diet has an average life span of twenty three months and a maximum span of thirty three months. White rats on a semi-starvation diet live for an average of thirty three months with a max of around forty seven months. The life span of a flea can be increased from thirty to fifty one days simply by restricting its diet! These observations are similar across the whole animal kingdom, even in the higher mammals. Not only conferring longer life, but also in remaining 'youthful' for longer too! Caloric restriction research on animals is showing benefits in relation to brain conditions like, Alzheimer's and Parkinson's, some cancers, diabetes and cardiovascular disease. For example: results published in 2009, showed that caloric restriction in rhesus monkeys, blunts ageing and significantly delays the onset of age related disorders such as cancer, diabetes, cardiovascular disease and brain atrophy. At the time of reporting (Wade 2009), 80% of these calorie restricted monkeys were still alive, compared to only half of the controls. Think of the headline if it was a pill that would do all this! Or, the reaction if this was more widely known, 'Hardly eat anything all day? What?

To decrease the risk of horrid diseases and extend my life by a third and make me maintain my youthful looks? Sorry, can't do that, you must be mad!'

So what's the evolutionary deal here – seems crazy? Well, one proposal is that during years of famine, it may be evolutionarily desirable for an organism to avoid reproduction; to up-regulate protective and repair enzyme mechanisms, to try to ensure that it is fit for reproduction, when better times come round in the future. It seems that starvation sensibly makes you infertile; but also puts ageing on hold!

For those of you wanting to live a lot longer (and are thinking about starving yourselves), I suggest you check out the calorie restriction related web sites; or maybe forget all that and go live on the island of Okinawa in Japan. The elderly of Okinawa enjoy what may be the longest life-expectancy in the world and are also known for enjoying relatively good health while doing so. The three leading killers in the West; coronary heart disease, stroke, and cancer do occur in Okinawans, but with the lowest frequency in the world. Compared to Westerners, the islanders age slowly and are about 80% less likely to get heart disease. They're also a quarter less likely to get breast or prostate cancer. In addition, they have half the risk of getting colon cancer and are less likely than Westerners to get dementia. On average they spend 97% of their lives free of any disabilities and there is a higher than average rate of centenarians there too.

I think most of us would prefer to grab these peoples genes rather than semi-starve, but looking at their diet and lifestyle is probably worth a bit of a gander too.

Detour over, you can make that stuff into a handout for your 'I'm-soon-to-die-and-ageing-paranoid patients!

Back to acute stress and cortisol. When there's an emergency, as we've seen, you want to get all the energy you need, ready and available and in the right places and, you don't want to waste energy.

So we've evolved a means of...

- shutting down sex and reproduction
- shutting down digestion
- shutting down healing, repair and biological turnover processes...
- shutting down the immune system which requires not only energy but also many vital nutrients
- conserving what resources we have, which includes not only energy but water too
- shutting down energy 'storage' biology

Cortisol and other stress-released hormones working along with the sympathetic system's effects are all involved. Thinking or blaming 'one chemical' is just not good biology, but it's what researchers and clinicians like to do!

If you study glucocorticoids and especially cortisol you'll realise it has far reaching effects on just about every organ and system in the body. If you're clinically awake you'll also know that synthetic cortisol, for example, drugs like hydrocortisone, dexamethasone and prednisolone, have far reaching effects and side effects too!

I will discuss a few more cortisol related issues. Now that we've dealt with its role in energy mobilisation it's all about the opposite, energy conservation management.

Cortisol/glucocorticoids are the most powerful anti-inflammatories known. For example, in the arachidonic acid 'cascade' (figure 15.5), cortisol can block it almost before it even starts! I like this 'cascade' – t shows what happens when cells are smashed up and how an injury area ends up containing a pile of prostaglandins and leukotrienes.

Arachidonic acid is a fatty acid found in cell membranes, so when a cell is injured, the phospholipid membranes de-nature and arachidonic acid is released. As you can see, from this simplified diagram, what follows is a 'cascade' of chemical changes that end up producing a variety of leukotrienes, chemicals called HPETE or HETE (for those who want to blow their opponent away at 'Scrabble', 5-HPETE stands

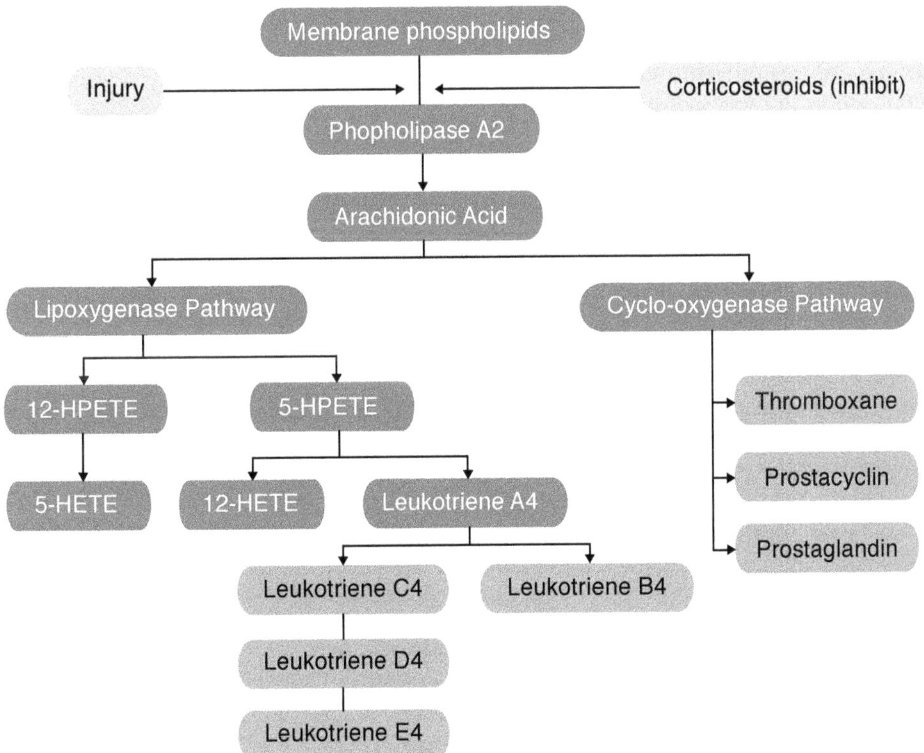

Figure 15.5 The 'Arachidonic acid cascade' Note how powerful corticosteroid is in that it can inhibit the whole cascade. Also, note on the right the 'Cyclo-oxygenase' pathway – which is blocked by NSAID's and 'Cox-2' inhibitors.

for 5-hydroperoxyeicosatetraenoic acid!) and the prostaglandins. Note the cascade divides into two; on the left, the 'lipoxygenase' pathway and on the right, the 'cyclo-oxygenase' pathway. You may have heard of Cox-2 (Cyclo-ox = 'Cox') inhibitor anti-inflammatory drugs (e.g celebrex or viox)? As you can see, this is the point in the pathway where they act to prevent prostaglandin formation. They're supposed to have less adverse effects than the more standard NSAID's that also work on this point of the cascade. This also includes good old aspirin! What you can also see from figure 15.5 is that these drugs are nothing compared to the potency of cortisol which targets and acts right up at the start of the chain and therefore puts a halt to the whole lot. No wonder synthetic corticosteroids are such powerful anti-inflammatories!

Sounds good, but if you consider that inflammation is a positive part of the early healing process, then what is really being observed is a sudden and very powerful inhibition of healing or infection control. A secondary effect of this inflammatory muting may be a reduction in nociceptive sensitisation and firing, hence a reduction in pain, which is a major requirement in an emergency that involves physical action.

Cortisol is known to be able to facilitate gene up-regulation (the switching on of appropriate genes), for the production 'anti-inflammatory' proteins/enzymes and to down-regulate genes, for the production of 'pro-inflammatory' proteins. It can also have a profound impact on the efficiency and workings of the immune system. You're quite rightly thinking that we're more prone to infection when stressed or when on long term steroid medication!
Cortisol inhibits collagen and bone formation too – as anyone who has been on

Box 15.1 - Stress and Immune Function

Further examples of stress and immune function... or the 'psycho-immune' response:-

Take one astronaut, measure their white blood cell count and the 'responsiveness' of the various cells, then send the astronaut up into space for a modest space flight... then re-measure and you'll find a significant decrease in the number of circulating lymphocytes and their responsiveness... and the astronaut is more prone to infection to boot.

I like one Norwegian investigation – these researchers investigated the reaction of the immune system in folks learning how to evacuate an oil-drilling platform. These guys have to climb a 60 foot tower get into a sealed lifeboat which is then tilted 35 degrees before being released and free-falling into the sea 60 feet or more below. They do this on four consecutive days and those who've never done it before find it none too pleasant and pretty stressful. Unsurprisingly, researchers found increases in our stress hormone cortisol, but also in prolactin and a couple of other immune 'indices'.

(Prolactin is most famous for its role in lactation – but is also an important immune regulating hormone and operates in many other areas too – in fact, as many as 300 different functions have been reported and include... effects on water and salt balance, growth and development, blood and vascular growth and development, endocrinology and metabolism, brain and behaviour, reproduction, and immune regulation and protection)...

What's brilliant is that, as many of you who've done scary stuff like bungee-jumping have found, – the more you do something scary... the less scary it becomes... (but it can still remain exciting) ... and the immune system reaction reduces in parallel with the amelioration of the 'scary' type of stress. This was found in the oil-rig evacuees.

At a more mundane level, a marked drop in cell-mediated and antibody-mediated immune function is consistently found in students at exam time. The drop in immune function again parallels the amount of perceived stress reported by the student subjects.

Even asking a subject to recall a stressful experience is enough to provoke brief reductions in immune function!

Though rather 'old' now, Paul Martin's book: 'The Sickening Mind: Brain, behaviour, immunity and disease is a must read.

long term steroid treatment can testify – you injure and strain, sprain and break more easily. Collagen and bone formation are biological 'turn-over' features and are important in relation to healing. Again, it's a 'stop-it-to-conserve resources' issue, that is fine in the short term but longer term, it sure isn't helpful.

Cortisol is one of the stronger players involved in muffling the efficiency of the immune system. Its message is basically, 'We're dampening you down guys, do your best on what you've got and when times are more favourable we'll let you get back up to speed again'.

Cortisol shuts down the reproductive system! (As you well know, you don't feel like sex when you're stressed /fighting/fleeing for your life!). Careful, it's a lot more complicated than just the one cortisol hormone. For example, you may remember in the male, the release of LH or luteinizing hormone which stimulates the testes to release testosterone and FSH, or follicle-stimulating hormone, which simulates follicles in the female, but promotes sperm production in the male? Both are released from the pituitary, except when there's stress about and the whole lot shuts down. And, as Robert Sapolsky puts it 'The testes close for lunch'! Stressors like injury, illness, starvation and surgery all drive down the male reproductive axis and that famous hormone of hairiness, muscularity and masculinity, testosterone! Think long-term stress and you can see why so many fertility problems exist. What's interesting is that the key inhibitory chemicals involved here are brain endorphins – which may help us to understand why male extreme athletes (40-50 miles a week!) have small testicles, low sperm counts and therefore aren't very good at making females pregnant. Sorry, that's a blanket statement, which is never going to be entirely true. There are bound to be a great many male super-athletes who are quite capable.

The female side of things is far more complex and I would highly recommend the reader devours Robert Salposky's book 'Why Zebras don't get Ulcers' for all the wisdom required in relation to stress biology and the human state. It's a must read. One note about females, is that it is wise biology for her reproductive system and sexual desires to go into temporary shut down when things aren't looking so good. According to Salposky, in humans the average pregnancy costs approximately 50,000 calories and nursing costs about a thousand calories a day – that's a huge investment. So, environmental stressors: like lack of resources, poor nourishment and hard work day-in-day-out to find nourishment; and in the modern female situation, things like exercising all the time, for example, serious dancers, runners; but also intentionally starving to lose weight (at worst anorexia) and on-going mental stress – all work against the likelihood of fertility. If you investigate any of these you're highly likely to find evidence of reproductive dysfunction.

It's important to mention that cortisol levels in the circulation are monitored by blood sampling sites in the brain (see figure 15.1, 15.2a, and chapter 15.2 next) which in the case of cortisol, will relay what's found to the nearby hypothalamus. The hypothalamus then scrutinises the cortisol levels and can adjust its' controls to get the level just right for the situation the brain and its body find themselves in. This is a good example of a negative feedback loop. Thus, when cortisol levels rise in the blood the hypothalamus gets to know and will decrease its activity. When blood levels drop it will increase again. That's what you learn in biology class anyway. It provides for a nice steady state. Unfortunately, life is just not like that. For a start there's day and night; normal humans have two very basic phases to their lives, awake and active and asleep and inactive. Cortisol is found to be at its lowest levels at about four in the morning and highest around eight am. I've never seen anyone put forward an explanation for this, but for me it fits nicely with the release, or 'disinhibition' of full-on healing, replacing, regeneration and immune system activity. Low nightly cortisol allows it all to run blissfully unhindered, then at around six to eight am, when cortisol levels now rise, it all gets turned-off to allow the body's resources to be re-focused and ready for the trials and tribulations of the forthcoming day... Numskull night shift manager on the tannoy...

'Calling all night workers please put healing, fighting infection and repair at low priority now lads, he's getting busy; resources are needed for the daytime shift. Cortisol will be along shortly to make sure you're all tucked up and in bed. Thanks for a good night's work, sleep well and see you all again tonight.'

What's interesting is that this nice steady diurnal fluctuation is easily disrupted by stressors. For example a loss of normal diurnal cortisol variation is found in; clinical depression, psychological stress, illness, fever, trauma, surgery, fear, pain, physical exertion, temperature extremes, rheumatoid arthritis and the list goes on.

These are all things that we meet in our day to day dealings with our patients (they're all 'stressors' and/or relate to on-going stress!). It underlines to me how important it is to try to help patients get back to a much better sleeping pattern and routine. Part of this is to deal far better with the stress/stressor if at all possible of course. Explaining this stuff to your patients is vital if they are to see the point of better sleep habits and tackling their main stressors.

We also need to acknowledge that there is a degree of variability in any one person's responses relative to another. A meditating yogi's cortisol level rise may hardly register when an unexpectedly sudden loud noise occurs, whereas it is likely to be massive in you or I, or beyond massive in anyone in a high anxiety state. The stressor's the same in each, the reaction certainly is not.

How responsive we all are is influenced by many things, here are a couple of them:

1. How high the response setting is in its normal resting baseline state. This has may have inherited as well as acquired components (e.g Pennisi 1997). Thus one can be born with a stress/HPA system whose activity causes baseline levels of cortisol to be continually above average or continually below average. This baseline can be further shifted up or down by environmental/ experience factors through early years and into adult life – like on-going unresolved stress, which I'll be discussing later (section 20).
2. How reactive or sensitive the response is. This has inherited and acquired components too. The system may have a relatively normal baseline level, but when provoked by a stressor, may respond massively or hardly at all. Environmental factors, like life experiences, may push it further one way or the other. Thus a novice yogi may have a hyper-responsive cortisol system but after years of meditating this becomes far less reactive. On-going stress may push the response further in either direction, thus a 'hypo' (weak) responder, may become even weaker and an over-responder, may become a mega-super responder. I will discuss this 'dysregulation' of the stress response further in the 'on-going stress' discussion (section 20).

Now, what I'm getting at is that because we are all so variable, the impact of stress on healing has to be variable too. For example, stress may have far more impact on slowing healing in those who are HPA axis hyper-responders, because of high levels of cortisol, whereas those who are 'hypo-responders', those with too low cortisol, may find that inflammation runs on out of control and is excessive – leading to messy tissue destruction! Either way, the result isn't good!

I hope you're all alert and thinking that this cortisol reactivity could all be reduced down to explanations involving 'receptor populations' and whether the receptor populations are in an active state. I've just thought of an interesting piece of mind-body type research. Would it be possible to take a highly reactive stressy person – measure their cortisol release threshold/sensitivity, then send them on a yogic meditation course for a year or two and then retest. The control group could just go on holiday perhaps? I'll bet it's possible to a greater or lesser degree to lower the stress response and create a calmer person without drugs. It's called 'conditioning' or perhaps 're-conditioning', if you think about it! The problem is that it may take a lot of practice and considerable time and effort. (What a great research project!).

Gulf War Syndrome next!

Chapter 15.2
Supersensitivity problems: the blood-brain barrier and Gulf War Syndrome

Masters Of War

Come you masters of war
You that build all the guns
You that build the death planes
You that build all the bombs
You that hide behind walls
You that hide behind desks
I just want you to know
I can see through your masks.

You that never done nothin'
But build to destroy
You play with my world
Like it's your little toy
You put a gun in my hand
And you hide from my eyes
And you turn and run farther
When the fast bullets fly.

Like Judas of old
You lie and deceive
A world war can be won
You want me to believe
But I see through your eyes
And I see through your brain
Like I see through the water
That runs down my drain.

Bob Dylan, 1963

I have been mentioning the blood-brain 'sampling' sites and thought it worth a brief excursion into a bit more detail.

As most experienced therapists know many 'chronic' pain patients have multiple problems: it's not just the pain, they have problems with digestion, with food intolerance, with various allergies, with tiredness and lack of energy and so on and so forth. I've observed this for years. We often say in our clinic that there is no such thing as a simple patient – if you really listen to their story; and the longer they've had the problem the more complex things generally become. Whilst reading about the blood-brain barrier, I came across some interesting research related to 'Gulf war syndrome'. I wondered whether there's a linking process here to the various hypersensitivities, allergies and energy related complaints that our chronic pain patients mention so often? First of all though, a more detailed look at the blood-brain barrier.

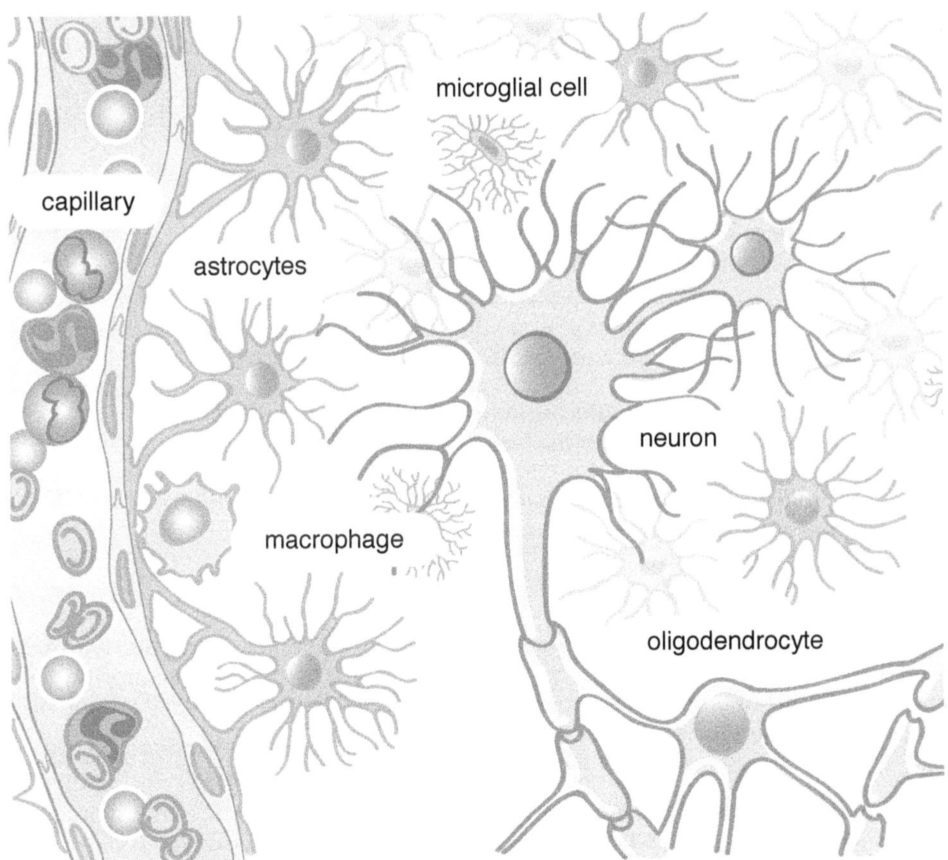

Figure 15.6 The wonderful but rather neglected Glial cells! An illustration of a few of them – especially the astrocytes and their relationship to the capillaries of the Central Nervous System. Redrawn from: Fields R.D. (2011) The Hidden Brain. Scientific American: Mind. May/June pp 53-59.

The brain is relatively well isolated from the blood and hence the rest of the body, by the blood-brain barrier. In order to do this, the vast majority of the capillaries of the brain and nervous system are unique in their ultrastructure and physiology. They are composed of a single layer of very tightly joined endothelial cells that are surrounded by a basement membrane and then invested by a continuous layer of astrocytic foot processes (they can be seen on the left of figure 15.6). What are astrocytic foot processes? Well, you may recall that the central nervous system contains not only nerves but also 'glial' cells, in the biology texts I studied in the early 1970's and up to the early 1990's, they were always described as 'packing cells' or 'glue' cells. Glial cells are now under great scrutiny, (and a big research topic that my friend and physiotherapist colleague, Dr Mick Thacker has been involved in). Glial cells are now thought to be vital; not only in terms of holding neurones in place, but also, in the supply of nutrients and oxygen to neurons; in providing insulation, in providing a defence against pathogens and in their ability to remove dead neurones. Most fascinating of all is that they have also been found to be involved in information transmission and neuro-modulation. In a recent Scientific American Mind journal article, Douglas Fields noted that:

- neurons make up only 15 percent of our brain cells; glial cells make-up the rest!

  Consider that the human adult brain has around 80 billion brain cells, that means there's around 480 billion glial cells! And consider this in relation to the number of stars in the Milky Way, estimated to be between 100-400 billion! Start travelling across the Milky Way at the speed of light and it'll take you around 120,000 years. Wow, Glia! How many light years would it take to follow every possible avenue that there is in one person's brain?

- glial cells control communication between neurons and play a central role in learning, but for years they have been dismissed as mere putty

- most neurological and some psychological disorders involve glia, so new therapies are targeting these cells

- keep your eye on glial research!

As you can see in figure 15.6, astrocytes send out long tentacle like arms that spread out into 'feet' around the capillary. So, the end result of all this is that for the most part, the blood-brain barrier is very 'tight', in that it doesn't easily let any old Tom, Dick or Harry molecule into the brain.

In the capillaries of all other organs there are pores and channels between individual endothelial cells, through which water and solutes and hence messenger molecules can easily pass. Indeed, when there's been an injury the endothelial cells contract and cause these pores to widen; to the extent that even cells can squeeze through and take part in the inflammatory and healing process. Because there are no pores or 'gaps' in CNS capillaries, for substances to leave and enter the brain, they have to actually pass through the endothelial cells, their cell membranes and the feet of the astrocytes!

The barrier is therefore not absolute, it's not a total barrier, essential substances can pass through the membranes and across the material of the endothelial cells. Think energy, glucose and of course, a great deal of oxygen which needs to get over easily and so too, any metabolic breakdown products leaving. Substances that cross easily tend to be small lipid soluble molecules (cell walls are made of lipoproteins and therefore allow lipid soluble molecules through). Large complex molecules, including most proteins and many drugs, because of the barrier, are completely excluded from the brain, under normal circumstances. However, smaller substances like glucose and many amino acids may be actively transported across the membrane. This means that they are grabbed by receptors lining the inner wall of the capillary, swallowed, spat out on the inside of the cell, transported through the endothelial and astrocytic cytoplasm and finally ejected from the outer astrocytic wall into the brain.

Messenger molecules in the blood that cannot traverse the barrier may still influence brain activity via second messenger systems (see figure 15.7). For example, messenger molecules like interleukin-1 interact with receptors on the lining membrane of capillary endothelial cells. This leads to a cascade of messenger system activity within the cell that ultimately influences neuronal cell activity on the 'other' side. In figure 15.7 you can see how interleukin-1 (IL-1) leads to the production of cyclooxygenase in the cell and then the release of prostaglandins into the nervous system. Prostaglandins act as neurotransmitters or 'messenger' molecules when in the brain. Try not to think they're just involved in 'inflammation'; unfortunately for the pharmaceutical industry and medicine, that relies on it, there's no such thing as a biological molecule having just one function. That's a joke and a nuisance to them.

Interestingly, this tight barrier function is absent from a few small specialised regions of the CNS, such as the anterior of the third ventricle (near the hypothalamus), the tuber cinereum of the hypothalamus, the pineal gland, and the area-postrema of the caudal fourth ventricle. It is in these selected regions that the blood has a far freer and more direct access to the brain than anywhere else – and the areas that I like to refer to as the brain's blood 'sampling' sites! It's where the brain sniffs and tests the contents of the blood.

Now back to Gulf war syndrome! Gulf war syndrome refers to a controversial illness involving a plethora of signs and symptoms that a great many returning veterans suffered following the war that ejected Sadam Hussein's forces from Kuwait after they invaded it in 1990. Typical symptoms include: headache, memory loss, diarrhoea, fatigue, muscle pain and cognitive problems. Suggested causes have included a raft of nasty chemicals that the soldiers may have been exposed to. These include muck like, depleted uranium, sarin gas, smoke from the hundreds of burning oil wells, as well as the vaccinations soldiers were given to try to prevent the ghastly effects of Saddam's various chemical weapons! It will be interesting to see what comes of the current situation in Syria and Assad's use of chemical weapons (I'm writing this in October 2013).

Research by Friedman and colleagues (see Crystall, 1996), found that the brains of laboratory mice that were put under stress, could take up drugs and other substances in the blood up to 100 times as readily as the brains of unstressed mice.

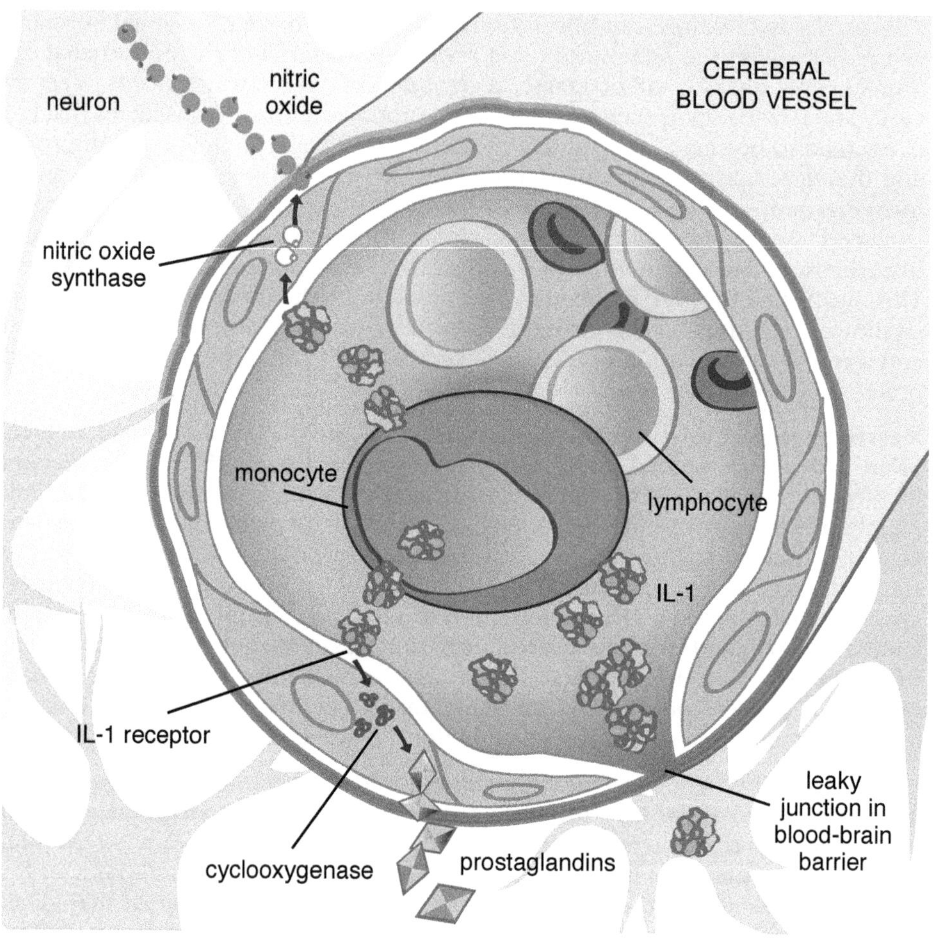

Figure 15.7 Capillary and the blood brain barrier. Redrawn from: Sternberg E.M., Gold P.W. (1997) The mind-body interaction in disease. Scientific American Special Issue: Mysteries of the Mind. June pp 8-15.

The researchers were looking into the effect of a drug used to protect Israeli soldiers from the effects of nerve gases. The drug, pyridostigmine, was thought to be unable to cross the blood brain barrier, but in the soldiers there were strong signs that it did. As a consequence, they suffered almost three times as frequently as expected from side effects that involved the CNS, such as headaches and drowsiness. In *stressed* mice, the researchers found that the dose required to protect against nerve gas was **1%** of the dose needed to produce the same effect in unstressed mice! The effect of the drug on a peacetime group of human subjects showed side effects, more related to peripheral nervous system, such as sweating and diarrhoea. As the investigators reported, 'The pyridostigmine was not getting through to their brains' (Crystall,

1996). The suggestion is that during the stress of combat, or potential combat, the blood-brain barrier becomes more diffuse and porous (Crystall, 1996). The Darwinian message is that this is a very adaptive activity: when a body is under stress, the brain wants to make all its sampling systems as acutely sensitive as possible, so that it can derive the best possible updates about what is going on. It's just the same as our pupils dilating when something frightens us. The other message is that if you want to get drugs quickly into the brain, get excited, wound-up or even better – get scared!

So, back to our patients: I hope the reader can see that the on-going stress of a pain condition may well lead to an increase in 'porousness' of their blood-brain barriers. To the extent that the 'normal' day to day toxins in our environment, relatively harmless to most of us, can actually cross it and get into the brain. The result: cognitive problems, memory difficulties, coordination and balance dysfunctions, headaches and generally increased sensitivity; not just to pain, but to a great many environmental toxins that are normally easily dealt with and have little or no deleterious effects.

Chapter 15.3
The Sympathetic Nervous and the Immune System

The sympathetic nervous system's 'schematic' is shown in figure 15.8 and 15.9. In the stress literature this system is often referred to as the LC-NE system, the locus coeruleus-norepinephrine system. Remember that epinephrine and norepinephrine are american for 'adrenaline' and 'noradrenaline'.

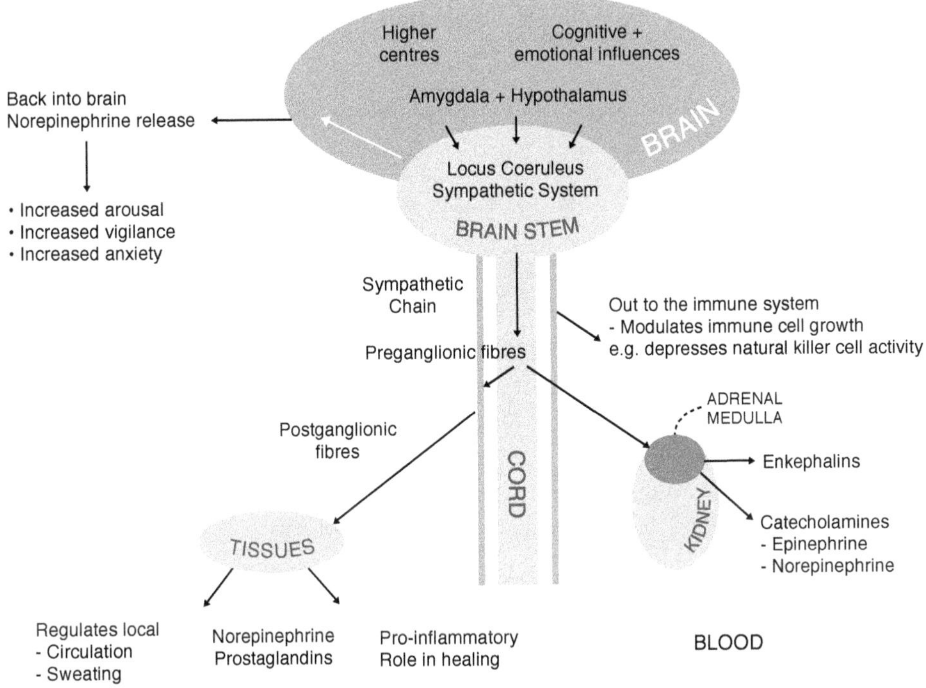

Figure 15.8 Stress and the Sympathetic Nervous System.

I don't know about you, but as a student, I remember finding the autonomic nervous system's anatomy and whereabouts almost sickeningly complex. So, I decided to sort that out and with my great friend and colleague Mick Thacker we wrote the first chapter in 'Topical Issues in Pain 3' (Gifford 2002, re-published 2013). Let me suggest that you study and read that chapter if you're the slightest bit nervous about the autonomic nervous system's weird wiring. It's yet another example of 'unintelligent design', or more correctly – of how evolution bodges along making do and adding to what's gone before. What's beautiful about it is that while it looks crazy and complex, it works and for that reason needs our appreciation! Try to get to know it a bit!

Let's say that you're walking home at night taking the short-cut through the cemetery – just a little bit creepy but you're OK, you've done it loads of times before. Suddenly there's this odd click-click noise and you instantly stop and peer about you trying to see what it might be. Your heart-rate's up, pounding away and you're pupils are dilated, trying to take in every little bit of light that's available. How did that happen? What's the wiring for pupil dilation?

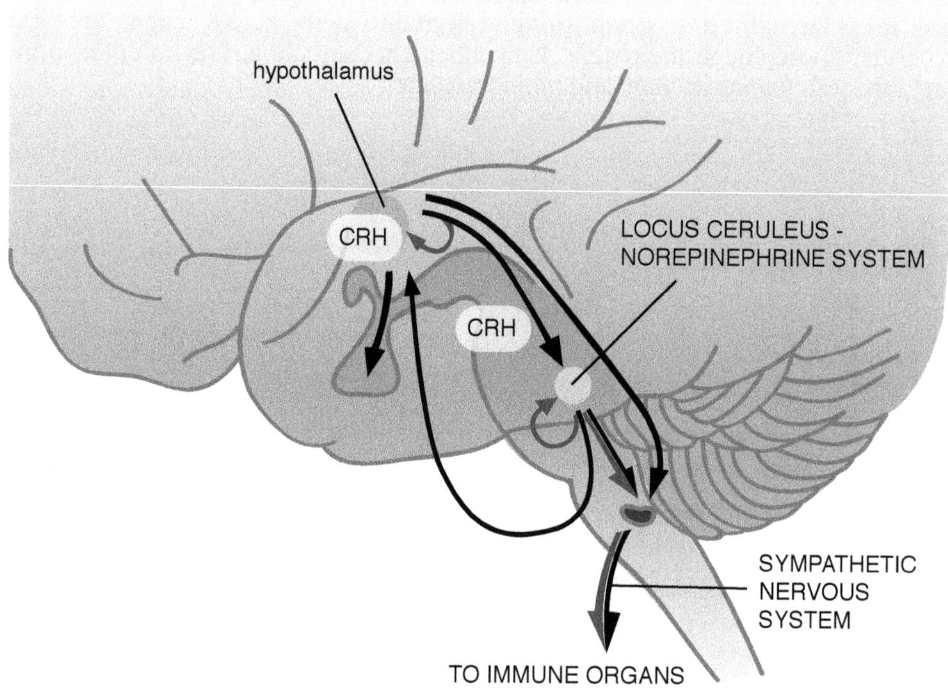

Figure 15.9 Illustrating the Locus Ceruleus-Norepinephrine System emphasising its links to the HPA axis (hypothalamus and pituitary), as well as output via the spinal cord to the immune system and the peripheral Sympathetic nervous system. Redrawn from: Black P.H. (1995) Psychoneuroimmunology: Brain and immunity. Scientific American Science and Medicine 2(6): pp16-25.

Well, your 'fear' modules have processed the situation and made you feel uneasy, your thalamus and amygdala (they're major threat processing centres deep in the forebrain) are just short of over-drive. Incoming signals, central fear and threat processing are not only making 'you' aware, but are also going straight out again to the hypothalamus, as well as on down to the brain-stem and the locus coeruleus, with the command which runs – 'Squadron, situation a little dodgy, let's get everything ready just in case!' And, amongst a whole pile of other parallel commands (heart rate up, respiration up, circulation to legs for possible running, etc.), there's also a sub-conscious message, 'I also want to be able to see better and take in everything I can, excuse me guys – could you dilate my pupils please.'

So, from the brain stem, impulses travel down the spinal cord in the neck to about the level of T1-2 in the upper thorax. Then, via the 'lateral horn' of the spinal cord, travel out of the vertebral column in preganglionic sympathetic fibres that course along the ventral (the motor) nerve root. Then, quickly branch off just outside the intervertebral foramen, to go, via the white rami communicantes, to join the sympathetic chain that runs up and down adjacent to the antero-lateral aspect of the vertebral column. On go the impulses following the chain upwards into the neck, to the superior cervical ganglion which is situated adjacent to the vertebral bodies of cervical vertebra 2-3. The impulses from the preganglionic fibres then neuro-chemically vault the synapses and move on in a posse of post-ganglionic fibres that go back up into the skull and eventually find their way to the papillary muscles of the eye! 'Dilation achieved, Sir! At ease, men...'

From a design point of view that's about the stupidest route to take to make the pupils dilate! Down from the brain into the spinal cord of the neck... then on to the upper thorax... then out of the cord and outside the vertebral column, to go back up to the head and to the eye. Think how far that would be in a giraffe! Compare how far it would be 'As the crow flies', in other words, from the brain stem straight to the eye (two inches maybe?) and the actual route (at least twelve!).

It's a crazy system anatomically – hey but it works and it probably works quickest in those with shorter necks! The thing about Giraffes is that they're not particularly frightened of much, because they're so big, so the need for instant pupil dilation isn't quite as urgent as in us smaller beasts!

Some of you may have come across Horner's syndrome – a condition caused by disruption of the sympathetic supply to the muscles of the pupils and eyelids. The end result is a droopy eyelid – 'ptosis' (from the Greek meaning to droop!) and a very constricted pupil, due to the loss of sympathetic supply, with subsequent paralysis of the muscles involved. The big deal clinically is that one should consider possible causes from the sympathetic chain in the neck and upper thorax. Think of it as a peripheral neuropathy affecting the sympathetic motor supply to the muscles of the pupil and eyelid.

I have seen Horner's syndrome several times in my career, most associated with whiplash, but one who presented with an acute upper limb nerve root problem affecting C8 with marked and rapid onset weakness of the C8 muscles in the hand. I saw the patient one week into his problem. I also noticed he had a droopy eyelid and constricted pupil – Horner's syndrome. He was actually the plaster technician at the old St Stephen's Hospital in London. Lovely fellow. I sent him back to our orthopaedic consultant with a quickly scribbled note:

Tom, RE: our colleague Derek

'Could we have an x-ray/review? Concerned something more serious as rapid onset of weakness in C8 distribution plus has Horner's syndrome. If thinking sinister... could it be a Pancoast tumour? He doesn't look too well to me.

Thanks, Louis, will do.

And so it proved. Sadly, two weeks later Derek died.

Section 12 discussed the role of the 'sympathetics' in the tissues at length and revealed that a lot of what goes on is not necessarily an-all-or-nothing type of response; but a very much controlled and focused one, dependent on local needs and conditions. It is also dependent on the 'general' needs and conditions too.

All I want to emphasise here is the role of the sympathetic system and of adrenaline and noradrenaline when we are mentally 'stressed'.

The sympathetic system, in contrast to the HPA system, is far faster because it is mostly impulse driven right to its targets. Hence, there's a sympathetic nerve supply direct to the lungs, the heart and all the blood vessels; with the result that blood, plus oxygen, plus nutrients gets quickly shifted to where they're needed most and diverted away from where they're needed least – places like the gut and your penis and so on...

In my 'aches and pains' lectures I always liked a little mention of the gut, because we often deal with pain patients who also have gut-related problems, like 'irritable bowel' syndrome. It's a big topic, but it's good to realise that when we are under stress the last thing the body should be wasting energy on is digestion and gut stuff. When we're relaxed, thanks to the parasympathetic system and a muted sympathetic system, the gut is happily writhing away (peristalsis!) churning, mixing and breaking down the gut contents. When we get stressed, there's a mega shut down of it all, the gut becomes motionless (pun slightly intended!) and digestion/absorption is also put to sleep. Then some spark in my lecture puts up their hand and says. 'Hang on a minute, when I'm nervous I get diarrhoea and want to 'pee' all the time – my guts are super active.'

Smart-ass is right. Think like this: lighten your load a bit (less weight to run with) or 'Don't-need-to-digest-but-do-need-to-dump', plus, we're all part skunk from time to time – not only are we a tad lighter, it also makes a pongy smell and a revolting mess, which may just put a predator off long enough to outsmart them and give you a good start. While the rest of your gut shuts down, the far end of it gets super active, but after that, the sphincters do clamp shut and allow you to get on with saving your bacon. Athletes love the loo prior to a race, but don't have to take a break after they get going. (I know, runner Paula Radcliffe managed a famously discrete and very quick p-wee in front of the telly cameras – but that was the marathon. It prompted the Sun newspaper to headline with, 'Easy peesy for Paula' – that was 2005). Take any animal by surprise and it usually deposits a quick one in your direction as it turns to flee. Don't pick up a toad... and there's a toadstool called the 'Stinkhorn' – smells of rotting flesh or dung and looks like a male phallus, hence the genus it belongs to, Phallaceae. I knew you were interested? Oh, a question from that man at the back... 'What's the smell for?' 'Good question, it's to attract flies. Who adore the odour, who go to investigate and eat the foul-smelling slime. At the same time, they pick up the spores on their feet and ingest a few too... and the fly henceforth provides a free and very effective dispersal service.'

As I think I mentioned in an earlier stress chapter, researchers measure stress levels in mice and rats by counting the number of poo-pellets they do. Also, to turn our attention to the front of the house, water in the bladder is of no use to you at all. It's actually out of your system, so you may as well get rid of it, it makes a nice smelly mess to go with the other and lightens the load a bit more. Your system thereafter wisely goes into water conservation mode, which means that our stress chemicals soon get the kidney to put the brakes on urinary excretion. Our body wisely holds onto as much water as possible while we're busy and may need it. Note that cortisol and hence steroid drugs are renowned for causing increased weight via water retention – the need for water-retention when running or fighting for your life under acute stress is the reason why.

Ongoing stress may shift the system either way. Take a patient with diagnosed irritable bowel syndrome and stress them while recording what's going on in their lower bowel. You stress them by sticking their hand in freezing cold water or another way is getting them to try and make sense of two conversations going on at once. Those, who have a tendency towards chronic diarrhoea, show a far greater bowel gastrointestinal response than healthy controls and those, with a tendency towards constipation, show the most activity in their small intestines and least in their large. How interesting is that!

What dictates the dysfunctional response, as always, is our inbuilt tendency to shift one way or the other and the nature of the stressor. For example, a stressed mouse confined to a cage will keep popping out poo-pellets, but allow it out of the cage and chase it around and it'll soon stop! As I said just now, you get the runs before the big match or lecture but once you've started, even though the stress continues, it all magically disappears! Got the runs? Get active, get chased! Got constipation? Get in a cage with a Rottweiler. Some say being in a lift that suddenly drops three floors makes you 'let-go' in all departments.

Back to the diagram (figure 15.8, 15.9). Appreciate that the sympathetic system, by forming and infiltrating a massive network of nerves and nerve plexi (including all the well known somatic nerves – like the ulnar, radius, sciatic, femoral etc. and all those in the abdominal cavity supplying the viscera – which makes it massively divergent!), reaches and supplies just about every tissue in the body. As we discussed in section 12, sympathetic release of adrenaline and noradrenaline influences local healing and pain chemistry. Sympathetic activity also controls the circulation by acting on the smooth muscle lining of arterioles and venules. It is a small and reasonable hop to see that, what is going on in the brain and what is going on in the mind of the individual, can easily and quickly influence, what is going on in the tissues – from inflammation and healing: to the gut, the cardiovascular system, 'to infinity and beyond[1]'...

One area of note is that like the HPA axis, the sympathetic system also stimulates the adrenal gland to release hormones into the circulation; this time to release adrenaline, noradrenaline and enkephalin (an endogenous opioid, like endorphin) from the adrenal medulla (see fig 15.8).

To some extent adrenaline appears to support the actions of cortisol. For example, it shuts down insulin production in the pancreas (which prevents glucose storage) and it stimulates glycogenolysis (breakdown of glycogen into glucose) in the liver and muscle and glycolysis in muscle. What's neat about adrenaline is that it gets to the targets quicker and then gets backed-up by the more slowly releasing cortisol. Adrenaline release is quick because the adrenal medulla is stimulated via preganglionic sympathetic nerves, whereas the adrenal cortex has to wait for CRH to arrive via the circulation, which takes minutes to occur. Remember, preganglionic sympathetic fibres are 'white', because they are myelinated – hence are fast conductors. Most preganglionic fibres, like those I described taking impulses to the muscles of the pupil in the eye, actually synapse either in the ganglia of the sympathetic chain, or a little nearer their destination in special ganglia. For example, the most famous ganglia outside the two sympathetic chains are the celiac and the superior and inferior mesenteric ganglia.

1 - Toy Story – Buzz Lightyear's catchphrase.

'Ganglia' are just sites of enlargement where synapsing goes on. It's where myelinated preganglionic neurones meet their non-myelinated postganglionic fellows who then take the message, but rather more slowly due to their lack of myelin, to the final destination.

Ganglia are thus like little junction boxes. It shouldn't be forgotten that, sensory afferent fibres relaying 'sampling' messages 'in', also pass through these ganglia and that they send little collateral branches to the pre- to post-ganglionic fibre synapse area. Evidence is mounting that a degree of modulation or gating may well take place particularly in relation to 'gut' reflexes like digestion, water conservation and peristalsis as well as inflammation or any threat to local homeostasis. Think bladder or gut infection and you're onto it.

(Read Gifford and Thacker's chapter: A clinical overview of the Autonomic Nervous System, the supply to the gut and mind-body pathways'. Chapter 1 in Topical Issues in Pain 3).

So the point I was getting to, before being distracted into sympathetic ganglions and the thinking-feeling-touchy-feely potential of the gut, was that the adrenal medulla is supplied, directly and quickly, by myelinated preganglionic fibres. What happened to the post-ganglionic fibres in this pathway then? It turns out that the adrenal medulla embryonically derives from post-ganglionic nerve tissue; thus the 'chromaffin' cells of the medulla are actually modified post-ganglionic cells, that then secrete our two friends adrenaline and noradrenaline, plus some dopamine too. This is a brilliant example of evolution needing quicker action to service 'fight or flight' physiology and finding that it can make 'do' with what's already there by modifying it a little.

Let's get back on track, well on and off!

Most interestingly is the relatively recently discovered finding that lymphoid and immune tissues throughout the body, plus tissues like bone marrow and the thymus, where immune cells develop, are innervated by the autonomic nervous system (see all the Watkins refs – note there are two Watkins's and both are stars of the psychoneuroimmune research world!). It seems that the nerve fibres of the sympathetic and parasympathetic system are able to modulate the development and activation of immune cells. Here then is yet another pathway that links the brain to the body. The birth of the science of psychoneuroimmunology or PNI, in the early 1970's, has been a major breakthrough for those of us interested in the effects of the way we think and feel on the health and healing of the body. It's good to have a few names of historical figures here and also to know a little of the progression to how it all came about:

Claude Bernard, in the mid 1800's, gave us his 'mileu interieur' – the internal steady state of the body and how any perturbation of it led to 'adjustments'. Walter Cannon coined the word 'homeostasis' in his book 'The Wisdom of the Body' in the early 1930's. Cannon is famous for earlier linking emotional state to changes in gut movement and the fight-flight-or-freeze response. Then follows my hero Hans Selye; with his stress research, the General Adaptation Syndrome and the focus shifting from adrenaline to cortisol/glucocorticoids. All good early 'mind-body' stuff, but the real start of it all was in the mid 1970's with Robert Ader who, with Nicholas Cohen, founded the science of PNI and coined the phrase. Ader sadly died in 2011, but their work is well worth reading still (see Ader refs). They were good at conditioning the immune system of rats and showed that the immune system could learn. Here's the story and like most discoveries in science, it was serendipitous!

Ader and Cohen were studying a form of behavioural conditioning called 'learned taste aversion'. In their research they gave rats a novel sweet drink (saccharin sweetened water) and then injected them with a drug called cyclophosphamide to make them feel sick. The rats soon learned to avoid the water, because of the consequences, but then it was noticed that the rats conditioned in this way started dying in quite large numbers – like Selye's story! The more sweet water they had drunk, the more likely they were to die. The key was that cyclophosphamide was also an immune suppressant, it often being used to prevent transplant rejection. They smartly rationalised that the neutral stimulus, the sweet drink, actually conditioned the rats' immune systems to be suppressed and then lead to ill-health and eventual death.

To test this hypothesis they conditioned a number of rats with sweet water at the same time as the drug injection. Three days later they gave the rats more sweet water, this time on its own. They then tested their immune function by measuring the number of antibodies they produced in response to an injection of red blood cells from a sheep! (Sheep's blood cells are clearly foreign and therefore will be powerful 'antigens'). The results showed a marked drop in antibody production compared to non-conditioned rats. The conclusion: that the sweet drink on its own, without the drug, could reduce the immune response. The finding that changes in immune function, both positively and negatively, can be brought about via seemingly psychological stimuli has been replicated time and again since Ader and Cohen's early work. Experiments have also shown that immune conditioning can alter the progress of arthritis, cancer and many other assorted diseases too!

Must read: Paul Martin: The Sickening Mind: Brain, behaviour, immunity and disease.

Best reference work: 'Mind-body Medicine: A clinicians guide to psychoneuroimmunology. Edited by Dr Alan Watkins

A final thought or two. Try not to only think of the immune system in relation to 'infection' e.g. coughs and colds. The immune systems cells and messengers work hard at; controlling and reporting, putting you back together, clearing up the mess from toxins and injury and maintaining your health; from the surface of your skin to the depths of your bowels. Just like the sympathetic nervous system, it's more than everywhere. From astrocytes and oligodendrocytes in the CNS, to leukocytes, monocytes, macrophages and mast cells out in the tissues. The immune system has fantastic, almost 'smart', sample-scrutinise and respond capability! Not only that, it informs the brain and the brain communicates back and controls and influences its activities too. That the way we think and feel can influence it is hardly surprising.

Let's now move on to look at some good hard evidence for brain-body links that are useful for our patient interactions.

Chapter 15.4
Stress, wound healing and surgery

'A lie gets halfway around the world before the truth has a chance to get its pants on.'

Winston Churchill

The mid to late 1990's saw a distinct surge in research investigating the effects of stress on wound healing. I'm glad I was there.

It's interesting and easy to explain to patients, when appropriate, so I'll outline a few of the findings and results found. I suggest you try to remember the basic gist of a few of these to relate to your 'non-healing/slow healing' patients when you want them to try and wind down a bit. Remember our phrase 'stress puts healing on hold'... or better, 'stress slows healing and it's proven.'

Let's start with rats and mice before moving onto humans. You can easily stress a mouse by sticking it in a clear plastic cylinder that only just fits round it. One end of the cylinder is closed except for a hole for the tail; the other end is open so the mouse can breathe. The mouse is effectively experiencing a similar feeling to what you get if you're pretty fat and you get put in an MRI scanner, but worse – because the tube it's in is slightly squashing it and it can't move its legs. It's called 'restraint stress'!

Researchers take a mouse, make a skin wound, stick it in the restraint apparatus every day for a period and then observe how long it takes to heal. They do this with several mice and then compare the healing rate to the exact same injury produced in control mice that are blissfully carrying on their simple lives in laboratory paradise; where there's not a care in the world, there's plenty of food and predators just do not roam and there's on-going in-house entertainment to fend-off boredom. There's even a daily cleaner to sort out the overnight mess.

So, they wound the mice in both conditions and then observe the healing. The wound is produced using a miniature punch, hence the term 'punch biopsy', which removes a thick-ish bit of skin tissue. They find that the wounded 'restraint-stressed' mice heal 27% slower than the 'non-stressed' ones. Not only that there's also an increased susceptibility to wound infection. Mice subjected to restraint-stress for three days prior to punch-biopsy exhibited 2-5 times greater growth of staphylococcus at the wound site compared to the non-stressed. Of course once infected this further compounds the healing rate and the result is more scarring at the end. Examining the site of the wound in restrained mice reveals far fewer neutrophils, monocytes and macrophages, all of which are essential for clearing bacteria early-on and providing essential enzymes and growth factors for new tissue deposition. Interestingly the stressed rats, as you might expect, had higher levels of circulating glucocortcoids (corticosterone); which as we know puts the breaks on healing and the immune response. Researchers found that if they introduced a glucocorticoid receptor blocking agent (to effectively stop the steroid from working), the healing rate improved to that of the control rats. It was also found that stress reduced the level of gene expression for inflammatory substances (cytokines) like interluekin 1 (IL-1) and tumour necrosis factors (TNF), chemical messengers vital to attracting and recruiting inflammatory cells (see section 11). Again, block the glucocorticoid receptors and the genes function normally!

Excellent stuff!

I'm sitting here now thinking that there's a sniff of irony in the atmosphere. What does medicine do when there's a wound? Immobilise, restrain and stop! Putting a mouse in a restraint tube isn't a lot different from tucking a wounded human up in bed for hours on end, or 'restraining' the wounded part in a splint or plaster! Hmm! I'm old enough to remember patients being put in trunk plaster-casts for low back pain! Don't forget doing nothing to a human (mentally and physically), let alone a mouse, can be a huge stressor in itself. Surely the same applies to a bit of a limb too and the trunk plaster-cast isn't far off a 'restraint device' either!

And on the same lines: I had a patient the other day who had a knee problem, a sharp very localised pain under his knee cap, it bothered him when he ran so he stopped running. Other than that he wouldn't know he had it and carried on doing everything most ordinary folk do. He can jump, squat, kneel, do the shopping and everything else you can think of. Is that a big deal? Well, for him, yes, he usually runs seventy or more miles a week, he's one of the country's top all terrain ultra-marathon athletes and being unable to run drives him nuts. As far as he's concerned he's restraint stressed! Checking out his 'at rest' cortisol levels might be interesting! I'm wondering if one day therapists will have a bit of kit that gives a continuous read-out of circulating cortisol or adrenaline levels? We could maybe then teach them to do 'biofeedback' to bring it up or down to their 'normal' (we'd have to know the 'normal-range' for that patient though, whatever that might be). For now, the best thing for my obsessive patient is to keep him going at something, so he's off on the bike (no pain – fire-apart-depart!). Surely, much better than going, there's an easy medical answer let's give the dude glucocorticoid receptor blocking agents, or some pain killer or anti-inflammatory and tell him to rest!

Now, stressing humans! Take a volunteer, make a punch biopsy wound and stick them in a tight tube with a hole for their tale! Well, nearly. Researchers take folks who live stressful lives, often carers looking after loved ones with Alzheimer's or dementia and compare them to age-matched controls that live in bliss. What they find in these chronically stressed individuals is that their immune systems are significantly dysregulated. Janice Kiecolt-Glaser's group (1995) revealed that **care-givers took nine days or 24% longer to heal a small standardised punch biopsy wound than did the well-matched controls**.

From the same lab of researchers (Marucha 1998): in a study of eleven dental students given mucosal punch biopsy wounds in the hard palate (ouch!), it was shown that **they healed an average of 40% slower during exams compared to when on holidays**.

These researchers (Kielcolt-Glaser et al 2005) also use what they call standardised 'blister wounds'. What's good about blister wounds is that they can easily sample the blister contents and check the levels of cytokines/interleukins being produced. They typically found that in parallel with slowed healing there were much lower levels of these bio-markers. For example, researchers 'blister' married couples and find that **those with consistently high levels of hostile behaviour towards each other heal at as much as 60% of the rate of couples with low hostility** and unsurprisingly, that their cytokine levels (IL-6; IL-1; TNF) are lower. Ha! Want to get that cut finger to heal faster? Get a divorce! The number of times I've heard fellow physiotherapists say that such and such a patient won't get better until they leave their home situation! Maybe they had a point!

- high levels of cortisol in morning blood samples predicts slowed healing too
- if you're a worrier and you go for surgery and that makes you even more worried, you're highly likely to heal more slowly
- if you're a worrier and you're in a lot of pain after surgery – you'll heal more slowly.

Janice K-G's group did a neat trial of punch biopsy wound healing and pain in women undergoing elective surgery. **What they found was that the healing was slowest in those women who experienced most post-operative pain.** In these it was shown that their immune responses were dysregulated – there was suppression of normal lymphocyte proliferation and increases in pro-inflammatory cytokine responses. **However, using adequate analgesia brought this response back to normal.** It seems that the stress of the pain had a powerful immune dysregulating effect and slowed their skin healing. The researchers were keen to point out that **pain medication in those who were not in pain actually suppressed the immune response and slowed healing** compared to those who were not in pain and didn't have the analgesia! The lessons from this are (useful to tell your patients):

- **use pain killers when it is hurting,** it reduces the stress caused by the pain which in turn allows the immune/healing system to work better. With the warning that if you use pain killers when it's not hurting you may be messing the immune response up. Unfortunately medicine/pharmacology doesn't like you to take pain killers PRN very much. (PRN is Latin, prō rē nātā and used in medicine to mean 'according to need')
- **pain slows healing** and that **pain plus other stress slows healing even more**
- **stressed humans heal up to 60% slower**
- Whatever you do don't go into the operating theatre having had an argument... with your partner, the surgeon, the nurse, the anaesthetist, or anyone of significance to you!

Over the years quite a few of my patients have either opted for surgery or I have recommended they consider it and seek advice on it for their problem. I'm talking of joint replacement surgery and even back surgeries like microdiscectomy and facetectomy; which if done well, will remove material that impinges on and compresses symptomatic and malfunctioning nerve-roots with minimal injury or disruption to the area, or that's the theory (and maybe another story for later).

I'm mentioning this because surgery is often a source of great anxiety and it is well known, though not by surgeons who should know it, that outcomes are strongly governed by psychosocial factors. For example in a fairly recent review of evidence for surgical outcome and psychosocial factors, Rosenberger et al (2006) stated (my bold added – because this is what I often point out to my patients who have been told they need surgery and are anxious about it, of which, more shortly):

> *'Results indicate that psychosocial factors play a significant role in recovery and are predictive of surgical outcome, even after accounting for known clinical factors.* ***Attitudinal and mood factors were strongly predictive****; personality factors were least predictive. The results suggest that preoperative consideration of attitudinal and mood factors will assist the surgeon in estimating both the speed and extent of postoperative recovery.'*

It also seems that if you're fearful of dying from an up and coming operation you're more likely too! (Ahhh, let your wish be fulfilled! Self-fulfilling prophecy is so interesting...) Anyway, such is the concern about this that some informed and wise surgeons are cancelling operations if they hear such premonitions from their patients. I found the following statement from a surgeon on the website 'Medscape today'.

> *'I have personally had the experience of a patient in the holding area for surgery state he didn't feel right before he went to the operating room for his gall bladder removal,' says a surgeon. 'I assured him things would be fine, and he would be okay. He coded on the table and died 3 days later. I have heard other patient's state that they think they are going to die and it happens. So, if a patient says that to me now, surgery is cancelled.'*

Over the years I've seen many patients who have OA in the hip or knee. I've helped to keep them going through the bad patches, as well as helping them to keep strong and maintain their activity levels and ranges of movements. The amazing thing is that large numbers who thought they were heading for surgery actually managed to put it off for a great many years and some completely. Eventually for many though, there's a point when surgery becomes a major option to consider.

Right now **Sylvia** has popped into my head. A very fit lady, a great walker and very active gardener who came to me with her right knee problem over twenty years ago. The knee had obvious early degenerate changes, with joint thickening and a modest loss of flexion (five inches heel to buttock distance on the right compared to about one inch on left) and extension (lift heel off couch while preventing the knee lifting = nil lift-off on right and about 1 inch on left), some movements were accompanied by a bit of noise. She was great, she diligently did all her exercises, she was chilled with flare-ups and keeping going – even continuing with badminton. With the help of my input and her regular 'keep-it-going' exercises she recovered about 80% of the ranges she had lost within about six months of first seeing me. Over the years she paid me occasional visits for what could be called 'top-up reassurance' sessions; plus a bit of good 'freeing' hands-on to get the knee range better and mollify any concerns! About five years ago she visited feeling very distressed and fed-up, with the knee not responding to her usual management strategy and that she was in need of help. She'd had to stop walking beyond the necessary round the house and shops and was finding herself resting and taking it easy more and more. I examined the knee and it was significantly stiffer and thicker than before. It was also noisier with clear bony crepitus as she walked. Pleasingly there was no valgus or varus deformity. Sylvia was 71 then, slim and otherwise in good shape, not on statins and had normal blood pressure. An x-ray of her knee done about three years previously showed 'marked degenerative changes' in both compartments of the right knee.

I treated her and gave her lots of advice and suggestions over three treatments spread out over about six weeks. This included all the standard NSAID's, good pacing, good non-aggravating joint maintenance exercises; easy cycling; heat and/or cold – if it helps – self massage etc.

At the third session she frowned and said she hated to say it but that while she did have odd good days overall she was going backwards. I want the reader to note here that with some patients like this I will persist for a lot longer – simply because OA flare-ups can last for many months. But for Sylvia I knew the joint was already bad, and when there's weight-bearing bone-on-bone crepitus things really aren't good, especially for someone so active. Her joint will inevitably get worse and worse and she will inevitably lose overall mobility and fitness. For someone so naturally active and healthy joint replacement so often makes a massive difference. My local Golf club is full of ex-patients who say that their joint replacement was the best thing they'd ever done, giving them a grand new lease of life. Back to Sylvia:

'How do you feel about getting a surgical opinion on it Sylvia?'

'Oh God! You know I'm don't want any operations, my Mum died on the operating table and I've got two friends who've had new hips and they now wish they'd never had them. I'm not keen to be honest.'

On further questioning it turns out that her Mum had multiple problems, wasn't at all fit at the time and was in her early 80's. Sylvia's two friends were physically rather slothful, always had some sort of pain going on, were always moaning about their health and were both significantly overweight at the time of their operations.

She then said...

'Are you thinking I need a knee replacement?'

Amazingly, the thought hadn't even entered her head. Most patients are at completely the opposite end of the spectrum, asking me if they're going to need a joint replacement when there are only very mild changes going on and I have to do my best to persuade them to stay well away from the surgeon and the thought of joint replacement.

I went on...

'Sylvia, no one has to have a joint replacement if they don't want one, but I'll give you one view that's maybe worth thinking about. It's this: that the best outcomes with surgery for joint pain, like knee replacement, occur when the recipient is fit, well and naturally active by nature and above all very positive about having it. I find that there is almost an ideal time to have a new joint and that's before it gets so bad that the sufferer gets significantly less mobile and as a result lose their general fitness. Those who are fit going in come out fit and do well. If your fitness is poor, your mobility is restricted, your fitness will be low and the outcomes are never as good – maybe that happened to your two pals?'

'Sylvia, you could have a very good outcome, you're a good candidate for a good outcome, but a key thing is to be convinced about wanting to have the operation and convinced that you're going to do well with it! I'm telling you this because when you compare those people who go into an operation feeling positive and hopeful, with those who are fearful and pessimistic about their outcome – it's the positive ones who do by far the best. Believe it or not, a posistive attitude is one of the most powerful predictors of how well someone is going to do. The other powerful predictor is actually the mood of the patient!'

She was smiling and nodding, I carried on...

'Let me give you an example of a good outcome of a patient just like you but older! This fellow was in his late 70's when he visited me with a knee just like yours is now. He was a keen golfer and played three times or more a week, so he was fit and enjoyed being active. However, he was really struggling with golf and he was using a golf cart rather than walking and he wasn't enjoying it! He then had his knee replaced, he's back walking the golf course and he's now 85. I saw him about four months ago for a shoulder problem and his words about the knee were, 'Brilliant boy, I wish I'd had it done ten years ago'. He's not a one-off, he's the rule rather than the exception, but that's only when the patient is well, fit and positive going into the whole thing.'

'If you feel you'd like to talk with a knee specialist at anytime I'll put you in contact.'

Syliva looked at me, paused and said, 'I'm going to discuss it with my husband Barry before I do anything.'

'Good idea, remember, you've only discussed this with me, I'm not the surgeon but you know I've seen many of these before. There's no obligation to have an operation but just getting an opinion from a good knee surgeon is wise action right now. If you decide you don't want to go anywhere near it... I want you to know that there are plenty of bloody-minded people out there carrying on perfectly well without having an op. They accept that this is the way it is and just get on with life with their limitations and cope fine.'

'Tell your husband if he wants a chat with me to phone, and if you have any questions, to phone, I mean it.'

Sylvia returned some weeks later after being reviewed by the knee specialist.

'I saw Mr Hackett FRCS like you suggested and he showed and explained the x-ray and a further scan he had done. He says the knee is badly worn and just like you he said I was a good candidate to get the most out of a new knee joint, so I've decided to go ahead with it.'

'Good! But tell me, are you feeling positive about the operation and doing well with the new joint?'

'I had a long chat with my husband Barry and we both decided that given your advice and Mr Hackett's I had nothing to fear. I guess like anyone would be, I'm obviously a little anxious.'

I offered her some more success stories and she listened eagerly – there was the 85 year old: who had terrible bilateral knee degenerative changes and incredible knock-knee (valgus) deformities in both; who could barely walk more than 100 yards with two sticks; her height increased by five inches after having both joints replaced because her legs were straighter and she could stand-up straight; who within one year of the second knee replacement was practicing getting down on the floor and getting herself back up; who then walked daily over two miles. Or the 65 year old who went back to skiing after giving up over ten years before.

I continued.

'Right, you've got six weeks before the operation – you mustn't give up on the exercises and you must also continue to keep the pain under control the best you can. We have a motto here which is, 'the fitter you go into the operation, the fitter you come out and the quicker you get back to normal activities.'

Luckily Sylvia found the cycling did her good and wasn't too demanding or upsetting to her knee. By the time she went for the operation she was actually able to cycle well for around an hour! I rang her up three days before the operation to ask how she was feeling and to wish her well. 'I'm good, naturally a bit anxious, but I'm looking forward to a new life with a new knee most of all,' – was the essence of the conversation. She did excellently and within six months was back to normal walking and by around eight months was starting badminton again. Five years on now and she's 76, still walking daily, still doing aqua-aerobics and still playing badminton!

The big point here is that the information I gave her was positive and realistic and she ended up being positive about the whole process – getting matching messages from me, the surgeon and her husband.

Spending time is worth it. But note my communication style is biased towards what's often termed 'information-giving', 'advice-giving' or even 'advice-dispensing' and not what's more formally called a 'patient-orientated' or 'patient-centered' communication style. Medicine always favours the first. It's almost as if patients have come to expect to be told what to do and the majority of Drs want to do just that, they dictate, they tell the patient what's wrong and what they <u>have</u> to do and so do we! Unfortunately dictating hasn't a good record. 'Stop smoking, give up the booze, go on a diet, or as with Sylvia, 'Don't be apprehensive, be positive', just doesn't often work for a great many patients. Here though, I had her respect, she trusted me and she wanted my advice.

Good communicators adapt the style of communication to suit the patient and the needs of the moment. Note that Sylvia was a compliant patient who required information and reassurance, who took advice on-board, who was comfortable enough with me to be able to challenge anything that didn't seem right or that didn't work and who had a generally positive outlook. I always try to go out of my way to be non-confronting and non-dictatorial. If on the other hand her problem had been more overwhelming, with plenty of 'yellow-flag' /psychosocial and behavioural issues, the communication would have to be adapted to stand any chance of being productive. The style required has to be patient-orientated, of which more in the 'communication' sections later.

I expect some of you are thinking about all the joint replacement disasters you've had to deal with, and yes, I have too. The notable thing about most of these patients is that they've often been badly prepared in the first place, they're often not at all fit – they have significant yellow flags. Gordon Waddell, the well known author of 'The Back Book' is the only surgeon I've ever come across who tries to triage patients prior to surgery (here spinal surgery) in order to rate them as likely or not likely to have a good outcome. I go into this in detail in chapter GE 3.2. For now, the key predictors that Waddell found were psychosocial. This is important, but I would add two other things: first, like I said above, be fit and positive about the outcome going in to the op and second, find a good surgeon.

A note now on bad behaviour!

As most of you know when you're fed up, a bit low, a bit stressed or a bit wound-up or tired out – you tend to behave 'badly'. In the old days it was grab a fag and a glass of sherry, these days it's grab a Jack-Daniels, roll a spliff or even snort a line of cocaine! Some of us just stuff ourselves with whatever's in the cupboard or fridge. Overload yourself with too much of anything and you're diverting the bodies resources to an unnecessary emergency, having to deal with and get rid of 'excess', plus the accompanying toxins too. No wonder those who indulge in bad behaviour have slower healing. In our clinic we underline the notion of 'create the best conditions for healing to be at its most efficient' and we list the following sorts of things (sometimes I tailor them to the individual and print them out):

1. Get stress as low as possible (stress slows healing dramatically, tell that patient about those experiments from earlier)

2. There are generally two types of stress; one is the stress related to this problem, the other is the stress from all the other things in your life!

3. If you are still worried about what's wrong or what's going to happen, let me know so we can discuss further.

4. Good balanced diet and avoid toxins. Why make your body work harder sorting out toxins when it's got plenty to do getting you healed! Sorting out toxins slows healing. Try to avoid over-eating, drinking, smoking and recreational drugs. Give your body a chance to concentrate on recovery rather than on having to deal with poisons that can be avoided.

5. Drink water, but don't overdo it, your kidney's can get overloaded.

6. Cutting down on caffeine is often helpful.

7. Good sleep is essential – you heal most when sleeping well (caffeine reduction can help here)

8. Exercise every day if you can. Make it more than you usually do if possible, but it must be relaxed and enjoyable. Start with the suggestions we've come up with?

9. Good social support speeds healing and recovery.

   Socialise! But try not to tell everybody about your ailments over and over again – that's boring (even if you're dying, the folks who keep listening to you going on and on will eventually wander off and you'll be left alone). Plus, if you keep talking about your problem your head doesn't get a chance to think about or do anything else.

10. ...and so on... to fit that particular patient.

Maybe have some of these up your sleeve to convert to easy messages...

1. A sample of twenty five women had a 'skin-barrier' wound created by stripping the equivalent of sellotape off their skin over and over again! (This removes a few layers of skin cells and disrupts the skin barrier). They were then deprived of sleep for 48 hours, examined and compared to non sleep deprived with the same wound. The wound healing was significantly slowed and there were easily detectable alterations in immune profiles as well as in growth hormone levels. Growth hormone aids healing, for example by stimulating monocyte migration, enhancing macrophage activation and amplifying bacterial killing macrophages. Growth hormone is released during sleep!

2. Nutrition: too low an intake of glucose, fatty acids, protein and certain vitamins may all affect wound healing.

3. Alcohol: heavy use of alcohol slows healing.

4. Smokers v non smokers – equates to slowed healing in smokers.

5. 'Slobbing' about doing nothing physically slows healing.

6. Try not to be anxious, depressed or lonely! The research tells us that if you're lonely you respond less well to vaccination, are at greater risk of developing high blood pressure and have poorer sleep. Combine loneliness with low mood, depression and anxiety and it's really not looking at all good (Bosch et al 2007)!

7. Even though temporary hypoxia stimulates the wound healing process early, as time goes on it really requires oxygen and any ongoing hypoxia delays things or slows it. For example, hypoxia is known to amplify the inflammatory response to maladaptive levels, hence causing tissue destruction.

8. The best way to improve oxygen supply to tissues in most of us is via exercise. For example in one study, older adults who completed a four week exercise intervention of one hour a day for three days a week healed a standard punch biopsy wound 25% more quickly than less active counterparts. This was despite levels of stress reported!

9. There's no such thing as being unable to do some form of cardio-vascular exercise.

10. Social contact and support – hamsters subjected to restraint stress who were 'pair-housed' (i.e. kept within sniffing distance of another restrained hamster!) had significantly lower cortisol levels than those who were isolated. Amazingly, the restrained and pair-housed hamsters healed just as quickly as those who were non-stressed. Maybe we should pair up our pain and stressed patients a bit more?

11. See the 'Pink flags' chapter (GE 4.9) later!

Check out any medication that's being taken:

1. Steroids: glucocorticoid steroids taken as anti-inflammatory agents are well known inhibitors of healing. As we've seen, the naturally produced hormone has global anti-inflammatory effects; it suppresses fibroblast proliferation and collagen synthesis, causes insufficient granulation tissue formation, reduces wound contraction and so forth. Paradoxically though, topical application (i.e. directly onto a skin wound) of low dose steroid on chronic wounds accelerates healing, reduces pain and exudates. Nothing in biology is as straightforward as we'd like it to be! As I said before, if you want it to be – become a dentist, or leave humans completely alone – try engineering or car mechanics perhaps?

2. The evidence for NSAID's isn't as strong, but remember the pain killer research earlier, if you're taking pain killers in the early healing phase when you're not in pain, the immune response is suppressed and healing slows. As discussed, this rather flies in the face of standard medical practice which is to take the pain killers regularly regardless of the level of pain: three times a day for two weeks being a common NSAID prescription.

Hopefully the reader will now have enough knowledge and ammunition to understand and explain to the patient the links between physical and mental stress and healing?

Section 15
Read what I've read

Ader R., Cohen N. (1991) Conditioning the immune response. Netherlands Journal of Medicine 39: 263-273.

Ader R., Cohen N. (1991) The influence of conditioning on immune responses. In Ader R., Felten D.N., Cohen N. Psychoneuroimmunology (2nd Ed). Academic Press. San Diego.

Ader R., Felten D.L., Cohen N. (1991) Psychoneuroimmunology (2nd Ed). Academic Press. San Diego.

Ader R., Grota L. J., et al., (1991) Behavioral adaptations in autoimmune disease susceptible mice. In Ader R., Felten D.N., Cohen N. Psychoneuroimmunology (2nd Ed). Academic Press. San Diego.

Bosch J.A., et al., (2007) Depressive symptoms predict mucosal wound healing. Psychosomatic Medicine 69:597-605.

Crystall B. (1996) Stress leaves the brain wide open to drugs. New Scientist: 12:21.

Fields R.D. (2011) The Hidden Brain. Scientific American Mind: 5/6: 53-59

Gifford L. S. (2013) Topical Issues in Pain 3. Sympathetic Nervous System and Pain. Pain Management. Clinical Effectiveness. CNS Press. Falmouth.

Jones S (1999) Almost Like a Whale: The Origin of Species. Doubleday. London.

Kiecolt-Glaser J.K. et al., (1995) Slowing of wound healing by psychological stress. Lancet 346:1194-96.

Kielcolt-Glaser J.K. et al., (2005) Hostile marital interactions, pro-inflammatory cytokine production and wound healing. Arch Gen Psychiatry 62:1377-1384

Marucha PT 1998 Mucosal wound healing is impaired by examination stress. Psychosom Med 60:362-365.

Martin P. (1998) The Sickening Mind: Brain, Behaviour, Immunity and Disease. Flamingo. London.

Medscape today - http://www.medscape.com/viewarticle/711634

Pennisi E. (1997) Tracing molecules that make the brain-body connection. Science 275: 930-931.

Wade N. (2009) Dieting Monkeys Offer Hope for Longer Living. New York Times 2009-09-10.

Watkins A. (1997) Mind-body medicine. A clinicians guide to psychoneuroimmunology. Edinburgh, Churchill Livingstone.

Watkins A. (1997) Mind-body pathways. Mind-body Medicine. In Watkins A. (Ed). A clinicians guide to psychoneuroimmunology., Churchill Livingstone. Edinburgh.

Watkins A. D. (1994) Hierarchical cortical control of neuroimmunomodulatory pathways. Neuropathology and Applied Neurobiology 20: 423-431.

Watkins L.R. (2000) The pain of being sick: Implications of immune-to-brain communication for understanding pain. Annual review of Psychology 51: 29-57.

Watkins L.R., Maier S. F., et al., (1995) Immune activation: the role of pro-inflammatory cytokines in inflammation, illness responses and pathological pain states. Pain 63: 289-302.

Weindruch R. (1996) Caloric restriction and aging. Scientific American 1:32-38.

Section 16

THE BRAIN

Chapter 16.1
What's the brain for?

'I will not let anyone walk through my mind with their dirty feet.'

Mahatma Gandhi

We all possess this organ that can somehow allow us to see, feel, hear, smell and be involved in making us able to think and talk about the world we live in and our unique experiences in it. That the brain we humans posess is probably the most complex thing in the universe is a humbling thought.

What's the brain for then? A very good question! For those who've done a bit of biology, a common reply runs: 'Well, it's sort of for organising things.' I agree, but it's also worth contemplating some examples of life without a brain or nervous system; little things, like bacteria, viruses and single celled organisms, but also fungi and then the whole of the amazing plant kingdom. Yes! So raise your hats to the massive Wellingtonia, the giant Redwood tree, each one serenely whiling away a life of several thousand years on the often cold but sun-drenched western slopes of the Sierra Nevada in the USA. Hail Wellingtonia! About the tallest (nearly 300 feet high) and most massive of life-forms that has ever lived on our planet and it hasn't even got a nervous system to 'sort of organise things!' Top plant it is: and along with the Bristlecone pine, the humble Dandelion, the garden Bramble and my favourite British wildflower, the common Toadflax; the giant Redwood tree has to be one of my favourite living, surviving and reproducing machines. The beautifully twisted and gnarled, but not quite so grand, Bristlecone pine is perhaps extra-extra special because it has the unique accolade of being the longest living of any *single* organism that has ever lived. One such tree the Americans called 'Methuselah' was measured by taking a horizontal core sample (they count the rings) in 1957 and they found it to be 4,789 years old. More recently (2013), a Bristlecone pine in the same area has been found to be 5,063 years old, meaning it was germinated in 3,051 BC! Top organism, I hope you agree? Just think of the history that tree could have witnessed if it had had a brain with a memory module!

Size is a big factor as far as nervous systems are concerned, but the main factor may just be movement or 'behaviour' which is what movement is called when we observe it. If you get much bigger than an amoeba and you want to move, you need a nervous system to coordinate it and make it happen. If you ever get the chance though, try and observe a paramecium under a microscope (see paramecium moving about on the YouTube link in 'Read what I've read'). Here is a tiny, single celled organism that zips about its environment at remarkable speeds. It bumps into things, reverses up and goes this way and that, all by using incredibly well co-ordinated waves of cilliary action. It turns out that the cilliary waves are co-ordinated via changes of ionic charge across its cell membrane, very similar to the waves of ionic movement that occur in all nerve impulses. This is primitive use of controlled electricity and it may well be where the nervous systems of the animal kingdom evolved from.

Most animals move and to move a 'big' animal requires pretty rapid co-ordination and control. When you need speed, you need electricity. If the thing chasing you has electricity and you haven't – you've had it dude!

Plants generally don't move actively, so they get eaten by organisms with electricity. OK, some plants do move, you've thought of the Venus flytrap! Oh and Mimosa, the sensitive plant (and there are many others too). The mechanism of their exceptional reaction/movement may just happen to involve ionic movements across membranes and even action potentials to kick them off, followed by a very smart interplay of hydrostatic and elastic factors. But for most plants communication via fluid flow and diffusion serves them well and is all they need. A great many just have to put up with being eaten from time to time and they've evolved ample ways to deal with this. It's a good job plants haven't got a nociceptive system attached to consciousness. That they've got some kind of threat sampling/nociceptive system, isn't in doubt, it's just not electrical and doesn't produce conscious awareness.

So, there are plenty of examples of immobile organisms like plants, that don't move and which have no electrical communication systems that could rightly be called nervous systems; and there are a very few rather quirky plants, that do have a bit of movement, who still really haven't anything like a nervous system.

Now, thinking along the same sort of lines. Could there be any animals which don't 'move', which don't have nervous systems to add weight to this 'movement/behaviour-requires a nervous system' hypothesis? Answer: yes, the sponges. Next question: are there any animals which don't 'move' that do have nervous systems? Answer: yes, the corals and sea anemones. But here, even though there's no movement typical of more obvious 'animals', there is actually Venus flytrap-like movement. If you stick your finger gently into the 'mouth' of a sea anemone, its body will withdraw and its mouth will rapidly close. This coordinated protective response is thanks to a rather primitive nerve network acting on muscle-like cells to produce the 'behaviour'. Time lapse photography of a rock pool soon demonstrates that anemones do physically move and do battle with each other. So they're out of this argument.

Lastly on this, my diversion-excursion and zoological indulgence, is to spare a thought for the humble sea squirt. In its adult form it is sedentary and can be described as a mere 'bag filled with sea water, plus a gut and reproductive organs anchored, in a similar way to the sea anemone – firmly on a rock' (see Dawkins 2004). But this deceptively simple creature has a larva whose structure changes your whole attitude to it. It rather elevates it because the larva looks like a tadpole (i.e. a vertebrate, which has a spine and a spinal cord). This larva has a segmented tail and swims in the plankton by thrashing its tail from side to side. Look closer, a primitive spine (called a notochord) and dorsal nerve tube with enlarged head-end ganglia are present. In contrast to the sea anemone, with a mere nerve 'network', this little fellow has quite an organised nervous system with many of the basic features encountered in its higher vertebrate cousins. Now when this larva eventually finds just the right rock, it sticks itself on head first and proceeds to turn into the simple, yet 'adult', bag of sea water described above. In doing so, it loses its tail, its notochord and most of its nervous system and there settles for life. The moral of the story is that if you need to move with any purpose and you want to be a 'real' animal, you need a nervous system, plus you need a 'brain' somewhere near the head end to keep control of what you do. Brains are all about organising responses to situations that are of benefit for the brains, the body they're in and the genes that must be passed onto the next generation. They're also all about homeostasis – organising and coordinating responses that keep the organism alive.

In the last section I introduced the basic three part brain structure – the forebrain, the midbrain and the hindbrain.

Take a healthy cat and damage its forebrain. It doesn't die, but it becomes a bit daft. Its purposeful, voluntary behaviour and problem-solving ability become impaired. Remarkably, even with quite massive injuries to the forebrain, there's still some semblance of normal coordinated behaviour remaining – the cat can orientate towards a noise or withdraw its paw from heat and can walk, eat and groom for example. It can even display full-blown emotional responses related to anger and fear... so long as the hypothalamus remains intact. Take away the hypothalamus and really that's it – the poor old cat can respond a bit, like bare its teeth or hiss, but can't get it all together in any semblance of coordinated behaviour. If the cat's midbrain was damaged it becomes 'essentially comatose', alive physically but not behaviourally or psychologically. When the hind brain is destroyed, life ceases (see Le Doux 2002).

So this is how it is, if you reason from a 'chopping-bits-out-to-see-what-happens' perspective (which is nuts really, but it does tell us quite a lot):

- the hindbrain controls very basic functions, those necessary for staying alive
- the midbrain is involved in maintaining wakefulness and coarse, isolated behavioural reactions
- the forebrain coordinates complex behavioural and mental processes.

Now, as Mick Thacker has pointed out to me, it's important to understand in 'brain-lesioning' studies (where bits of the brain are destroyed and subsequent observations of the 'loss' of function that result, are used to ascertain the exact function of the part destroyed), that the functioning brain which is left, alters its function in response to the lesion. That's one thing, but it also appears that parts of the brain that are left intact, often at a good distance from the intentionally-made lesion, may fail to function normally too, it's called 'diaschisis.' The big point is that a lesion in one area of the brain causes massive changes that give rise to novel functions and malfunctions in other areas of it. Thus, what the researchers observe, after their 'precise lesion', is likely to be a great deal more and a great deal different from the actual function of the area – if indeed it has a precise function. The problem is with researchers wanting anatomical regions of the brain to be like individual organs with fairly distinct and discrete functions; the reality is that individual functions are dispersed throughout the brain. Dang, it's hard!

Here's an example of the type of reasoning that goes on... Tissue injury creates nociception, impulses go to brain and there's conscious awareness of pain. Researcher comes along and cuts nerves that go from tissue injury to spinal cord. The pain goes completely. The researcher writes up a paper to say that the nerve they cut is therefore the source of pain consciousness.

Most 'brain-centric[1]' researchers and writers would deem this conclusion ridiculous,

1 - Brain-centric – a word I coined to mean an over-focus on just the brain and its various parts. Well, I thought I'd coined it but I soon found that it's a word that is Google-able!

but if we think about it from an 'embodied consciousness[1]' perspective, it isn't as mad as it may seem. What's bad about it is the allocating of function solely to the area lesioned and removed, in other words the loss of pain consciousness could just as easily come from many other areas involved in its processing.

From here on, for the next three sections (17-19) and all the chapters they contain, it would be good for the reader to have in mind the notion just discussed: that observing the effect of brain lesions doesn't necessarily provide a clear indication of the function of the area lesioned. The reason this is so important is that a great deal of what we know about the workings of the brain are the result of brain lesions and subsequent observations.

Let us continue...

In the animal kingdom, it could be said that, if you observe animals to be capable of what appears to be thinking and problem solving – **look out for a forebrain**. If they haven't got one but they're still smart, you might be observing a cuttlefish, a squid, or an octopus! Cuttlefish, squid and octopi are Cephalopods which are invertebrates that have evolved smartness in quite a different way to the vertebrates. Complex communication, thinkers, problem-solvers, even tool-use, they are to be marvelled at.

I originally wrote 'look out for a **decent-sized** forebrain' in the last paragraph – but thanks to Mick Thacker, who gave me a book called 'Do Fish Feel Pain?'(Braithwaite 2010), I've been reading about the thinking, feeling and problem-solving capabilities of fish and I've been impressed! Fish don't have a large forebrain and neo-cortex as we do, but they do have basic forebrain 'limbic' structures like the amygdala and hippocampus and research shows that fish have surprising mental abilities.

For example: imagine that you are a tough male and in order to win a female you need to take on and fight all the local male contenders to assert your dominance. Think Friday and Saturday nights down the local village square after the pubs close.

There are five males in contention this season. Day after day you smartly observe the other blokes fighting each other and you note that Dave always beats Edward; Edward always loses to all the others; so does Dave, he can only beat Edward. So, these two get beaten up by the other three: Colin, Brad and Ash. Ash can beat the lot, no problem. Brad's not bad, he only has a problem with Ash, but Colin has a problem with both Brad and Ash. Now, suddenly one day you come into the village square and there's three of you; the other two are Edward and Brad. Which one are you going to go for? Yes, you've watched them all, remembered and know that Edward always loses and that Brad is pretty good. You go for Edward and steer clear of Brad. Think about this for a minute, it's quite something – apparently it's called 'transitive inference' by cognitive science. You've noted and remembered who beats who and worked out the hierarchy; in a split second you can make a decision about the weakest and therefore who is best to turn on and assert your dominance over. Mayhem at midnight in the village square, but the chicks watching are impressed, you've won your first fight!

1 - Explained briefly, at the end of the chapter – wait until you get there.

This hierarchy stuff seems easy but children under four years old are hopeless at it. As Victoria Braithwaite (2010) says:

> *'It wasn't that long ago that transitive inference was thought to be exclusive to humans and indeed to humans over 4 years old'.*

What's amazing is that this sort of intelligent thinking, reasoning and behaviour has been observed in Cichlid and Siamese fighting fish that live in the Great Lakes of Africa and which we all commonly see in home aquariums. The researchers who did this clever bit of research on the fish didn't just put Ash (the strongest) and Edward (the weakest) together with the fish that had been observing all the fighting... they also used Brad and Dave. They reasoned that Ash being a 100% winner and Edward being a 100% loser would be easy to discriminate. However, Brad has wins and a loss and Dave losses and a win, that's more complex. Yes, our fish can quickly sort out that they'd be better-off tackling Dave than risking it with Brad! These tiny little fish brains are doing some marvellous remembering, problem-solving and hierarchy recognition that would put any three year old human to shame.

My point in this aside is that there's a surprising amount of thinking and consciousness going on in the animal world and we are not unique. Then, do fish feel pain? Yes, they probably do. Will that stop me fishing? NO! Sorry, but I do use barbless hooks!

What are brains for then? I'm hoping I've answered the question really, but in a nutshell, the main thing is that they 'look' at all the options, weigh them up, make the most appropriate choice and then 'do it'. Brains produce and co-ordinate behaviour, moving and doing. Brains are all about cooly being the ultimate and ongoing sample-scrutinise and action-coordination processors.

If you think about life and all the basics, then you have it. I see it like this:

Divide life into two: survival and reproduction.

1. For survival, an animal generally needs to bring about and co-ordinate moving or behaving. That means moving and behaving to feed; making the best of the resources available (eat like hell and get fat, skimp and save, make a food stash somewhere); find and drink water. Moving and behaving to find shelter and to outsmart, escape, fight, hide, out-wit, run away and generally do very clever things to stay alive in the face of 'macro-adversity'! That's being chased by a lion, a thug, a neighbouring village warrior and so forth. I'm now watching a squirrel and thinking of it hiding away a stash of acorns in various secret places, but also of the smart lazy squirrel who secretly stalks the stasher and when they've turned their backs does a bit of pilfering. Remember the great rule of survival – 'get as much as you can for as little effort as possible?' Ah ha, cheating is cool for survival, but not nice for culture. Know it and overcome the urge and you'll be a better human for it, but sadly, when the chips are down, you'll not be as good a survivor! If you like this theme, try 'Dark Nature' by Lyall Watson.

   For survival, the brain and CNS also needs to help in maintaining and controlling the physiology and health of its own body. That means playing a quite subtle, coordinating role in some of the very complex physiological processes discussed: mending, repairing, strengthening and dealing with micro-organisms via its communication with the immune system. But it also means responding behaviourally too. Think pain and sickness behaviour. Think smartly avoiding 'bad' food and drinking water, or avoiding others who don't look too good and might pass some killer disease on to you. Let's hear it for 'revulsion'.

2. For reproduction, the brain is there again, co-ordinating mate-finding, courtship behaviour, the reproductive act, the birthing process and all the stages of nurturing – as well as looking after the physiology and biology that allows it all to happen. From the egg and sperm production, right up to the more visually obvious side of things, the brain is surely involved!

The big message so far, is coordination of various deeds and actions, as well as of body biological processes. There are good words in there too, out-wit, out-smart, cheat, deceive, impress (think smart Cichlid fish) and so forth. That many individual organisms and different species have, to a greater or lesser extent – memory, the ability to think and work things out, the ability to know their surroundings and what might happen in the future, are all a big part of what's bound to come about – given the nature of nature and the evolutionary survival rules we have.

So, a next level might be that nervous systems and brains in particular, all need to produce some kind of sense of the situation, a sense of what needs to be done, a sense of meaning perhaps. It's all very well having all the apparatus to run from an approaching thug but there has to be some sense of meaning and feeling of danger, in order to then motivate you to do something about it.

While I've been writing I've been watching two pigeons on my front lawn, a male and a female. The male keeps fluttering all over the female and trying to get on top of her back, she flips away every time and he looks pretty pissed-off. Like most successful males though, his persistence wins and she remains still for him to do his thing. A pile of hard work; for about ten seconds of bliss. In a month or two and throughout the whole winter, I won't see this behaviour again. What's going on in those pigeons' brains? If the answer is 'the reproductive urge' then those pigeons are highly likely to be 'feeling' something that motivates them to do their thing. As far as I can see when we whittle it all down, feelings drive behaviour. I'll discuss this further in the following chapters and I have a little already in the discussion of homeostasis in the MOM chapters. For now, think about feeling hungry, thirsty, wanting a pee, wanting sex, wanting to sleep, feeling pain. Somehow and this is one of the biggest challenges for neuroscience, the interaction of the individual, with its nervous system, its brain and its body, contrive to produce motivational *feelings* that drive or motivate appropriate behaviour. Most consciousness thinkers and investigators are focusing on the human brain, but I have a feeling they'd be better-off going back to fish, insects, slugs, snails, all those simpler organisms that show more limited and less complex behaviours, if they want to start to understand it at its most basic level. The trouble is – you can't ask those creatures anything!

Going back to nervous systems and brains of simpler organisms means accepting that most of them, where quite complex behaviour can be observed, have nervous systems that can actually produce feelings. Feelings too, are a part of what consciousness is all about and as the brain physiologist, thinker, writer and now Baroness, Susan Greenfield suggests:

> *'A more plausible scenario, however, is that consciousness is more like a light on a dimmer switch that grows as the brain does. The more complex the brain, the greater the consciousness. If you go along with the idea, it circumvents many of the problems we normally have with animal consciousness. Think of a continuum of consciousness, ranging from minimal through to very profound, and that in turn will be reflected in the sophistication of the brain. Such a continuum of consciousness would help us understand child consciousness, and indeed potentially that of the foetus.'*
>
> Greenfield (1998), How might the brain generate consciousness? In: Rose S (Ed) From Brains to consciousness: Essays on the new sciences of the mind. Allen Lane The Penguin Press, Harmondsworth.

Consciousness is a big subject, so is how the brain works. I've made a list of books in the 'Read what I've read' section. The next sections will hopefully help you get a little bit of a handle on it and, it's all hugely relevant to understanding pain.

In my recent discussions with Mick Thacker, I realise that I have been too 'brain-centric' in my rather dismissive thoughts about consciousness. To make my excuse, it seems understandable when you read all the mainstream and current literature on 'consciousness explained' and read paragraphs like the one above from Susan Greenfield – whose sole focus seems to be on the brain and particular regions of the brain. You soon come to realise that consciousness cannot be easily explained. To me it's like trying to imagine and understand what's out there, beyond the end of the universe. For most, the easiest way to think about consciousness, is to place it in some as yet undetermined part of the brain, most likely the forebrain and use words like 'emergent' to explain how it comes about. Mick's view is that to understand consciousness, we need to see it from an 'embodied' perspective. That means including not just the brain, but the inputs to the brain, the rest of the nervous system, all the sensory and motor systems, the scrutinising systems and ultimately the whole of the body and its interactions with the environment. It's a perspective that has been around for a good while (and properly referred to as 'Enactivism') and what seems quite nice at this moment in time, is that it neatly fits with an MOM view of looking at things!

Chapter 16.2
The quick and dirty low-road

'Illegal aliens have always been a problem in the United States. Ask any Indian.'

Robert Orben

The following four chapters are simply my way of understanding the brain which I have found useful and have helped me to understand pain. I hope it helps you too? I warn you now that I touch on the rather 'brain-centric' anatomy of consciousness, but hopefully I do it in a way that is easy and enjoyable to follow. My advice, in the one or two of the more difficult bits, is to spend time pondering the diagrams. And, note that if I was teaching this material figures like 16.3 and 16.6 would be built up in gradual stages.

The chapters in section 17 flip back to 'real patients' to illustrate how useful this brain related understanding can be to them. It's more or less a 'how I use it with patients' chapter.

The section 18 chapters review the 'Mature Organism Model' in relation to the nervous system, the brain and pain processing. To me, it's an extension of MOM thinking and reasoning into a quasi-reductionist perspective on the brain of which shyly, I would like to admit I'm rather proud. I would be very interested to know whether this way of thinking about the nervous system and brain is of any value to those who think about and investigate it. I suspect I may be naively dreaming though.

Section 19 is 'for me' chapters; I researched and wrote it primarily to help me get a better handle on 'Sensory cortex area 1', or 'S1 mania' that has been 'all the rage' in the last few years. I also wanted to understand the underlying mechanisms of all the treatments on offer and give my opinions on them. I hope the section 19 chapters are as helpful for you as they have been for me?

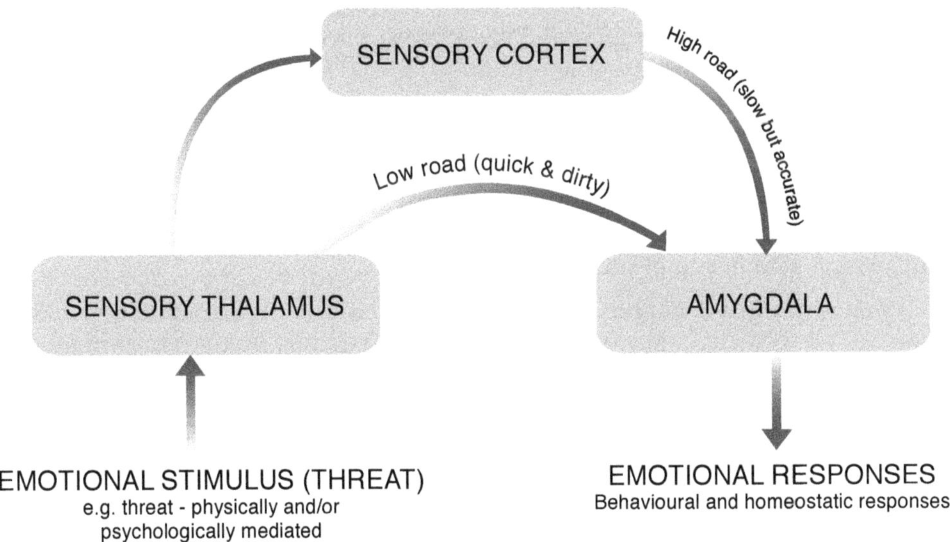

Figure 16.1 The Quick and Dirty Low Road and the Slow but Accurate High Road. Redrawn and modified from: Le Doux J. (1998) The Emotional Brain. Weidenfeld & Nicolson, New York

The quick and dirty low road

To start with I'm going to lean moderately on a brain hero of mine Joseph LeDoux (1998, 2002) whose two books: 'The Emotional Brain' and 'Synaptic Self' are very special. If you want to get to know how nerves and brains work? Then these two books are very good places to begin.

LeDoux came up with the diagram in figure 16.1. He uses the term 'emotional stimulus' (bottom left of figure) because he's interested in the emotional side of the brain and in particular, fear. I prefer the term 'threat' or 'threatening stimulus' instead and have added it in brackets. It's simply because I use this term when explaining things to patients. Substituting the term 'threat' for 'emotional stimulus,' makes the whole thing easier to understand when talking about and explaining things in relation to pain. If you've followed the earlier chapters, you could also replace 'threat stimulus' with 'stress' related stimulus – in other words, a stressor, or anything that challenges homeostasis.

In the diagram, you can see that an incoming threatening or potentially threatening stimulus has a rather smart 'quick and dirty' route, with quick processing and a quick response. This is channelled by the sensory thalamus straight over to the amygdala and then out to all the various 'action' modules that go on to produce, the quick physiological and motor responses that save your bacon. You will also note in the figure, the 'slow but accurate high-road' involving the sensory cortex – this will be discussed in the next chapter.

This 'quick and dirty low road' is happening before conscious 'you' even registers it. It's the brain's equivalent of a simple spinal reflex – like the reflex withdrawal response you get when you step on a thorn or a sharp object. But think about it, even here, messages go on up to the brain and involve the mobilisation of defence physiology, as well as conscious appreciation of what's going on.

So, what's the 'quick and dirty' all about? Well, the key features of any suddenly threatening situation and you can include any actual or potential physical injury here, are stereotyped behavioural responses or strategies. Withdraw, avoid, move away from, run, 'flight' or, stay and give a good account of yourself, make yourself look big and nasty and 'fight.' Then there's immobility or 'freeze' and finally good old give-up, submit and plead.

It's been noted that if you put animals, including humans, in threatening situations that they all respond in any one of these ways, depending on the situation they're in. The response wisely seems to be pretty much 'hard-wired' into the adult brain. It should be pretty clear that while these responses are superficially easy to describe, they are in fact extremely complicated and require an incredible amount of co-ordination and organising to produce. Hence being far too hard for the spinal cord alone to take on and manage. Step forward, the sampling, scrutinising and response organising brain!

Think about the key features of something unexpected happening, like the weird 'click-click' noise heard while walking through the cemetery in the dark, mentioned in section 15 chapters. You stop what you're doing, you orientate towards the source of concern, you focus your attention on it, you 'respond' as per the options above and it all happens in less than a moment.

Now think of a sudden pain in your back, you stop what you're doing and perhaps you 'freeze'? You also stop what you were thinking about; you immediately orientate your attention and focus on the area of pain and you change your behaviour. You might stop what you were doing, sit down for a bit or just stand there, frozen solid clutching your back and speechless. A great many patients report that it made them 'drop to the floor' and that they were unable to move for half an hour or more. Locked in pain, or maybe, in fear of pain too.

Keep the odd cemetery event and the sudden back pain in mind for now.

The 'quick and dirty' processing – via thalamus and amygdala, rapidly gets onto the various action systems. Hence, autonomic/sympathetic; HPA axis; pain on or off system; motor/tension/movement/behaviour systems and all the appropriate arousal systems, that are so vital for that instant survival process to be able to happen, should it be necessary. This system works on the wise assumption, given the 'is it good?' or 'is it bad' choice discussed in the MOM, that it's best to go with the 'it is bad' option – at least to start with! It makes survival sense to react and be ready rather than get nabbed. Quick reactions in evolution have been embraced by a great many as a smart option because those that have them, are better at survival. Think about swatting a housefly – now they're quick to react! Ah, but also think about other strategies too, like the Bittern's, a heron-like bird that lives in marshy and reedy areas, it freezes stock still, pointing its head and beak upwards. The Bittern is very hard to spot because it is so beautifully camouflaged and almost impossible to see when not moving in reeds. It makes itself look like a reed. It's a good strategy and it's obviously worked, otherwise the Bittern would no longer be here.

Temperament

This discussion about opting for the 'quick and dirty low road' and the fight-flight-freeze type reaction to a situation, leads nicely to a little aside on 'temperament'. Let's face it, some people react to a situation more readily than others. There's a nice long spectrum that runs from the super jumpy and stressy – those who flinch at the slightest provocation, to the languid and docile who never seem to get the slightest bit bothered.

Think of the animal kingdom. I like the housefly, which is a good example from the jumpy and fidgety end of the spectrum. In the grass and shrub-lands of South Africa, you might think of the small flighty antelopes like Duikers and Springboks, whose very lives depend on being able to suddenly jump clear of the predatory leap of a cheetah or leopard. Or, at the other end of the spectrum, the laid back life of a sloth who has about one quarter as much muscle tissue as other animals of similar weight.

We all know human springboks and human sloths. If you're a 'prey' animal, no doubt about it, it's best to be jumpy. If you're a predator at the top of a food chain, you don't have to be jumpy, or do you? Evolution doesn't like waste. Why be jumpy and waste energy, when you don't need to? Top predators' 'jumpy' circuitry has rather dulled. Being jumpy all the time not only wastes energy, it prevents you enjoying sitting still, you just can't get anything done. Have you been there when you're really wound up?

But even top predators still need that jumpy circuitry, they save it for threats from their own species. Think of male lions or baboon troops with a dominant male and think rivalry for food and females. The lower ranked adolescents get beaten up all the time and they're like, super edgy, wound-up and nervy most of the time. Are you low in the pecking order in your little family unit or community, at home, or at work? Many are!

Read Sapolsky's book, 'A Primates Memoirs' and also discussed in his book of essays 'Junk food Monkeys' (now called 'The Trouble with Testosterone'). He found low ranking male baboons to be loaded with glucocorticoids – they're super stressed! But surprisingly, so was the alpha male. He had to stay edgy and alert to keep his foothold, at least he had to inside himself but outside, just like in humans, he presented a rather fake facade of being laid-back. The truth is in the glucocorticoids!

Some of us may just be born nervy perhaps and some of us have that enviable 'cool under pressure' way. All our pain patients are on this spectrum somewhere too.

I hope you can see that the very nature of being human is adaptability. We have the capacity to chop and change, to mould and adapt relative to the circumstances we find ourselves in.

You may have heard of the 'open-field' experiments that researchers looking into rat or mouse behaviour do? Rats and mice generally don't like to be in open spaces; which is wise, because owls, hawks and any opportunistic predators get an obvious and easy catch. Note how quickly a shrew or a mouse scuttles across a road when it has to. Researchers stick a mouse in a big tray (the 'open-field') with nowhere to hide and note what happens. Stressed mice, as we've noted previously, show their anxiety by doing do-do's (droppings!) and researchers note that some mice do more than others. The low do-doers are less stressed than the highs, obviously. If you then start breeding the lows together for a few generations, you end up with an army of 'courageous' mice! Likewise, inter-breeding high do-doers give rise to very timid mice. Traits vary and as seen here, have a genetic or inherited component that can veer an individual towards a particular temperamental characteristic. It seems that evolution has given a 'variation' tag to just about every characteristic you fancy observing. Variation in: height, weight, sexual preference, pain sensitivity, jumpiness, broad and narrow mindedness, caring/not caring, honest/cheat (I'm writing this around the time of Lance Armstrong 'coming out' or rather being 'outed' for his years of drug abuse). You name it and you'll find there's a spectrum with extremes at either end, but the great majority around about 'average in the middle'. It's evolutionarily wise for a given population to have variety, simply because if some environmental condition suddenly changes, there'll always be a few of us who happen to be approximately 'just right' in our attributes and we'll be the ones who survive and keep our species going.

Temperament – genes or environment!

From the human point of view and the pain point of view, it's pretty obvious that some people 'react' to an injury or a pain situation far more than others. It may be that some people are born destined to be more jumpy, uptight or wound-up in response to stressors like pain than others, but there also has to be environmental factors too. As far as I can see there is a big 'learning' component involved in how we react to pain. If you're brought up with parents who showed high concern to pain and react strongly to your (and their own) injuries and pain, who then let you go on to play football where you learn to cry and roll about when you get the slightest bit of physical contact, you may shift towards being a high 'reactor'. On the other hand, there's the more 'robust' family who haven't got time for whinging and who see all cuts and bruises as part of normal growing up. For boys (and more recently girls too), they might encourage them to go on to play rugby! Note the difference! It's called 'learned behaviour'.

On the other hand, it seems that we often note that our kids are slothful, lazy, sensitive, jumpy, cry-babies, un-feeling bruisers and fighters, insensitive, tough or some other attribute... from 'the moment they were born'. Further, we can breed strains of rats (see chapter NR1.6) that show heightened sensitivity to injury or that are more timid or slothful, which all points to the potential of genetic influences.

However, what follows is an important warning that highlights the danger of assuming things like being jumpy, having high sensitivity and heightened pain responsivity are all 'inherited', 'genetic' or 'nature' rather than ***nature via nurture*** (see Ridley 2003). It comes from the brilliant Robert Sapolsky again.

This is from one of his essays in another great book of his called 'Monkey Luv' (Sapolsky 2005). Take two strains of rats, the first strain is characteristically anxious and skittish and researchers label them 'timid'. These rats are slow to enter and explore a scary or novel environment and have more trouble learning during a stressful task than a second strain, who are designated 'relaxed'. It was noted that when they were mothers, the relaxed-strain rats were observably more nurturing, doing more licking and grooming of their offspring, than the 'timid' mothers. Geneticists, as you might expect, were pretty convinced that the two characteristics were governed by genetics. Indeed, if you take the offspring of relaxed-strain rats and have them raised by timid-strain, you find that they still end up 'relaxed' regardless. Seems proof that it's genetic! Ah, but by using IVF type kit, they implanted fertilized relaxed-strain eggs into timid-strain females who carried them to term (plus did all the correct controls too). The interesting result is that when relaxed-strain embryos go to full term inside Mrs Timid and are then brought up by her – they become timid too! As Saplosky points out ... 'Same genes, different environment, different outcome.'

The big point here is that environmental influences don't begin at birth, as most would assume. To start with, genes are in the environment of the materials that go to make the rest of the egg (that's mostly from the ***mother's egg***) then, in the materials of the developing embryo and all this is in the environment of the ***mother's*** womb. And then in the neo and post-natal periods, every environmental thing out there in the world, gets thrown in too! If you ever get labelled from the moment you were born that you were 'wound up, stressy and jumpy' or, that you were 'a lazy, slothful, can't be arsed bastard', I think you now know who should take the brunt of the blame – sorry Mum! Read Sapolsky, but also what has to be one of my favourite books: Nature via Nurture by Matt Ridley (2003).

So, is modern life rather too soft? Are we nurturing hypersensitivity? It may be politically incorrect, but if you think about it with a little flavouring of biology and neuroscience and a nod to the environment of the developing embryo and the womb, we must be.

Let's do a bit of research that requires a time machine. We start by going back say about fifty years and look at the prevalence of cuts and bruises in 5-10 year olds and then compare them to the kids of today? Am I wrong or has the real rough and tumble of life been superseded by non-interactive, non-physical virtual computer based sport and violence? The young of today may rarely need a plaster or experience a nettle sting.

I predict that there's going to be a new disease called 'SCARRED' that's: 'Screen Activated Reclining Recreation Excess Disorder.' I might just be advocating a bit more rough-and-tumble in early life and a lot less screening! **As I have pointed out many times, our pain inhibitory systems need practice.** If you never get the experience of injury and pain, cuts and bruises, as in play time when you're young, you're system is never going to get the chance to practice in dampening or turning off pain. But wait a sec, what happens when you get shot in the video game you're playing?

Everyone reacts differently and everyone, even though they may have a similar basic wiring loom, is wired up in their own unique way. Environmental influences and life experiences, especially early on but also through to maturation, are vital to normal brain development. What happens to the naive-growing-learning-organism surely matters?

One point here patient-wise, is to be aware that pain patients may be of the slothful or jumpy variety, or anywhere along the spectrum. (But please don't stand there and blame the mother or what may have happened in the womb!). I'm particularly thinking of the chronic pain patient example, you touch them and they flinch. Where every input from you is processed as a threat and every movement you explore with them is 'Arghh' and the primitive defensive 'tension/freeze' module is stuck in place, when it should have left-off long ago. My examples in section 17 should help here.

So, a gentle appeal to be careful with apportioning blame to a patient's past experiences (like spending times on screens!), even though what other humans do in their lives and as they grow and mature, may wind you up! It's not as if you can re-run any given individual's life-history and make things in their past disappear. I have had so many patients over the years that have been made to feel bad or worried by a variety of practitioners, because they've dragged up and blamed things from the past. 'I was told my back pain and disability was due to my strict and cruel stepfather; my therapist is regressing me to my childhood and I now know why I hurt when the weather changes.' 'My psychogenic massage therapist is working me back to early days in the womb.'

As I just mentioned, the past cannot be changed or re-run, but sometimes an understanding of the impact of the past on the present, on how and why we react and behave in the way we do, or why we think and reason the way we do, can be productively analysed with some patients. The key is that looking at the past has to be done in a productive way and with the sole intention of helping the present, not providing yet another cause for concern, worry, or worse – to feel guilty about. Right now I'm thinking of patients who have an on-going pain problem and who have a past history of pain problems. One conclusion is that their pain-on system is well primed and easily engaged, even by relatively minor strains. In the light of a good explanation of pain processing, some of my patients have found this helpful to understand. It provides a good basis on which to see that hurt doesn't necessarily have to mean harm, that it may well be their well primed pain system turning itself on and staying on far more easily than others might.

A reasonable understanding of the past helps you understand the present, but you still have to deal with the patient in front of you. The tragedy is that many of our chronic pain patients are maladaptively stuck in a 'quick and dirty low road' kind of way and many needn't have been. We can't do anything about the past necessarily, but we do know that the 'slow but accurate high road' can modulate the 'low road'. So there is quite a bit of hope in this biology. That is coming next!

Chapter 16.3
The slow but accurate high-road

'The best way to find out if you can trust somebody is to trust them.'

Ernest Hemingway

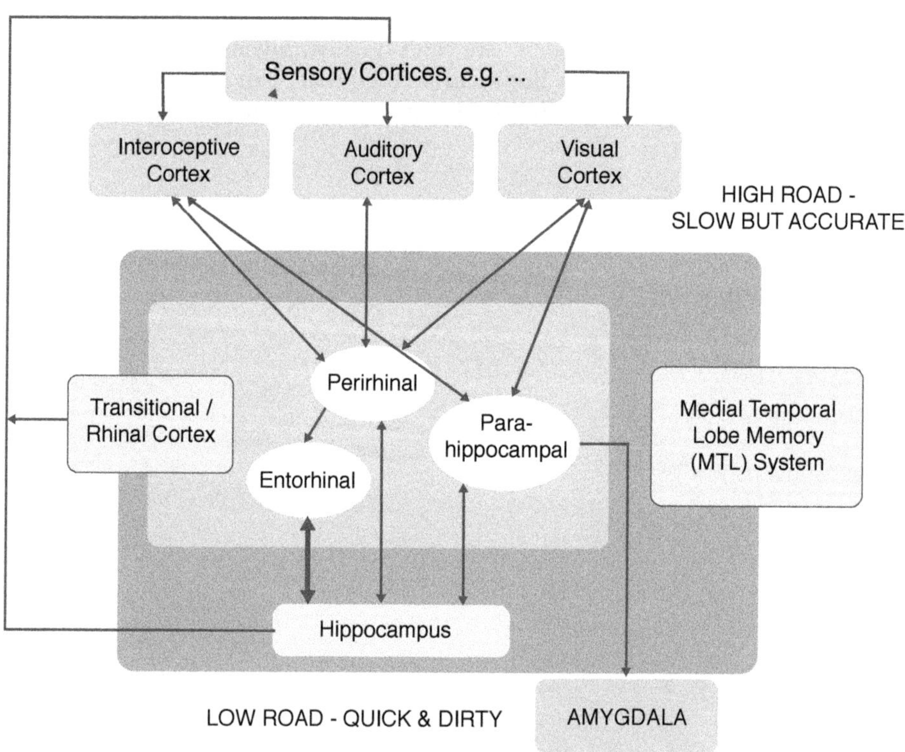

Figure 16.3 The Sensory Cortices and the Medial Temporal Lobe Memory System. Modified, expanded and redrawn from: Le Doux J. (1998) The Emotional Brain. Weidenfeld & Nicolson, New York and Le Doux J. (2002) Synaptic self. How our brains become who we are. New York, Vicking Penguin

This chapter is about how our cognition and thinking, via the 'high road' (if we get it right) can help change the 'low-road' processing for the better. Thinking of the patient, it's all about reducing the perceived level of threat of their condition and situation. I may have already mentioned the phrase 'reassurance is a painkiller'? This chapter adds credibility and anatomy to that statement.

Note this chapter and the next (as well as the chapters in sections 17-19) are occasionally dominated by standard brain area allocations of function, which, as I argued in the last chapter are challengeable. Therefore, what I want the reader to keep in mind is that although function is allocated to specific areas of the brain the eventual story may turn out to be quite different. I am also guilty, given the brief note at the end of the last chapter on 'embodied consciousness', of allocating anatomy and location in the brain to aspects of 'consciousness'. My excuse for now is simply that it is difficult not to, but also, via vehicles of explanation like the numskulls it occasionally makes it easier to visualise and understand.

Scene: that odd 'clickety-click' you heard in the cemetery on the way home...

Let's bring in some numskulls – 'the quick and dirty team'. They're all down there in the sensory thalamus and amygdala; slaving away getting a bombardment of messages from the eyes, the ears, the nose, the body. They're sorting it all out and pressing the various response buttons, then some bright spark in the thalamus goes, 'Hey, can someone tell 'him-up-there'... blimey, so busy, almost forgot.' Off goes a flow of impulses from the thalamus to the visual, auditory, olfactory and somatosensory cortices to now bring in, what LeDoux (1998, p 164) terms, the 'slow-but-accurate-high-road' (see figure 16.1 and my additions in 16.2). Simply, this is the where conscious awareness, scrutinising and appraisal come in. It's where in

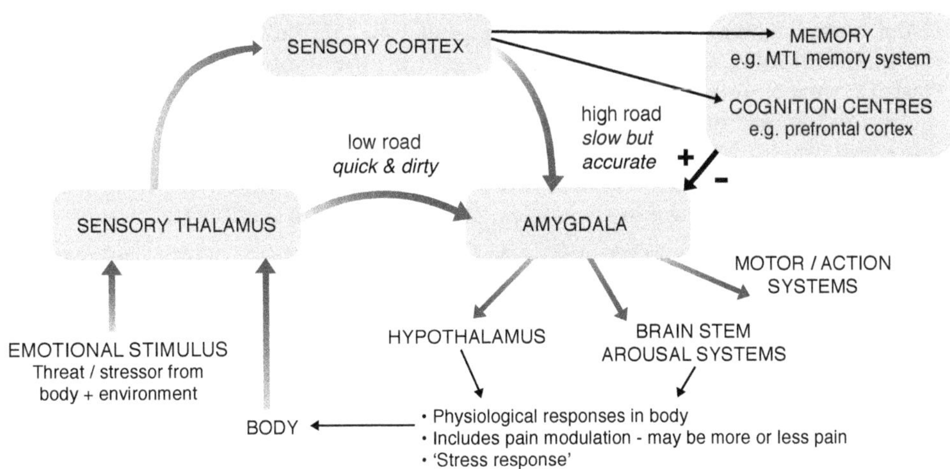

Figure 16.2 The Quick and Dirty Low Road and the Slow but Accurate High Road. Redrawn, but expanded and modified from: Le Doux J. 1998 The Emotional Brain. Weidenfeld & Nicolson, New York and Le Doux J. (2002) Synaptic self. How our brains become who we are. New York, Vicking Penguin

MOM language 'the brain samples itself' or at least that's how it can be seen. Rightly or wrongly, I think this way of thinking makes it easier to follow and understand, especially when you go on to read real 'brain' books! I've changed and added a fair bit onto LeDoux's original figure (16.1). Hence, in figure 16.2 the bubble up to the right containing 'memory' and 'cognition centres' are added to allow for conscious appraisal element and also to see how it all draws inescapably on things from the past – our memory banks and files. It also shows it's not just about the 'sensory cortex' part of the brain, there's much more to it than that. Note that 'MTL memory system' in the top right bubble of figure 16.2 stands for medial temporal lobe memory system, more on this shortly.

Two things need to be clarified.

First: the 'cortex' of the brain or more correctly the 'cerebral cortex', is the folded outermost layer of the brain which we see when we look at a brain in a picture or in a preservative jar. The term 'neo-cortex' is sometimes used and usually reserved, incorrectly, for humans and a few primates, but it's found to have a presence or semblance of a presence, in more lowly creatures on the ladder of evolution like birds and reptiles. It's certainly got a good presence in all mammals and an amazing one in the primates (see chapter 16.5 soon).

Second: the term SENSORY CORTEX is often used to refer to the famous 'Somatosensory cortex' or 'S1' area. Thanks to the fame given to it via the weird out-sized little man 'sculpted into' the brain, the 'sensory homunculus', this area is probably what's immediately thought of when the term 'sensory cortex' is used (dealt with in more detail in section 19). More accurately, this area is the primary area for the processing of the sense of touch; it's mostly about skin and our body surface's sensitivity. The way which I wish the term SENSORY CORTEX to be used here is as an 'umbrella term' for the cortices of all the different senses. Hence: the visual cortex which is found in the occipital lobe, the auditory cortex found on the temporal lobe, the olfactory cortex, again on the temporal lobe, the gustatory (taste) cortex found on the insular lobe/cortex and the somatosensory cortex just mentioned, found on the parietal lobe. These areas cover all our 'common senses' and they correspond to the environmental stimuli we are all able to receive. The area of the cortex primarily used for our more 'bodily' senses is called the 'interoceptive' cortex and is found in the insula cortex, more of which in section 18.

Let's now move to figure 16.3! Up at the very top you will note a box with 'Sensory cortices' in it and underneath I've illustrated only three of them – the interoceptive cortex, because it's so important in terms of pain and what's going on in the body and the auditory and visual cortices. To avoid clutter the others have been left out.

Let's get back to the cemetery scene.

The various cortical areas responding to environmental stimuli (say the visual, olfactory and auditory cortices) in a fair, but rather over-simplistic way, can be seen as giving us conscious and precise information about our surroundings. Thus, we're getting an immediate picture/snapshot (graves, old Yew trees and creepy silhouettes in the difficult light), plus a sound-bite (clickety-click) and perhaps a little whiff of smell of something. These three cortices are basic processing or scrutinising centres, which to be of any use at all need to liaise and combine with parts of the brain responsible for 'what-does-what-I'm-perceiving-now-actually-mean' centres. If they don't we'll hardly be able to make any sense of the situation.

If it all works out and what we perceive at this moment is seamlessly integrated with what we already know about similar combinations of sights, sounds and smells, we enter a state of even more heightened awareness in our zone of focus/attention than we had as a result of the 'low-road' thalamus-via-the-amygdala numskulls already doing their thing. For example, we now 'know' about the location and nature and possible meaning of the threat – 'There is someone over there and to me that means 'really odd' for this time of night.' The 'low-road's' already made me feel uneasy and got my heart pumping (take a bow interoceptive cortex!) and now I've managed to work it all out. I'm really not happy – time to think about what to do about it... Well, that's what happens in slow motion.

So, our attention is drawn inescapably in to assess the situation (unless you're a yogi in a trance). Quickly, all these separate inputs from the sensory cortices get ferried to an area called the '**Transitional**' or '**Rhinal Cortex**' (Figure 16.3). As you see, it consists of the 'perirhinal cortex', the 'parahippocampal cortex' and the 'entorhinal cortex'. These 'transitional' areas bring all the information together from the various sensory cortices to make a more integrated representation of the situation. This could be where, or how, we 'perceive' the 'whole' picture that we are in at that moment. Think of the various sensory cortices as providing a conscious awareness of only parts of a picture, i.e. the clickety click (auditory cortex), various bits of the 'cemetery scene' (various processing sub-modules of the visual cortices), the awareness of unease from the body ('interoceptive' cortices – see later chapter) and feedback from the body following changes to it brought about by the 'quick and dirty low road' autonomic responses and – like heart rate racing, tense muscles, dry mouth, gut feelings etc...

'The Fighting Temeraire' painted by Turner in 1839, has been voted Britain's favourite piece of British art. If you don't know it simply 'google-image' it, or better, go and see it in the National Gallery in central London. Or you may just have spotted it in the film 'Skyfall' when James Bond met Q in the National Gallery? The two of them actually briefly discussed it, true to form and very British! It is one of the most famous 'atmospheric' paintings and depicts the battleship Temeraire, a distinguished veteran of the battle of Trafalgar, being sorrowfully towed to her final berth before being broken up for scrap.

To appreciate what I am trying to explain, focus on small parts of the picture and block out the rest – say the upper right hand side of it. It's a hazy British sunset; now take in the tugboat – decrepit old craft with its massive blackened smokestack belching out putrid smoke; now the Temeraire, just behind, weirdly contrasting with the harsh and unromantic outline of the tugboat, the condemned and ghostly looking square-rigged battleship and so on. Now bring them all together and view the whole – get the 'full-picture' of what is going on and appreciate the difference! Yes and to quote the rather trite but still useful Gestalt – the 'whole is greater than the sum its parts'. Or to be rather pedantic and more correct – 'the whole is other than the sum of its parts! This is 'Holism' – putting all the parts together and getting an extra impact from a 'whole' that is far more than each component bit that goes to make it up. Unfortunately a great many alternative therapists have latched onto the word 'Holistic' in a rather too queasy way for me. I find if I use it when discussing pain or health it seems to rather uncomfortably super-glue me to some force field, lay-line or extra-terrestrial harbinger, so sadly I've shied away.

See it like this perhaps: the sensory cortices attend to the details of the 'parts' of the painting/situation, while the transitional cortex is the 'holistic' place that starts to pull them all together to form a whole picture. The collective bits of the painting (or the situation we are in), once drawn together and made overall sense of, can simultaneously be linked to other similar experiences squeezed out of appropriate 'files' in memory centres and systems. This in turn can have a threat 'value' attributed to it, provided by an 'MOM style', 'Is it good is it bad?' spectrum of possibilities. The outcome is that the object or situation is given a quality or emotional rating that motivates an 'action' or response to be carried through.

Start here: a simple thing like a painting, even though having no intrinsic threat, may still be given emotional valence and be remembered, or it may be just cast off to be discarded and vaguely remembered, or gladly forgotten. Think about going to the museum of modern art with your best friend who's into Formula One racing and has an 'anyone can paint this crap' type leaning towards modern art, or going with a tugging kid on your arm. The kid just wants you to play and isn't really ready to be told to be intellectual about a fuzzy mess on a wall. The petrol-head friend says he'll catch you in the coffee shop. Pleasure comes in different guises, so does fear, although there is a point when most of us would agree the level of 'threat'. The pleasure end of the spectrum is far more open to variation.

So, there can be feeling and action or reaction attached to just about everything. 'Dad, I'd rather be in solitary confinement than be in here looking at boring paintings.'

My point is that this transitional cortical region (the inner rectangle in figure 16.3), is considered a major area of the brain that brings-it-all-together to form a 'holistic' representation; to be assigned a 'holistic' meaning, upon which appropriate feelings can be produced to motivate and drive a behaviour or reaction. The reaction to the painting may be purely internal, a feeling of amazement, wonder or pleasure that makes you remain there for a while. The feeling derived from amassing the cemetery information is likely to be one of anxiety or fear and it is this feeling that drives, or 'motivates' an action response to move quickly on your way.

To make sense of any novel situation or object we need help and this comes either, from sampling our own past experiences (i.e. our memory) or, if we happen to be a young 'naive' organism with little life experience in our memories, we have to rely on other peoples' experiences/memories. Most often that's our parents or guardians. Naive organisms, youngsters, learn mainly from their parents in those very early months and years. They learn what their parents think is bad, to be feared, or is dangerous, just as much as they learn what is useful, good and desirable. So, it's little wonder that the young human brain is such a good learning machine and little wonder it takes in and tends to believe everything it is told by those it knows and trusts; youngsters are credulous. In survival and biological terms the young human organism has to believe what it's told in order to survive. Imagine being in the cemetery situation with a toddler, more than likely he or she will be totally unaware of any potential danger, but hugely influenced by the way you look and respond. Children pick up on the subtle indicators of concern and anxiety very rapidly.

In cultural terms this may give rise, via parental indoctrination, to quite irrational beliefs about the workings and ways of our world. Thankfully modern culture, via rational thought, open scrutiny, scientific investigation and good education, has given us the opportunity to challenge, rework and make better sense of our world than our immediate and more distant ancestors were able. It's a work in progress though and is up against a very stubborn human trait that human beliefs, once established when young, are very hard to change. Think of some of your patients entrenched beliefs! Think of some therapists! Think of some consultants! Think of some gurus!

Do you ever think that some of the stuff you were told by your parents was a load of rubbish? For example, my parents told me that I would get piles if I sat on a cold radiator or a cold floor! I never really understood what they were on about, piles made me think of dog poo, so I pretty much dismissed it. The other one was eating chocolate gives you spots. Luckily my Dad countered this one with 'drinking Guinness gets rid of them'. I liked my Dad. I bet if you went and interviewed a few 'clever people, like university professors and judges – you'd find that they, just like you and I and everyone else, still hang on to some nutty 'old-wives-tale' type beliefs. Even Richard Dawkins might be caught off-guard!

I also always find it astonishing what some Drs and many therapists believe as far as musculoskeletal pain is concerned. Stuff like spinal joints being 'out' and mal-alignment, Chinese acupuncture meridians and all the rest of the pseudo-scientific flim-flam that burdens and contaminates a more rational and better understanding. I rationalise it all by seeing this stuff in terms of 'cultural beliefs' (memes), while not necessarily scientifically valid, are part and parcel of what makes us colourful humans and therefore, when I'm not feeling too grumpy, can be tolerated! I once treated a Professor of physics who loved a good argument about religion. How could he, as someone who understood the innermost workings and origins of the universe, keep coming back to a divine hand in all this? Being unable to fully explain why the universe started isn't a good enough reason to jump to some divine-hand doing the business, sorry, that's scientifically lazy and a terrible cop-out! I'm also very friendly with a consultant haematologist who insists that if you cut the ends of an onion off in a particular way, they won't smell the house out! Where did that belief come from? Ah, her Mum when she was a kid, she believed her and it stuck, firmly! Point made.

I don't get cross; I pompously sit back and marvel at the sometimes strictly compartmentalised and unshiftable beliefs and reasoning of which humans seem to be capable of. But don't you agree that we can often observe in each other a great deal of inconsistency, for example, people saying they believe in this or that and then demonstrating behaviour that completely flies in the face of what they've just told you? 'I'm a strict vegetarian'... 'Come on, we had fish and chips last night...' All lies and hypocrisy sadly, but come on we all do it and we don't realise we're doing it sometimes. Try, 'I'm not racist, 'I'm not a bigot' and 'I'm always open-minded!'

Thankfully there are people and patients whose compartments can be challenged, educated and harmonised for a better life/pain perspective. Different compartments can often be linked and, given the right sort of tactic and diplomacy, be adjusted for the benefit of the patient. That means new pathways are being formed most probably. I like that idea. But there are limitations. For example, I can get my mother-in-law to think 'left-wing' politics, even 'Green' on a good day and also be much more humanistic. I do this by quietly and peacefully backing up the opposite to her arguments with what sounds like proven 'facts'. She enters our house as a dyed-in-the-wool Tory and leaves as a hearty tree-hugging, Guardian-reading socialist with Tony Benn's memoirs in her hand. But when she gets back home, shazzam, she's straight back to her old ways. You don't trip an oldie up that easily. It's the same with patients, they often leave you with a brilliant new perspective on pain and you're patting yourself on the back for a great 'explanation' performance, but when they get back to 'Tory' headquarters (I mean home!) it's all to no avail – 'I got what he was on about at the time, but he didn't seem to really understand that the pain was in my leg. It was all a bit talk and no do for me, sounds like, well, he's not going to even try and help me I don't think...'

So, as therapists we're up against many patients with firm and long held beliefs about pain, like the causes of it, what they believe they should do about it, or what medicine should do about it! Ahhh, the human being and its old-wives-tales, the love of the simple, most easily accessible and usually most absurd explanations over the more complex but rational and correct, is where most seem to want to go. Philosophers call it 'Naive Realism', which is defined as, *'An intuition held by most people that the view of the world that we derive from our senses is to be taken at face value.'* 'Yeah, look, the world has to be flat. I can see it's more or less flat, that's it. It's flat.'

How many hundreds of years did it take to get everyone to feel comfortable that the earth was a globe! Here's a quote from Patrick Wall the famous pain scientist we met in earlier chapters: *'It is almost impossible to replace widely accepted medical dogmas, especially where the paradigm being challenged has to be replaced with a more complicated one.'*

The folky thing that you were told seems so obvious and much easier to go with over that complicated science way of seeing it. Here is an example from the top of the hit parade of trash that I've heard through my career, 'My chiropractor told me that I had three vertebrae out, my pelvis was out and that my right leg was longer than my left.' It is the 'go-to' diagnosis for anything from chronic headaches to sciatica to irritable bowel syndrome. The public believe, chiropractors seem to believe it and a great many Drs seem to believe it too. I'll come back in a couple of hundred years I think and see if anyone's moved on at all!

No wonder explaining a different perspective on pain can be so damn trying with some people! (Please find time to read Richard Dawkins, 2003 letter to his daughter in his book of essays: A Devils Chaplin, it is beautiful; but also Stuart Sutherland's book 'Irrationality').

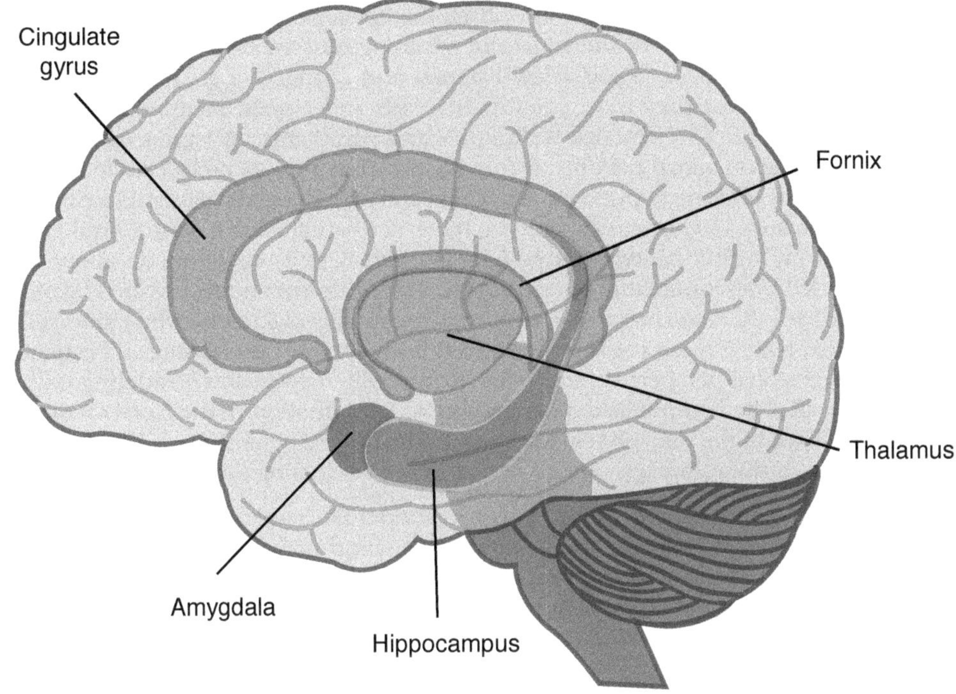

Figure 16.4 Important brain regions.

The most difficult patients are often those who have the most stubborn and entrenched beliefs. If you can't change a patient's belief about their pain it can be hard to move on: for example from the belief that something's badly wrong and needs to be fixed, to one of pain being maladaptively amplified, out of proportion to any damage done and which is safe to start loading and get fitter.

'The tendon is out of its groove.' 'My back is hypermobile and keeps going 'out' ... 'Look Louis, you're saying I've got pain out of proportion to the damage done, that it's all to do with processing in my computer or something. Look, I'm not trying to be funny or anything, but the pain is right here in my thigh, I know it's coming from here, it even feels tender, there's something wrong right there. You're never going to fix it if you don't find out what's wrong in there, I know.' (I have to say, this last statement is a very understandable stance.)

If you can't change a patient's beliefs and attitudes, you're task with recovery and rehabilitation may be much more difficult. Stubborn beliefs! Stubborn circuits! Brain compartments not communicating. Blame evolution! Blame culture, blame the parents, blame the educators, blame history!

No, NO! Don't go there, recognise this whole thing as a human trait and there are ways round it using behavioural and cognitive techniques, patient orientated skills and slowly and subtly **getting the patient to challenge their beliefs via experience.**

I had exactly the same problem with many in my own profession when I was giving my lectures. I was trying to get the physiotherapists who attended to see the need for a change in attitude to the causes of on-going musculoskeletal pain and a need for change in practice. While a few listened and changed, a great many just went back to doing what they were comfortable with and a great many found it far too challenging to their treatments, techniques and paradigms. It wasn't until I started demonstrating on actual patients in front of the class that therapists started to really grasp what I was trying to put over. They saw and experienced what I was trying to tell them. I am sure David Butler would be the first to admit that it wasn't until he later witnessed me with a patient that he fully grasped what I was going on about in my long-winded intercontinental fax messages. That shift from being a skilled 'Maitland' manual physiotherapist hugely focused on nerve mobilising, to one who embraced the notion that a great many pains were derived from aberrant processing and required a multidimensional perspective was to his great credit. Especially considering it wasn't that long after he had published his first book, 'Mobilisation of the Nervous System.' That was back in the mid 1990's, when we both enjoyed being a part of the early pain revolution in physiotherapy. For all of us it was a fascinating time of change.

The massive point here is, don't expect to suddenly change patients with on-going pain problems just by giving them some explanation or knowledge, it rarely works. Ultimately patients need to find out, with care and guidance, that they can move again and get fitter. It's a massive skill to learn, getting the context right, but it's hugely worth it.

I'm back! The point of all that was to shake hands with the stuff of memory and what's in it and why it can sometimes be a problem with regards to facilitating or inhibiting of the 'low-road'! Top-down may hinder, but, if it can be changed, it can start to help. Note the big 'plus' and 'minus' signs at the end of the arrow from the bubble up on the right to the amygdala/low road in figure 16.2!

So, clinically as far as I can see, there are two options with getting the 'high-road' to help dampen the on-going unhelpful activity (processing pain as a 'threat') of the 'low-road'. The first is by challenging the patients' beliefs and attributions about the pain via information giving and helping them re-conceptualise the problem. The second, especially if it's a waste of time giving the patient a different perspective on their situation, is to get on and start a graded exposure and behavioural experiments approach (see later). In most patients, both are combined.

Let's just clarify some terms and relationships. I already mentioned the addition of the top right hand bubble to the basic 'Le Doux' figure in 16.2, and that it contained on the one hand, cognition centres, and on the other, the 'medial temporal lobe' (MTL) memory system. If we now take our attention to figure 16.3 again you can see that the MTL memory system consists of the whole of the transitional/rhinal cortex PLUS the hippocampus. I hope that's understood and visualised. No? You want to know where the hippocampus is? OK, check out figure 16.4 with a warning, the brain's easier to visualise in unidimensional boxes than in real anatomy, even so, it's still good to have a three dimensional perspective of all this!

What's in an individual's memory modules is what the brain samples when I talk about the 'brain sampling itself' in the 'Mature Organism Model' from earlier chapters. What we sample from our memory library, our understanding, our beliefs, what Mum told us about spots and chocolate, is what can then strongly influence the responses we make to a given situation.

The 'slow but accurate' high-road (fig 16.2) involves the bringing together of reasoning, memory and the planning parts of the brain to produce not only knowledge but also 'feelings' and to then bear some influence on the 'quick and dirty' low road. Hence in the cemetery/back pain scenario we suddenly 'feel' an awareness of fear/uneasiness/concern, we are soon 'aware' of what's going on – the kind of threat, where it is and most importantly what it might mean in relation to what we might know from previous experiences. This may either support what the 'low road' instinctively is trying to do, or may negate it and calm it down. Note again, the arrow in figure 16.2 with the plus and minus sign going to the amygdala! This, albeit rather simply, represents the biological and clinically important 'top-down' pathway where big changes to lower levels of processing and 'bottom-up' activity are distinctly possible. This may be via knowledge and reasoning, via information that reduces the level of concern or threat, via the more experiential 'cognitive-behavioural' methods mentioned and highly likely, via the placebo or nocebo top-down pathways too!

So in the figure (16.2) the high-road, 'slow but accurate' (but quite often inaccurate too!) plays its role down below. In the cemetery, it may be the realisation that there is someone in the shadows is pulling a trigger back and about to shoot; or for the back pain, it's 'Oh God, this agonising back pain is going to lead me to losing everything, if I move now I'll do something I'll really regret', both of which support and facilitate the low-road. Or, the high road may just suppress it, 'There's a fellow just over there trying to light a cigarette, his lighter made the click-click noise, bit weird doing that here, think I'll just up the pace a bit, but blimey for a moment there I thought I had a big problem.' Or the back pain: 'This back pain will soon be better, I'm not going to let it be a problem, let's see if I can move a little.'

By way of its screening and scrutinising, the 'high road' modulates the reflex responses of the emergency 'low road'. By 'sampling' themselves in this way, our brains modify the response to the threat, or, as I said in section 10 using different terminology for what amounts to the same thing – it modifies the stress response intensity and may even stop it in its tracks.

To underline once more, one of our most powerful therapeutic tools may be our influence on the low-road processing via the high-road. This is done via, for example, good examination and handling, good explanation, reassurance, changing beliefs and attributions, decreasing fear/concern about the problem/the pain; helping the patient see that they can do more, getting them moving, using graded exposure and behavioural experiments and maybe, even the use of caring and confident hands-on treatments and, why not squeeze this in too – medical interventions including surgery! Through these sorts of skills the patient can come to see that a positive brighter future is more than possible. A big factor though is to get the patient to learn how to modify their own low road, using behavioural techniques, graded exposure, a little clear information giving; but not 'lecturing' or 'telling', unless the person is particularly receptive and, via the amazing skill that is cognitive behavioural therapy.

Chapter 16.4
Memories and cell-assemblies

'Right now I'm having amnesia and déjà vu at the same time. I think I've forgotten this before.'

Steven Wright

Early on in my explorations of pain understanding, I found that the neurological mechanisms of memory in relation to maladaptive pain mechanisms were a fantastic revelation. It wasn't until I'd experienced quite a few 'blank' and awkward patients, that it dawned on me, that the actual contents of an individual's memory was so important to the way they might respond and react to a pain situation! Beliefs and knowledge about pain, about treatment, about cause, about recovery, about the future, about other people's experiences, about what they think should be done; the list could go on and on. Memory of itself is a massive part of what makes us human too. Take away an individual's memory and they become virtually non-functioning and dependent on carers, as we will see.

Where's memory? Where are my life's recollections? Where's my knowledge of pain and physiology and of patients and bones and ligaments and nerves and so on, all stored? Where's me? Ha! Amazing, makes me smile at how incredible our nervous systems, brains and bodies are.

As you've already seen in the pain memory chapter earlier (chapter 6.1), back then, in the mid 1990's, I quickly latched on to the 'pain-is-simply-a-circuit-of-neurones' analogy – a mere Hebbian 'cell assembly', whose neural connections had been facilitated and welded together by the process of long-term potentiation (chapter 5.3). The notion that our memories and hence pain could be likened to some kind of recording or 'imprint' in the nervous system and brain, was perfect for explaining maladaptive pain to patients. This seemed to be powerfully supported by examples of patients whose previous pains could be reproduced using brain stimulating electrodes. You may recall the lady who was having an operation to implant deep brain stimulating electrodes to try and help alleviate her chronic leg and perineal pain caused by arachnoiditis? Whilst the surgeons were trying to place the electrodes to do this they inadvertently reproduced her old angina pain (chapter 6.1)! They were probing around in her thalamus somewhere. Could it be that just as the brain seems to hold the memories of a lifetime, it could also hold all the circuits or cell assemblies relating to the pains of our lifetime too?

But where is our pain/nociceptive 'circuit' or 'cell assembly'? Could it run from the very terminals of nociceptors in the tissues, whose original distress caused the flow of nociceptive impulses, right through the very same neural network that involved the processing and eventual feeling of that very specific quality and location of pain which occurred in the first place – and then somehow back out to the tissues again? Well, from an embodied consciousness perspective, it most likely does. Thinking this way about the ladies angina, from the example above, means that it could also have been reproduced by stimulating peripheral nociceptive fibres that were involved originally, or anywhere else in the brain that was involved in the original processing – not just the thalamus, but the interoceptive cortex and many other areas too. Later, in section 19 I will be discussing how research into motor maps and learning motor skills show how the representational maps of a newly learnt skill may get larger to start with, but when the skill becomes more automatic, they get smaller and may actually be moved from one motor cortex to another! This may also be the case with pains too – in other words, the longer a pain remains the more likely its representational maps will become more efficient, smaller and be moved! So, the notion of a pain memory or for that matter any memory 'representation', remaining as exactly the same neural assembly as the one that originally gave rise to it may not be quite the full story.

Let's start by taking a rodent example apart for a minute or two:

Put a rat in a metal cage that's wired so that the rat can be given a shock through its feet. Let's call the cage a 'shock-box', just to lighten this rather macabre tale. Set a buzzer off for a few seconds and then give the rat a shock. The rat doesn't like this one bit and immediately shows its fear response – freezing, crouching low, maybe a poop or two. Now set the buzzer off again for few seconds, pause and then give the rat another shock. No need to repeat very often, the rat very quickly learns and shows the fear response just to the buzzer. It learns that the buzzer means that the shock is coming. You would too and so do many much more lowly creatures. The rat can be congratulated on becoming 'conditioned' to the sound of the buzzer. Now, take the rat, put it into a different cage and give the buzzer a blast – but don't give it a shock. Repeat a few times. The rat after a bit of early tension, very soon relaxes and ignores the buzzer, the learned fear response is now extinguished – it seems that the rat has forgotten. But it hasn't, because if you put it back in the original shock-box and do the buzzer, that old wise rat is straight back to the fear response – even when there's no shock. The rat learned about the buzzer in the shock-box situation, realised what it had learned didn't apply in the no-shock-box and stopped acting so stupid, but it immediately remembered what the buzzer meant when brought back to where it all began. Seemingly extinguished memories can be quickly reinstated given the right environment or context! If a circuit is inappropriate – it's still there, but it gets switched off and archived!

(If you're thinking pain and you're thinking context triggering pain, you're bang on the right track!).

Think about it and what's happened to the nervous system. The environment of the shock-box, plus the buzzer sound awareness, plus the fear response (input via ears, processing in thalamus/amygdala and output to hypothalamus and all the stress response centres that include not only all the autonomic and HPA physiological responses, but also the 'freezing', 'crouching' and 'pooping' motor responses/ behaviour too), have all wired themselves together. The buzzer perception circuit plus the shock-box (the environment of the shock) circuit get quickly learnt, imprinted and linked to the ready and waiting 'fear-response' circuits. Now it's more than cells that fire-together-wire-together, its **circuits** that fire-together-wire-together! However, change one part of it (the environment) and it appears that the circuits can quickly depart and fire apart. Have you ever had patients with on-going pain who have a few weeks off, go away and come back saying they did things on holiday they haven't done for months or even years, and that they felt so much better? What's the catch? No catch, it's called remove one of the important circuits – the home environment (the CONTEXT) and all the habitual stress responses and pain circuits to which it's attached. It's just like my mother-in-law shifting her politics and outlook on the world to the left while she's here with us, but as soon as she's back in the her 'home' environment, it all goes back to her well engrained reflex Tory status quo – maybe she should move in with us! So, the patients' pain soon comes back when they return from holiday to the triggers from the 'same-old-environment'.

LeDoux (2003) has a neat figure to explain this which I've redrawn and altered a little in figure 16.5. It shows, enclosed in the circle, a neat circuit representing the wiring that produces the response. It's a ready and waiting wired-up 'cell assembly' circuit doing nothing; just like one in your brain that represents, say your telephone number, or even an old back pain or for the rat, its fear response behaviour. On the left are several arrows representing neurones that convey messages from stimuli that have triggered the circuit in the past, for example, 'What's your telephone number?' Or if it's the rat; that particular buzzing tone, or a shock to the feet, or the frigging shock-box torture-chamber, or a combination of the buzz and the shock-box.

In figure 16.5 I hope you can also see that the triggering input, the 'cue', to any given cell assembly can have origins from the environment and the body, as well as from within the brain itself. For example, I can ask myself, 'What's my telephone number?' and quick as a flash, this triggers a neuronal pathway to my telephone number cell assembly, switches it on and outputs it to 'consciousness' giving me the answer. An external trigger for my telephone number is when someone else asks me for it. It comes in via the ears in the form of a meaningful sentence!

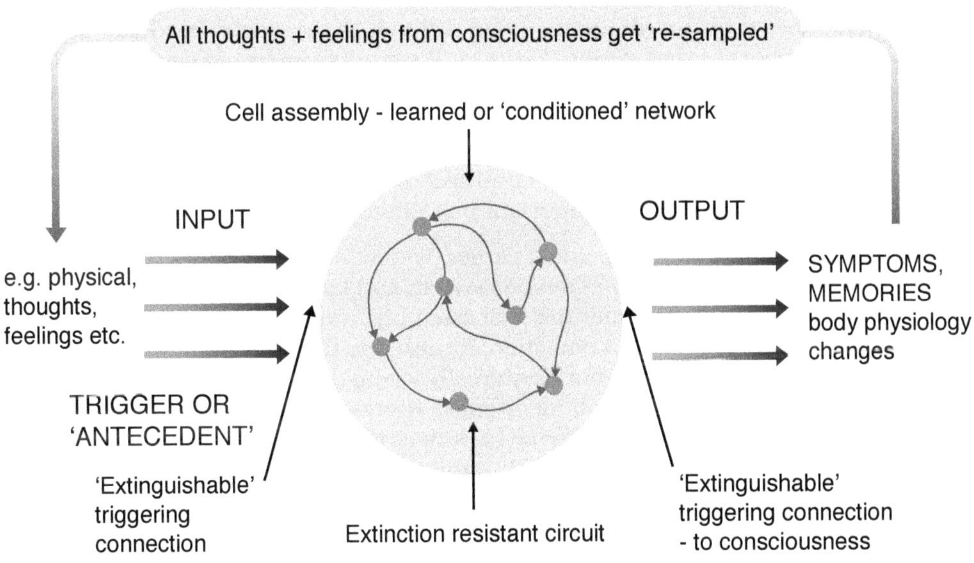

Figure 16.5 Schematic to help explain a 'cell assembly'

As an aside, figure 16.5 has had great clinical utility for me when helping patients get a handle on all the possible triggers there may be to their problem.

Now, this may be important for pain sufferers and at this moment I have those who suffer from office related repetitive strain injury (RSI) pain in my mind. Their various pain representational circuits or cell assemblies may be activated, not only by the computer/typing 'activity' (i.e. from the firing of sensory nerve endings in the moving and contracting tissues that hurt), but also by the often despised office environment (just like the rat knowing they've been put back in the shock-box again). Or maybe even just by watching a film of someone else typing in an office! Looking at it in this way also helps us to see that even merely thinking about using a computer can easily trigger the 'pain' output to occur.

So, are you mischievously wondering what would happen if we could move the RSI sufferer and their computer to a sunny paradise, paint happy, hippy graffiti all over it and figure in a 'lotto' win? Change the context of the problem, would the pain go away? Well, you're certainly changing a few possible triggering factors... Compare the result and the biology of the result, to the outcome following an office 'ergonomist' consultation resulting in a big spend on new office equipment, seating, mouse, keyboard... the lot. Well, again, you've changed some of the triggering factors... but perhaps the ergonomist should also include a picture of paradise up on the wall, a more pleasant and agreeable line-manager and a tasty pay rise!

Seeing a pain in terms of conditioning, context and environment is massive leap from the old manual therapy perspective of upper limb tension tests and nerve mobilisation. I hope figure 16.5, by reducing pain to a mere 'cell assembly', can help the reader see how these 'softer' issues can be so important.

As I mentioned, even the thoughts going through the patients' head can activate the cell assembly. 'If I start typing, I know it'll start playing up' or even the feelings that are there and are already associated with it; 'I just dread the computer and all that ghastly number-crunching, I feel so tense and wound-up right now.' Or is it the thing that most clinicians think about, the actual physical input that goes on with the keyboard and inevitably, the patient's posture? Boring? Not at all, but to be a good all-rounder, it still has to be an important part of the holistic overview.

I am now back to the question asked earlier, whether a memory is a cell assembly-circuit from the tissues into the nervous system and back out again? The answer I like is: yes to start with, but later the 'cell assembly' way of looking at things makes you realise that it's likely to become more localised in the brain somewhere, casting its mooring lines adrift a little, but never really losing the capability to stay in touch. It becomes more like your telephone number representation, isolated! As you can see in figure 16.5 I've drawn an arrow back over the top for the 're-sampling' arm of the overall circuit. That may go back within the brain or right back to the dorsal horn, or even back to the tissues. Don't get confused, but if you want to try, think of the 'Wheel within a wheel' song again, last verse:

> *'Like a circle in a spiral*
> *Like a wheel within a wheel*
> *Never ending or beginning,*
> *On an ever spinning wheel*
> *As the images unwind*
> *Like the circles that you find*
> *In the windmills of your mind'*

Lyrics by Michael Legrand (original French composer);
from the 1968 film 'The Thomas Crown Affair'

Input from the tissues is just one of many possible 'inputs' that can trigger it to fire and output. One of the arrows on the left of figure 16.5 may represent the inputs from the fingers and arms. Other triggering arrows may represent for example: the office, the keyboard, the thoughts about typing, thoughts about typing causing pain, the dread and associated feeling you might have about doing it or of it causing yet more pain, the other people in the office, the line-managers face or even their silhouette and so on. Psychologists often call indentified triggers 'antecendents'. Most patients will volunteer physical antecedents and if they can't find any reliable ones, they often start to blame things like changes in the weather. In my experience it's relatively rare for a patient to immediately volunteer that it might be a thought or a feeling of some kind, but when you've explained it all in a similar way to as I have here, the more 'feeling' and 'thought' related triggers usually start to come.

Appreciate that, just like the rat in the shock-box and the buzzer, there's a whole pile of different triggers and plenty more potential triggers too! No wonder a single treatment modality isn't very effective!

'Sally, I'm using ultrasound today, it'll stop you're line-manager triggering the RSI pain forever!'

We know that mood/emotion and memory are closely linked; when you're down it's easy to bring to mind all those horrid things; when you're up and chirpy, you tend to ping-out more pleasant experiences. Memory circuits often get linked to the emotion circuit that happened to be going at the time of the experience memorised. It seems that strong emotions can help to strengthen memory formation. It's hardly surprising therefore that whenever you feel strong emotions you're more likely to bring things to mind that were laid down as cell assemblies during those very same emotions; the facilitated connections are already in place. Emotions and feelings are on the 'input' side of our 'cell assembly' representation and emotions can trigger pain; they are common antecedents of pain. Using figure 16.5 to point this out, among many other things, can be hugely helpful with some patients. It is always best to get this and other antecedent material out of the patient rather than 'telling them', and I sometimes do this using 'star-charts' which I discuss later in the 'Graded Exposure' section of the book.

On-going cell assembly activity

It seems likely to me that activity in some cell assemblies may just keep on rolling along, never stopping and always trying to play their unhelpful and pointless tunes up into consciousness. In effect they've cast-off from the mooring lines to any triggers or controls and remain in a state of constant activity and output giving the sufferer on-going and unvarying symptoms. There's no 'stop-button' and because it's on-going there's virtually no 'start-button' either. Ah, preoccupation – more on this later when I discuss the Australian 'sand-rag' experience. Ah, that annoying tune!

As I mentioned in section 6, I have tinnitus, I've had it for about five years now and as far as I can tell my tinnitus cell assembly representation is banging away 24/7, constant, totally. The trouble is when I think about it like right now – it's there, when I don't it isn't, I don't notice it! So is the thought about it being there and my spotlight of attention picking it out – the actual trigger to switch it on? Or, is it on all the time and I just don't happen to be focusing on it because it doesn't bother me? Tricky! I think it's on all the time and the on/off with it that I experience is a feature relating to gating-to-consciousness processing. It's just like me turning my attention to what's going on in my foot right now. I merely start listening to what's coming in all the time anyway, for example, the pressure, the tingling and the temperature of various parts of it. The attention shift simply opens the 'gates' to consciousness. The problem of the analogy with the foot is that what I'm getting varies over time. Right now my toes are a little cold, later they might be hot and sweaty. My tinnitus does not vary at all, which makes one figure that there's no peripheral drivers having any kind of modulating effect – it's cast off its ties to the tissues where I notice it, the inside of my ears!

Attention is rather like a sentry's spotlight moving around the environment (and your body) as well as inside your own head looking at your past memories, any little thoughts and even emotions, homing in here and there to pick up on something. Unless you're dreaming, the only time it really rests is when you sleep.

This tinnitus anecdote and thought may be one of many little keys to chronic pain management!

Here are a few things (that can sometimes be useful examples with your patients):

1. ***The pain maybe like my tinnitus, it just won't go away, the circuit*** is on all the time and if your attention drags back to it, as it invariably does with chronic pain sufferers, it's always there. Maybe the trick is to not process it as anything bothersome and so, like a good meditator, you note it when it comes, quietly and calmly acknowledge it and let it pass when it's ready. Avoid the amygdala and the low-road! That's easier said than done for a great many, but it may well be key to living with pain. I once had a patient when I was working at Geoff Maitland's practice in Adelaide, whose tinnitus was making her suicidal. That's how bad pain, or 'symptoms,' can get if you let them. (It's rather like my neighbour's dog barking – sometimes I could kill it! But I have developed a relaxation strategy and it remains alive!). The other thing that often really bothers me are the kids who do hand-brake turns and rev the living daylights out of their cars at 1.00am on the beach car park near here. I have this masterplan to purchase a massive fire-shooting bazooka rocket launcher – like the one that the 'mystery woman' (Carrie Fisher) had in the film 'The Blues Brothers' and go frazzle the little shit-bags and their swanky revvy cars. Interestingly, my neighbour Roger, likes to hear them having a good time, he wishes he was down there with them! Bloody hell. So, how, do I re-process this? 'Just like you would get a chronic pain patient to Louis!' 'Ah, I see, what, you mean. I better wander down there and say hello then!'

2. If pain is upsetting to the patient it is processed as a 'stressor' by the brain.

3. Another way of putting this is to say that the pain is being processed in the 'threat' centres of the brain and hence:

    a. Because it's a threat, it's given high priority in consciousness and easily bumps other more mundane stuff out. To get it out of consciousness, the individual (and hence their brain, nervous system and body) may need to be doing something that is a little more exciting than mere 'mundane'. That's easy, think of an individual with chronic pain and what might be being processed when they're in the middle of a bungee jump, or doing something they love doing – which might be as simple as socialising, playing chess for a while, or getting the flame throwing bazooka out of the garage at 1.00am! Recent suggestions in the media have been to join a knitting group for chronic pain and join a baking group for depression. I'm sure both are interchangeable. Hobbies and interests often get side-lined by pain and stress, but it can be a good strategy to start graded re-introduction of them when appropriate. As the evidence says, try to keep doing normal things. I would add, try to start doing a few <u>new</u> things sometimes too. <u>Novelty</u> works better than an ultrasound machine, that's for sure! Swimming with dolphins has just popped into my head and so has magic mushroom collecting!

    b. By activating 'threat' responses in relation to pain – the brain is bringing or 'orientating' attention to come to bear on the pain. Giving something strong attention amplifies its intensity – recall that cemetery clickity-click? Here your eyes and ears are quickly programmed to see/hear more intensely and when there's 'threatening' pain your pain monitoring senses do the same; think about it in a similar way to pupil dilation when something exciting is going on. For the male brain this might be the three 'F's: Food, Females and Fishing! Big point: <u>Attention amplifies</u>.

    c. If pain is scrutinised as a threat, it is likely to increase local muscular tension with any movement or even the general muscular tone. Good therapists quickly pick out tension in posture and movement. For most chronic pain problems the ability to do smooth relaxed movement has largely disappeared, or requires huge concentration to overcome and has to be re-learnt. Long ago, a significant leap in my pain 'management' and treatment was when I eventually managed to leave the manual therapy obsession with pain response and range of movement to look more closely for relaxed floppy movement – in all patients, acute or chronic. That also meant overcoming the on-going, 'Where's your pain?' 'What's happening to your pain?' 'Where's the pain?' 'What's happening to the pain?' Needle-stuck-on-the-record problem, while assessing standard movements. As I've already mentioned in earlier chapters, observing movement and learning to say absolutely nothing, or using minimal but appropriate communication as reinforcement techniques was a massive move in the right direction. Hint, it can take ages! THINK PINK! (That's explained in the treatment sections of the book, chapter GE 4.9).

d. If pain is perceived as a threat, it is likely to increase other 'stress' responses. For example, those related to autonomic/sympathetic and HPA and hence to influences on immune system, circulation, healing and so forth.

4. A significant leap in treatment/management can often be made if the patient can be helped to stop processing the problem as a threat. Easy to say, hard to do! There will be more about how to set this up in the management later – it can be very brief, or, as in section 17 almost dangerously lengthy! For now, one of the key things is to get the patient to try and 'make friends with the pain'. Sounds mad, but given the right knowledge about their pain (with them understanding and believing it!) some patients can make this giant step. Think about it, if you change your relationship to the pain – you'll change where it is processed and how it is processed. Get it out of the threat processing system! Stop that 'low-road's' madness!

5. Repeat: <u>accept it</u>, make friends with it and don't let it bother you so much and you'll shift it from being processed in the 'threat' circuitry!

6. Like my tinnitus, when you don't let it bother you, you don't think about it and for all intents and purposes the circuit is off – even though it may not be. The thing here for the patient to realise and find out, is that whenever you concentrate on it, your spotlight picks it out, it gets attention, you then visit it and it all returns.

7. If the patient finds an on-going pain intrusive, annoying or bothersome, it will be being processed as a threat and it will 'be in mind' a great deal of the time.

8. Any form of pain relieving inputs that really work and preferably ones that are not reliant on a therapist for long, can be hugely helpful (fire-apart-depart). Keep practising and when one method stops working find another. You can condition pain-off just like you can pain on. Just draw some more circuits to follow the 'extinguishable' arrows in figure 16.5 and you've explained it.

9. See the case history and figure in chapter 14.2

10. If a patient's only way of coping with the pain is to be careful with what they do all the time – they have to be processing it as a threat and again, it is more than likely to be in their mind virtually constantly. Ask them about it! Invariably they'll tell you it is. Graded physical exposure, challenging and experiencing higher levels of activity and movement that doesn't make it worse overall, can very effectively help the patient realise that it is possible to do more and is often a key process. The goal, I tell my patients is: 'Thoughtless-Fearless-Movement' (TFM!), or 'Thoughtless-Fearless-Activity' (TFA!).

Lastly, before moving on to looking at yet another interesting aspect of memory/consciousness, is to see that the 'Inputs' or triggers on the left of the cell assembly 'representation' in figure 16.5 are actually cell assemblies themselves. Appreciating this makes the terms 'circuits-that-fire-together-wire-together' and 'circuits-that-fire-apart-depart' become 'cell assemblies-that-fire-together-wire-together' and 'cell assemblies-that-fire-apart-depart'. Easy? I think it is and many of my patients have found it revealing, useful and easy to follow too. Note also, that 'output' from the cell assembly activity on the right is what gives rise to body biology changes, as well as consciousness and awareness.

Chapter 16.5
Three types of memory and a bit on consciousness!

'You can no more explain mind in terms of the cell than you can explain dance in terms of the muscle'

'Conscious is not something that happens inside us. It is something we do or make. Better: it is something we achieve. Consciousness is more like dancing than it is like digestion.'

Alva Noe

Next: a bit more about memory; and some of the areas of the brain that may be involved.

There are two types of 'long term memory' – the first is called declarative or 'explicit' memory; the second is 'implicit' or 'non-declarative' memory. There is also 'short-term' or 'working' memory. I'll have a brief look at each.

A great deal of what we understand about memory has come from brain injury and the sad side- effects of well-intentioned brain surgery to specific brain areas. Many of these patients are said to be 'amnesic'. They're unable to remember anything for more than a few moments, but strangely often have clear memories of the past well maintained, for example, they can recall events and people from their childhoods.

Long term memory is divided into two forms: firstly those memories we 'know 'about, often called 'declarative memory' because we can 'declare' the memory details, but sometimes also called 'explicit' memory. To make it easy think 'facts' and 'experiences' and you've got it.

When I ponder memory and what I can recall, I come up with this sort of thing: a wonderfully vivid memory of Jimi Hendrix on stage at the Isle of Wight pop festival in 1970, at about two in the morning, playing his version of 'God Save the Queen'. I can see some scrappy bits of it in my mind and get a 'visual' flash of a frame or two of what I must have seen (think, visual cortices in cohorts with the medial temporal lobe memory (MTL) system). I can also re-play it a bit in my mind too. So have a rather 'bitty' memory of the music, presumably coming from the auditory cortices and related sound processing modules in the MTL cobbling it together. These two neural cell assemblies, the auditory and the visual, are therefore linked and have the trigger cell assembly words: 'Isle of Wight' in-putting them. I also get rather disturbing flashes of the toilets too. They were bad!

I have quite vivid memories of flying over the top of that car, after hitting it from behind on my motorbike (see earlier chapter), but no memories of any pain. I do remember grazing and bruising my knee cap and my Mum treating it with ultrasound when I got home. It was swollen, but the pain I remember, wasn't at all bad. I was full of endorphins probably, thankful to be alive!

So we seem to have a word-based memory which drives life's narratives – hence recounting stories of things that have happened, how to do things, how to get somewhere, or of one's life history. What I note here is that when I try to remember say my infant school, I get visual flashes at first; the playground, the teachers, the classrooms, my mates and then their names come and possibly some incident like when my friend Sarah ran into the boy's toilets whilst I was having a pee! Sometimes though the names come first and they're followed by a visual and so on. If I smell something it can be familiar, so smells are in memory – but for most of us smells don't 'come to mind' like sounds, visuals or words and narratives. For example, if I say 'cinnamon' I can't suddenly sense its smell. If I were to smell cinnamon when it wasn't there, I would be hallucinating!

But there are some people who can remember smells as if they were really there. Here's what Gordon C. wrote to Oliver Sacks in 2011:

> *'Smelling objects that are not visible seems to have been a part of my life for as long as I can remember... If, for instance, I think for a few minutes about my long dead grandmother, I can almost immediately recall with near perfect sensory awareness the powder that she always used. If I'm writing to someone about lilacs, or any specific flowering plant, my olfactory senses produce that fragrance. This is not to say that merely writing the word 'roses' produces the scent; I have to recall a specific instance connected with a rose, or whatever, in order to produce the effect. I have always considered this ability to be quite natural, and it wasn't until adolescence that I discovered that it was not normal for everyone. Now I consider it a wonderful gift of my specific brain.'*

Could it be a similar thing for people with persistent post-healing pain and chronic pain? Instead of being able to recall smell, they have a unique ability to recall pain? Note that Gordon C can't just bring any given smell to mind, he requires it to be in some kind of context. Can we think of this in the same way as the RSI patient whose pain returns or significantly worsens when their attention is given to work, the office and all the many other cues, it is associated with. The context triggers the cell assembly into activity and their unique brain has the ability to bring the pain to consciousness – in the same way that Gordon C's thoughts of his grandmother triggered the recall of the smell of her powder. Perhaps it's those who have the 'pain recall' capability are the ones most likely to suffer on-going pain problems?

My brain can think of the injuries I've had and it can remember that it hurt at the time, but I don't get the actual feeling of the pain coming back to me at all. What I'm saying is that maybe some brains can do that, or get good at doing that? Thinking like this has led me to wonder whether on-going chronic maladaptive pains could be considered to be hallucinations. I think this idea should be taken seriously. The word hallucination, in tandem with the example of smell given above, I have found to be a useful metaphor for explaining on-going pain in some patients recently. One has to be very careful though. The important thing about hallucinations is how exceptionally 'real' they are to the person who has them.

If you're ever brave/daft enough and have the opportunity, the experience of taking LSD may be well worth a visit! It allows you to see that the brain can be capable of giving you a perceptually distorted, novel and rather bizarre view of the world for round about twelve hours and sometimes a lot more. Well that's how long it lasted in the early 70's when I took it!

You'll soon see, with only a little chemical help, that the brain can get things awfully wrong and awfully distorted, yet it feels incredibly real. When I did it, I could smell the strong fragrance of odourless paper flowers, I could hear music in incredible detail – when there was silence and I could see people and objects that weren't there at all.

Would anyone, with a memory like mine that has no past pain recall ability, like to volunteer for a trip to see if they can go and visit the painful situation they were in and then see if they can recall some of their past pains? (Rather than just having the memory that you had awful pain at one time). Care though, because a bad trip isn't a nice place to get stuck in.

I'm now wondering if anyone has tried LSD as a pain treatment. LSD trips get easily directed by suggestion – maybe a trip with some pain-fun or pain-manipulating suggestions might help a bit of re-processing? It'd be like hypnosis by LSD perhaps?

If you're worried about taking LSD you're probably right, but be aware that Oliver Sacks in his younger days took a great deal of it and so did Baroness Susan Greenfield of Ot Moor, the brain physiologist. So did Louis Sebastian of Falmouth and that's probably why I've only got 'bits' of memory left from the Isle Of Wight pop festival in 1970. It can't have been too bad, I've still got plenty of bits of Leonard Cohen, The Who, Joni Mitchell, Jethro Tull, Ten Years After, Chicago, The Doors, Emerson, Lake & Palmer, The Moody Blues, Joan Baez, Free, even Kris Kristofferson, Donovan and John Sebastian and the maestro of jazz trumpet Miles Davis. I tingle to remember, but the fact is there isn't really that much left now! They say if you can remember the 1960's, you can't have been there! Well, that was 1970!

The second type of memory is less obvious, hence it being termed 'implicit' or 'non-declarative'. The easiest things to think of here are motor skills, or 'procedures' – actions we do and repeat day in day out and give not one jot of thought to. Other things 'implicit' include emotions and responses we have, that are the result of conditioning. When the clinic phone rings in the house at the weekend or evening, I always get a sudden 'pang' of anxiety in my stomach. No matter what I try to do to stop it, it won't go away. I just accept it as a rather annoying and unpleasant reaction.

If you read any of the memory literature it is almost bound to mention patient H.M. In the early 1950's H.M's brain was operated on in a last ditch attempt to help his very severe and uncontrollable epileptic fits. The surgeons removed large parts of both temporal lobes on either side of his brain (remember, that's where the MTL memory system resides). His epileptic fits were successfully quelled; sadly though, H.M lost his memory and as a result became a subject of much interest and study. From the time of the operation and recently, some forty years after his surgery, he does not know his age, the current date, where he lives, whether his parents are dead or alive or his own history. Although his fits have been controlled, he accomplishes little, if any new learning, to such an extent that he has required constant supervisory care ever since the operation. He has been unable to learn the names and faces of those who see him regularly and doesn't respond to or recognise photographs of himself. As quickly as the daily events of his life occur he forgets them.

H.M is described as 'amnesic'. He not only lost his long-term memory, he also lost his ability to hold anything for very long in his 'short-term' or 'working' memory; that's the place, for example, that you stick the flow of these sentences momentarily, in order to understand what I'm on about. It's also the place where you try to keep hold of the directions someone might give you when you're lost and have to ask the way. It's the place where you know what happened to you, who you've just met and where you've just been – it also may be a vital part of being conscious.

Short-term or 'working' memory also contains the stuff that can go into long-term memory.

In H.M's surgery, the surgical notes revealed that the main temporal lobe areas removed were the hippocampus, the amygdala and parts of the surrounding cortex. From this and the results of other subjects with specific brain area damage, it seems that the hippocampus is the area most consistently associated with memory deficits. Note that in figure 16.3 there are very strong connections from the transitional cortex back and forth with the hippocampus.

When researchers looked more closely at H.M, they found that he was still capable of some memory tasks. For example: with practice he learnt and got a lot better at the mirror drawing test. If you don't know this test, what you do is trace round a star shape with a pencil; but you do it by viewing the star and your hand with the pencil, in a mirror. Because it's all back to front it's quite tricky when you start, but with a few practices speed and accuracy improve and this is exactly what H.M did. Sadly though, because of his difficulty with short-term and explicit long-term memory, he was unaware that he had been practicing and was getting better at it. He got better at it even though he didn't realise he was! H.M was also able to improve his ability to mirror-read, for example, *noil* is lion and *elzzup* is puzzle (and *siuol naitsabes* is my secret code name!), but again without being aware of it.

This tells us that some forms of learning are independent of the temporal lobe and the hippocampus. They're processed and stored elsewhere. Even so, if our 'medial temporal lobe' memory areas are intact, we can still know that we've learnt things that are peculiar to these 'implicit' forms of learning. If I practice mirror-reading, I get better at it (the skill is stored in implicit memory circuits), but unlike H.M, I know I've got better at it – that 'knowing' is stored in the explicit memory system.

Recall from earlier that the 'integration' of information from the sensory cortices ('The Fighting Temeraire'!) occurs in the **transitional** or '**rhinal**' cortex, which is situated in the medial temporal lobe near to the **hippocampus** (figure 16.4). To remind you again, these two areas are considered to constitute the 'medial temporal lobe' memory system (see figure 16.3 and 16.6). LeDoux 2003, feels that the integrated picture formed in the transitional cortex is then passed on to the hippocampus, which, as we've seen, is an area of the brain known to be important in memory formation. The hippocampus is also known to be vulnerable to the detrimental effects of stress (cortisol is known to cause degenerative neural changes in the hippocampus in particular). No wonder memory suffers when you're long term stressed; and no wonder patients with on-going pain report poor memory and concentration. Stressful levels of pain can hijack consciousness, screw up concentration and leave you forgetful – so can stress, without pain.

It's not all negative though, short term stress and controllable stress actually enhances memory formation. I like the rule: a little of something bad is bound to be good for you. That's why smoking about three roll-ups a week will one day be shown to keep your immune system on its toes!

Pathways taking information from the sensory cortices via the transitional cortex to the hippocampus are said to be 'mirrored', hence information can flow back again (see figure 16.3). In this way it seems that all areas involved in processing information can actually become involved in the formation of long term memories. I find it easier to understand if I imagine that there's a 'reverberation' going on between all the areas and it's this that goes on to form a part of the neural network specific to the experience being processed. Ian Robertson (1999) used the term 'trembling web' which may help. It's simply lots of neural activity going on, round and round, back and forth in specific circuits related to what you're conscious of at that moment. Every time something new happens, space is found for a novel neural network to represent it and if it then reverberates, having been switched on by attention, context, physical and environmental triggers, antecedents, cues, feelings etc. It has the capacity to 'come to mind'!

Now, care is required for us to not be lazy and think that a given memory is a mere neural network or circuit of firing neurones in some nicely insulated little location in the brain. The plea from the embodied consciousness position, as I mentioned at the end of chapter 16.1, is to think more interconnecting circles-on-circles-on-circles and to always be inclusive of the body, the nervous system and brain, all the relevant inputs, the central processing and all the outputs back to the tissues and on in again.

Could this be how consciousness might work, that whatever we 'have in mind' is a switched on and far reaching network of 'firing' cell assemblies? Well, maybe, I'm not qualified to say and here I'd just like the reader to get as much of a handle on it as I have and then maybe think about finding out a bit more. Certainly getting to know the various 'bits' I'm mentioning should make any exploration you do a little less painful!

I have to say that I find it hard to imagine that we'll ever understand how neural (and more/other) activity can give rise to conscious awareness and to thinking, planning, imagining, feeling, dreaming, scheming and a whole lot more. We'll know the anatomy and wiring that's for certain; in fact we're getting there now at this sort of gross level. To me, working out how consciousness emerges from the activity of neural networks and the myriad of bio-physiological interactions is a similar sort of challenge to thinking about what's out there beyond space, or how our universe may have started. Bill Bryson in his book: A Short History of Just About Everything does the best job on this front that I've ever read. He's a master, an absolute master at making complex things easy to understand and be amazed at. Hero, yes, as a master explainer, why not! Maybe he could take on the brain and consciousness next?

Onwards! Let's do our best and take this conscious thing a little further. You hate it? I love it! At least I love the idea of being able to make it understandable to a pretty average brain like mine and then to try it for size with Mr and Mrs-interested-but-don't-make-it-too-difficult-please. I'm going to try all this out on my son Jake soon. He's foolishly showed some interest after answering this question correctly first time: 'What's the main function in nature of the abdominal muscles?' It's a question I used to always ask at my lectures and never got the right answer straight away[1]

1 - Abdominals, in most creatures who have them, are primarily used for expelling air from the lungs – not core stability, or sit-ups! Want a toned up flat tummy? Go on a 'calorie restricted diet' and get out of breath regularly and for good long periods; not only will you develop the abdominal looks and tone of a whippet, you'll live forever.

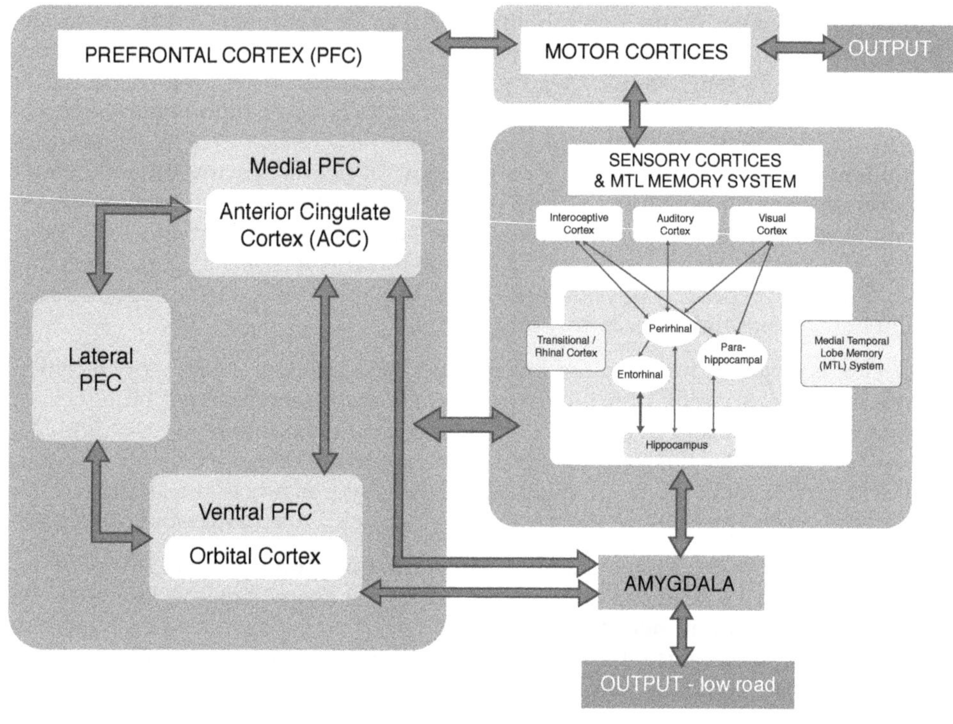

Figure 16.6 My own diagram but in the spirit of Joseph LeDoux – to show the relationships between working memory/prefrontal cortices, the medial temporal lobe memory system and the various sensory cortices. Explained fully in the text.

Working memory and consciousness

Let's now move from the top, side and back of the brain (figure 16.3) to the front (figure 16.6). Slightly technically, we're moving forward from the **Temporal lobe** (put your hand on the side of your head over your ears with elbows pointing forwards – as you would if you were shielding your ears from a loud noise), the **Parietal lobe** (hand on side of head above ear, fingers upwards) and the **Occipital lobe** (back of the head), to the bit at the front of the front that is particularly massive in humans, the **Frontal lobe** (put your hand on your forehead like you would when you're at the end of your tether with the kids!). Not unreasonably the front of the Frontal lobe is called the prefrontal area!

Why did I mention all those lobes? Don't forget like I said earlier, the 'sensory cortices' are not all in one place on the cortex. The **visual cortices** are in the Occipital lobes, which are more to the back of the brain, the **interoceptive cortices** are generally concentrated deep in the temporal area, as is the **auditory cortex**, and the **somatosensory cortex** is in the Parietal lobe or area (more of which in section 19).

The **'prefrontal cortex'** (PFC) has strong connections to all the sensory cortices just listed, as well as to the medial temporal lobe (MTL) memory system (as a reminder, that's the transitional/rhinal cortices combined with the hippocampus) and also to the motor cortices too (it's all in figure 16.6). There are three areas of the prefrontal cortex that are thought to be key to 'working memory' or, to take a nice LeDoux based leap – to consciousness! (Take a smack for being too 'brain-centric' and reductionist, but live with it. It helps to pop in there from time to time).

If you think about it, what's in our working memory is really what's in our mind and that is consciousness! Not only that, these frontal areas are also key to attention, planning , meaning and doing something about the situation we 'consciously' find ourselves in or, more mundanely, simply being aware of the thoughts we are having and what we might want to do in a minute.

The important prefrontal areas for 'working memory' are the lateral, medial and ventral prefrontal cortices (PFC's). To be a bit nerdier, because the areas crop up in nociceptive processing and we should know them, the ventral PFC contains a special zone called the **orbital cortex** and the medial PFC a special zone called the **Anterior Cingulated Cortex**. The anterior cingulate cortex, or ACC, is very commonly referred to when you read about 'pain' processing in the brain. Now take a quick break to check, by following the arrows in figure 16.6, the relationships between: the Sensory Cortices and MTL memory system; the Prefrontal Cortex; the Motor Cortices and the Amygdala. You could put the whole lot, barring the Motor Cortices, in the upper right hand 'bubble' in figure 16.2. Also, note the connections from the prefrontal cortex **direct to the Amygdala** from the medial and ventral prefrontal cortices. This allows a direct controlling effect from what you might have in your mind, to what the quick and dirty low-road is trying to do. A mind-over-matter type connection, perhaps?

Easy! Lighten up for a second. No, 'on second thoughts', don't!

Try imagining something with a bit of emotion attached to it if you can. I can think of that motorbike crash I had where I went over the top of a car; I can also think of the time I had 'clot retention' while on a canal boat holiday in South Wales. Clot retention, if you don't know, is when a blood clot blocks the urethra and you can't pee as a result. It's the most horridly painful experience and you think you're going to die, no you don't – you'd like to die. Not only that but the pain involved in clearing it, at Abergavenny Hospital A & E department, was even worse. Think chimney sweep! It's the one experience in my life that if I think about too deeply, can bring a strong emotional reaction out in me. Don't go there Louis! Perhaps you're better-off thinking of a situation that has strong positive emotions associated with it, like that romantic sunset moment when you first met your loved one? Ah, novelty and yup, biology tricked you! Stop it, we don't go there!

Having questioned a fair number of friends about remembering and getting emotions to well-up at the same time, it seems that some folk find this task a lot easier than others. I'm not good at it at all, hence the clot retention memory being one of only a very few I've ever experienced that 'gets-me'. Actors/actresses seem to be able to well-up the tears as easily as Wayne Rooney manages to find his spit, or do they sniff an onion just before the cameras roll? The best examples are families of victims' following a court case, or some kind of inquiry – often many years after some ghastly tragedy. They front up to the cameras fine and get asked all sorts of questions, then there's one slightly deep one and they lose it emotionally. I'm thinking of the Hillsborough football stadium disaster right now. That disaster was 1989, a long time ago, but recently (2012-13) the long awaited and terribly delayed enquiry has finally exonerated the Liverpool fans who were gleefully blamed by the police, the press and the government of the day. Those who were there knew otherwise. The recent enquiry revealed that none of the Liverpool fans were responsible and that the authorities made massive attempts to conceal what happened. Apparently over one hundred witness statements were altered by the police and a great many believe that Prime Minister Thatcher and her government colluded with police to keep the focus of blame on the fans.

The key thing is that emotions run deep and last a great many years, if not for a lifetime. As the recent Hillsborough enquiry revealed its findings, the aggrieved families of the victims still had great difficulties during interviews. When will someone come forward to say they were responsible? When will those terribly wronged families get what they are due – a fair trial and investigation into who was responsible? I find it amazing. If I was guilty of something, I couldn't hide it or live with it. Or should I somehow admire the ability of humans who have done a 'wrong' to someone else to then be able to concoct a narrative that completely alleviates their personal sense of guilt? A great many seem to be able to convince themselves that they are guiltless, when they are blatantly guilty.

Anyway, bring whatever memorable moment you like to mind and hopefully you can see that the image you get is quite vivid, perhaps even as strong and powerful as a Turner painting or your favourite view, or maybe some loss or love in your life.

So, by asking you to think about something, I've cued your prefrontal cortex working memory areas to connect up with medial temporal lobe memory system and the cortical visual centres that hold the slide show of your life, which in-turn activate the neural 'cell assemblies' that are relevant to the cue. The prefrontal areas, in activating the medial temporal areas will give the broad overall picture, but will also get added detail direct from relevant areas of the visual cortices in the occipital lobe. Then, with grand reverberations back and forth, the frontal lobe working memory circuits, fuelled by the memory networks all come together in some wonderfully conducted and co-ordinated kind of concerto, to fill consciousness with the scene selected in all its details and dimensions.

This visualisation, may, if you've delved right down, like I can if I really let myself go 'deep' into my 'clot-retention' narrative, bring along with it some quite powerful emotional feelings and qualities, but, there's not only the emotional feeling, there's the physical tension, the raised heart beat, the gut feelings and the sweaty bits too. Much of this stuff comes from the 'implicit' emotional memory circuits that surround the 'low road' and hence from regions like the amygdala (see figure 16.5, bottom right), the hypothalamus, the brain stem, the spinal cord and on out to those tissues and organs involved and all the way back in again... and again...

Just now I mentioned three pre-frontal cortex brain areas and I would just like to add some 'brain-centric' functional aspects of them. Firstly, together, the lateral prefrontal cortex and the anterior cingulate cortex (ACC) are thought of as important attentional networks but also important in decision making and voluntary movement control.

... 'Clickety-click' in the graveyard via the amygdala and its close links to the hypothalamus and brain stem sympathetic, as well as appropriate motor pathways – the 'low-road' ramps up the overall somatic and physiological tension and readiness. The autonomic and HPA systems kick off, hence appropriate heart rate and cardiovascular responses and the dulling of anabolic (repair and growth) physiology. Moments later, the 'high road' grabs it all too, conscious attention drops what is was doing and gets heavily focused and interested in the potential threat. Working memory and cortical sensory systems start begging for and getting every bit of detail that it's possible to have. It samples the here-and-now of the environment and anything from the past that may be relevant or may help. Thereupon planning consciousness takes to the floor to deliver its grand verdict: 'I have all the facts now, I have dwelled on what is now – I have dwelled on my knowledge and wisdom and I have decided that I agree with the low-road... Get the bloody hell out of here!' Or maybe it thinks, 'I know that bloke, that clickety-click was a cigarette lighter, he lives over the road in the housing estate, he often comes over here for a fag and to check his wife's grave.' The prefrontal working memory ponders whether the low road's response needs to be modified. 'Yes it does, calm down it's only that old fella' having a fag by his wife's grave.' The low road is dampened down but a degree of adrenaline remains just in case!

The third prefrontal area – the orbital cortex is my friend, in that it's a kind of 'MOM central' place. It's associated with what's good and bad at that very moment and therefore is likely to play a role in making us feel 'bothered' – which in turn drives a chosen behaviour. Patients with damage to this area show indifference to emotional cues that may well come directly from the amygdala (see arrow figure 16.6).

'Oh, it's a threatening bloke with a flick knife and a gun, am I bothered? ... Nah.'

Evolution deals any given population a spectrum of 'botheredness'. As I've said before, some of us are up and running at the slightest sniff of danger, others may be more laid back. It's the 'Springbok' temperament at one end and the 'Sloth' at the other. That we can move along this spectrum will be reviewed in section 20 when I look at chronic stress.

You may have come across the commonly used term 'limbic brain' and associate it with the more primitive and anatomically 'deeper' parts of the fore and midbrain, whose main concern is with emotional processing and our emotional life. As a result, the limbic brain has always been separated from the so-called more 'advanced' neocortex, the outermost layer of the brain. The neocortex, the outer 'crust' or 'rind' of the cerebral cortex, is generally described as consisting of six, cellular layers and notably present in mammals, but not given the time of day in more primitive vertebrates like the birds and our reptile ancestors – hence the 'neo', meaning 'new', prefix. However, since evolution is renowned to be a slow plodding process and not given to the sudden appearance of 'new' structures it is unsurprising that with a closer less anthropocentric look, rudiments of a neocortex are indeed present in birds and reptiles. It's a bit small and a bit hidden, but it's there, and it isn't really 'new' after all.

The point though is that we wouldn't be quite what we have come to be, if it wasn't for the massive increase in size of the mammalian neocortex. Humans have the most awesome one, so awesome that we can only fit it into our skulls by having it carefully and accurately folded up. The relative size of the neocortex between chimps and humans is nicely illustrated using what's called the 'neocortex to medulla' size ratio. In chimps the ratio is 30:1, whereas in humans it's 60:1! We have the mother of all neocortices – double that of a chimp in these terms. That a chimp has 96% the same genome as a human is often quoted to show how alike we are, but this lesser known ratio perspective is far more revealing to our differences in brain power!

LeDoux (1998, 2003) goes to some lengths to dispel the notion of the limbic brain and its strong historic ties to the so-called 'emotional brain'. For the simple reason that the neocortex is inseparably involved in emotions and in turn, the classic limbic parts of the brain are inseparably involved in thinking, memory and consciousness. The example of the orbital part of the prefrontal cortex (i.e. neocortex) being involved in working memory/consciousness as well as in processing and acting on emotion is one of many that can be used to support the limbic/neocortex/whole brain and nervous system functional overlap! The 'limbic brain' term doesn't look as if it's going to go away any time soon and I have to say I don't mind it, but I do like LeDoux's perspective.

The 'high'... 'slow and accurate'... get-the-situation-into-consciousness-and-make-sense-of-it-in-terms-of-what-the-brain-already-knows-and-then-decide-what-to-do... 'road', is vital for humans to be adaptable and flexible. It allows us to feel that we're in control (but note, if you've time and the inclination some day, read the last chapter in Satel and Lilienfeld 2013).

As far as therapy is concerned, hopefully the perspective on the brain, briefly discussed and reviewed here and the last few chapters, will give added credibility to aspects of our interactions that impact processing via 'bottom-up' and 'top-down' inputs.

Behaviours and emotions when we're in pain...

Lastly, though this may not be quite the place to do this, I'm quite randomly going to throw in a bit about pain and what we 'do' when we're in pain. It's easy.

When I used to lecture about brain 'outputs' it used to go like this...

1. Conscious awareness of 'pain' can be seen as an 'output' of the brain.
2. We can see it like this:
   a. The CNS and brain **samples** the incoming 'help me' nociceptive messages from the tissues of the body (or even the messages it might be receiving from some old and now meaningless or over-active pain representational 'cell assemblies').
   b. The CNS/Brain **scrutinises** the incoming information – not just the nociception but everything that might be going on in the body and

environment at the time as well and may produce or 'output' pain if circumstances allow. Clearly the pain itself can then be sampled too, thinking 'sensory dimension of pain' – there's plenty of information from pain that can be scrutinised; the location of the pain, the intensity of it and its quality for example and it all begs for some kind of immediate response. For example, go and have a look see what's happened and do something appropriate to help.

c. While all this pain is going on, the brain also samples itself – for things like past experiences; what it may know about this sort of problem, what it knows about what others have done in order to make sense of the pain and come up with some kind of understanding or assessment of the situation and from there plan an appropriate response – this is part of the 'cognitive' dimension of pain.

d. The outcome of the basic scrutiny is that the individual comes up with an evaluation of their situation with the pain – which is crudely somewhere along a spectrum from 'It is bad' at one end to 'It is fine' at the other. Whatever is decided the person ends up with a 'feeling' about the situation and this feeling relates to the 'Affective' dimension of pain. Feelings can be seen as yet another 'response'.

3. In this way it can be seen that after all the complex sampling and scrutinising we end up with two categories of response to pain:

   a. **Those involving 'efferent' or motor pathways, i.e. behaviour**, which are supported by appropriate physiological changes; well co-ordinated thanks to 'stress response co-ordinating centres' in the brain to produce appropriate efferent autonomic and endocrine activity for example.

   b. **Those involving 'emotional' processing and output.**

I'll make a list of each, but if you teach get your students to make the list – see if they're thinking broadly like this. It's fun too.

a. **Those involving 'efferent' or motor pathways/behaviour:**
   - do nothing, rest
   - get restless, don't stop moving
   - limp, use antalgic movement and posture
   - illness behaviour
   - groan and moan
   - tense and clench
   - decide to never move normally again
   - fill in a claim form
   - ring a law firm
   - handle and hold the painful area all the time
   - wimp out
   - gesticulate
   - talk incessantly about what happened and the whole problem
   - stay inside
   - go walk about

- go to bed
- read the holy scriptures
- call for a holy man to help
- relax and enjoy a day-off
- seek help... Dr, therapist...
- get on with life and ignore it, go to work
- take drugs and medication
- get smashed
- cry a lot
- phone a friend
- blame someone or some organisation, especially the government
- get cross
- book a holiday
- read a book
- take an overdose... etc. etc.

b) **Those involved in 'emotional' processing and output:**

- annoyance
- anger, pissed-off
- drained and deflated
- 'Oh, no' not again...
- dread
- fear
- anxiety and worry
- concern
- frustration...
- wound right up
- really pleased
- elated
- sick feeling
- puzzled
- why me feeling
- blame
- retribution
- hate
- distaste
- disgust
- anguish.

I'll leave it there.

Final thoughts: you now have my twist on LeDoux's; 'slow but accurate high-road' and 'quick and dirty low road', two types of long-term memory, short-term or working memory and, a tiny insight into all I feel I've ever needed to understand about consciousness. Although and thanks to conversations with Mick Thacker recently, I'm changing my mind a lot here! In the 'Read what I've read' section at the end, I've listed a few of the good consciousness books that are worth trying. The main thing is an appreciation of how the brain deals with 'threat' – especially in terms of how the 'threat' of pain is perceived and evaluated by the patient. That 'top-down' related inputs are a very significant part of our therapeutic input and have a sound and rational biological foundation, should be powerfully evident. I hope you agree?

The main thing is that change is always possible!

Section 16
Read what I've read

Braithwaite V. (2010) Do fish feel pain? Oxford University Press. Oxford.

Bryson W. (2004) A Short History Of Nearly Everything. Black Swan. New York.

Blackmore S. (2010) Consciousness: An Introduction. (2ND Ed). Routledge. London.

Dawkins R. (2003) Good and Bad Reasons for Believing. Letter to his daughter, In: 'A Devil's Chaplin', Weidenfeld & Nicolson. London.

Dawkins R. (2004) The Ancestor's Tale: A pilgrimage to the Dawn of Life. Weidenfeld and Nicolson. London.

Edelman G., Tononi G. (2001) Consciousness: How Matter Becomes Imagination. Penguin. London.

Greenfield S. (1998) How might the brain generate consciousness? In: Rose S (Ed) From Brains to consciousness: Essays on the new sciences of the mind. Allen Lane The Penguin Press. Harmondsworth.

Le Doux J. (1998) The Emotional Brain. Weidenfeld & Nicolson. New York.

Le Doux J. (2002) Synaptic self. How our brains become who we are. New York, Vicking Penguin.

Paramecium moving about. http://www.youtube.com/watch?v=YtRie9sDE-8

Ridley M. (2003) Nature via Nurture. Genes, experience and what makes us human. Fourth Estate, London.

Rose D. (2006) Consciousness: Philosophical, Psychological, and Neural Theories. OUP. Oxford.

Sacks O. (2012) Hallucinations. Picador. London.

Sapolsky R.M. (2001) A primates memoir: Love, death and baboons in East Africa. Jonathan Cape. London.

Salposky R.M. (1997) Junk food monkeys. Headline. London. (It's now called 'The trouble with testosterone')

Sapolsky R.M. (2005) Monkey Luv and other lessons on our lives as animals. Vintage books. London.

Satel S., Lilienfeld S.O. (2013) Brainwashed: The seductive appeal of mindless neuroscience. Basic Books. New York.

Watson L. (1995) Dark Nature. A natural history of evil. Hodder and Stoughton. London.

Robertson, I. (1999) Mind sculpture. Your brain's untapped potential. London, Bantam Press.

Section 17

WHAT'S THE BRAIN GOT TO DO WITH PAIN?

Chapter 17.1
Arousal, attention, pre-occupation, tension and expectation!

What's all this brain stuff got to do with pain? Perhaps it's all about some of the unfortunate spin-offs due to the way our brains work. The main thing is that it should help us to improve treatment and management outcomes, as well as understand pain a great deal better. For management it's all about top-down before and during bottom-up! In other words, top-down can modulate or change bottom-up. The 'high-road' can change and influence the 'low-road'.

Here we go.

Thanks to the way we have evolved, we're saddled with a well entrenched and ancient system, that when there's a threat about is biased towards the 'it's bad' choice (recall the 'Is it bad?' or 'Is it good?' choice discussed in the MOM, section 10). This is even stronger the more uncertain or novel the situation appears. Thinking 'brain-centrically' this is all about 'threat-processing', with the amygdala and the 'low-road' dominating in parallel with the 'high-road', that's agreeing and therefore egging-on the 'low-road'. A new and unexpected pain, the pain that comes on with injury or illness and immediate pain relating to changes in our muscles and joints, will all be 'low-road' processed before anything else. An ascending nociceptive message should wisely register as a threat because its very nature is to selfishly seek expression in consciousness, cause pain and then demand our attention and get something done to help. You could see a nociceptor as a philanthropic messenger that cares for the tissues it supplies. Ultimately though it is a selfish tissue based message, a 'me, me, me, look after me... only me, forget the rest, me, me', thing.

Our default setting for pain, is to quickly mistrust and be careful, to avoid and pay attention and to tense and become aroused. A result of this, is that there are much stronger upward, conscious bound connections (between the somewhat automatic 'low-road threat' circuitry and the sophisticated 'high-road' processing components) than there are in the opposite direction, trying to impose some control and dampen things down. That may be why 'mind-over-matter' and 'will-power' are so hard and why we have such difficulty in trying to get patients to change their habitual modes of thinking and behaviour. A lot of top-down effort and practice are required to overcome the default 'reactivity' of the 'low-road'.

Arousal attention and preoccupation

Clearly, it doesn't take much of a dispassionate look at the way humans behave, to realise that emotional reactivity powerfully dictates what we do and how we respond. There are only a very few who are really good at stepping back in threatening situations to let their high-road cognitive processing take charge, in order to weigh-up the options of the situation before responding! The result is, that it's often hard to over-ride the default 'threat response' setting. It seems that the amygdala circuits are very capable of capturing or hi-jacking control of consciousness, manipulating it so as to force attention, perception and memory towards the thing it is selfishly concerned with and wants to react in its way to. Not only that, it can also collar the **brainstem arousal system** to then impose and maintain **the interest of working memory circuitry**.

In this respect, pain or nociception, when processed as a threat, is very much a 'bottom-up' and formidably dominant force for any high-road cogitation to contend with. As most of us know, especially when intense, it's often easier to go with it or give in to it rather than sit back think about it, weigh up the various possibilities about, then act upon a fair assessment of them all!

Arousal systems revolve around specific neurones, that project to cortical areas and which are endowed with specific 'arousal' neurotransmitters. Hence: acetylcholine, noradrenaline, serotonin and dopamine containing neurones. If you get a bit focused on something, it's these chemicals that keep the concentration and preoccupation going! They help to hold your attention to the task in hand. If there's pain, it's the low-road and its naturally cosy relationship with the arousal system that helps keep your attention glued to it. Attend to pain and you feel it more because the arousal system sharpens the response of the pain processing modules.

If you're a bit of a hunter-gatherer, like me, you'll know, that if you've ever been out foraging you 'get your eye in' for what you're looking for. Your attention gets 'zoned in' to your quarry. Pain may be the same. You are bound to have plenty of patients who admit that they find their heads have become almost obsessively 'preoccupied' with their pain, they're 'zoned-in' to the pain, try asking them, their responses are interesting! For someone with longstanding and pain the easiest way to word the question starts with a statement and runs something like this:

'Others with on-going pain like yours report that they find the pain is constantly on their mind and that they seem to be always thinking about it, some say it almost becomes a 'preoccupation'. I'm interested whether you have any experience or thoughts about this?'

In my experience most patients report that this is indeed the case and they find it drives them mad, being constantly distracted from the task they're trying to do, even when the pain's not there, they find themselves looking for it! This admission often leads into a useful conversation about what actually does distract them and that can be very useful in management.

I'm now thinking of a recent patient, his wife had accompanied him and was listening to the story unfolding and my questions. I asked him the question above about preoccupation and he answered, 'That it just drove him mad'. We then started discussing whether he'd noticed any times when he was distracted and it didn't bother him. He looked puzzled and was shaking his head, but then his wife popped up with...

'Glen, you sit and watch the football for a whole match sometimes without flinching. There, that's an example. You know he tells me he's in constant hell but when the footy's on, he looks normal and you wouldn't know it.'

Well, Glen looked and frowned at his wife, but it opened things up wonderfully. There was the footy; there was when his mates were round; there was when he was having a smoke out the back... He did well in the end. A big thing was when he understood how he could influence his pain processing. He also grasped the need to get going again quickly too.

A story relating to attention and preoccupation has popped into my head.

If there's a skill involved in catching your dinner it's well worth practicing hard until you've got the knack. I guess I've learnt a mass of skills through my life, but one of the most entertaining things I ever tried to learn was how to catch sand-ragworms on the pacific beaches of Morton Island, just off the coast of Brisbane in Australia. This was around 1987-88. We were with Dave Butler, his wife Juliet and Juliet's brother-in-law, Bruce.

Sand-ragworms live in tunnels in sand and they're good fishing bait. This is how it goes. You gather a few little cockles by raking through the sand with your fingers and feeling for them. You then smash the shell of one the cockles and go and crouch on the beach at the tide line, where the waves washing up pass you a bit. As the water runs back down the beach, you waft the smashed cockle in the receding water to add a bit of scent to it and at the same time look out for a raggy's head popping up out of his hole (it senses the cockle smell and detects that a bit of a feed might be nearby). The trick is to deftly grab the head of the worm and pull it out in one quick, but smooth movement... Watch Bruce, yup, looks easy, out comes the worm about two or three foot long and we all laugh, bloody thing's massive. Bruce quips, 'Mind the pincers, the buggers bite.' Fifteen minutes later and Bruce has enough ragworm to start fishing. We're all struggling; it takes me an hour or more to get three! The point is, that there's a tad of fear involved, which makes you hold back, as Bruce said for a laugh these ragworm have a bit of a nip to them. So while you try to go for it, there's this little gremlin called 'fear' holding you back!

The moral of the story is that becoming preoccupied with pain can, at least for some people, be as inevitable as getting preoccupied with learning to catch sand-rag! Preoccupation is a useful brain module for training hunter-gathering and learning useful skills, but it sometimes costs in the context of pain and maybe obsessive-compulsive behaviours too. 'Well, it was like this Doc, I got this terrible fixation with sand-rag!'

The pain message is simple, it's a threat report from the body. It's easily processed, with a strong bias to threat/danger/get focused and get aroused, it grabs your attention and your attention gets locked into it, becoming preoccupied, forcing you to stay with it and to try to do something about it!

Being 'locked-into' a pain problem can mean more than just the pain, it can be the whole input-processing-output expression of the experience. For example, when people have musculoskeletal pain many are poor at relaxation, they habitually and almost sub-consciously hold their muscles tense when they rest and more so when they move Their faces grimace, their whole body moves with an underlying expression of caution and tension. The output causes the antalgic tension and the input, from the tense muscles and pressured joints, then ferries this information centrally. The subsequent scrutinising of it promotes yet more 'threat' related processing.

'Hey mate, you've lost control of your threat-on system...!'

'I know, I know, I'm in a bit of a mess....'

That feedback from the body plays a part in emotional expression, has long been mooted by the well known neurologist and writer, Antonio Damasio. He called his theory the 'somatic marker hypothesis' (see refs). LeDoux quotes some neat work done by Paul Ekman, who had subjects move parts of their face so as to produce various facial expressions, characteristic of different moods. For example, they might be asked to follow the instruction: 'Furrow your brow strongly and clench your teeth,' rather than being asked to make their face look concerned or puzzled. In other words they avoided any mention of emotional expressions. Afterwards, the subjects had to answer questions about their mood and it was found that the way the subjects felt was significantly influenced by their facial expression.

The massive point for us clinically is, that the way a patient moves their body, or the painful part of their body, not only influences the pain but also influences how they feel and their mood. No wonder bottom-up, for example, good quality relaxed movement – helps lift a patient's mood!

I work hard with all pain sufferers to get relaxed movement and relaxed demeanour. Here's a quick example.

Tension and 'top-down-during-bottom-up': Jude

Jude has had on-going back pain for six months. She walks very stiffly and cautiously, her face is not at all happy – it's screwed right up! (Appreciate that I've done a full assessment, explained the findings and a few other things to her etc.) I'm now looking at walking quality and doing something about it at the same time.

I ask Jude to walk up and down the treatment room while I watch.

'Jude, let's stop walking for a minute. I want you to walk again in a moment, but this time I want you to concentrate on your face!'

'What's wrong with it?'

'It's all screwed up, you look like you've seen a ghost! Look at me...'

I smile.

'Smile a minute.'

She does something pathetic but her expression really looks like she thinks I'm nuts...

'Stick your tongue out and see if you can touch your nose with it like this...'

I do it. Now she's smiling.

'Go on have a go.'

She tries and she's starting to giggle...

I keep looking goofy with my tongue sticking out and touching my nose...

'Walk towards me and copy what I do with my face... look at my face...'

She starts walking and I get her to raise her eyebrows with me, then tongue out, then mouth open, then a sickly stupid smile... now sneer... now bored... now...

'Swing your arms and relax as you walk, stick your tongue in and out with every step...'

So it went on, cajoling, playing and mucking about to try and trick the processing to access the happy emotions and turn off those associated with the tension and concern – the threat modules!

We work on shoulders, face, trunk-swinging, arm-swinging. I ask her about her levels of concern...

'Scale of 1 to 10 now Jude, what's your anxiety rating score? A ten score is the worst anxiety you've ever had.'

'It's about a six right now.'

After another five minutes of 'mucking around' and playing with her tension and her expression while moving around it came down to zero. I didn't expect her to change quite so rapidly, so was rather pleased. She sits down and we have a rest.

'Jude, why do you think I've been doing all that stuff just now?'

'Because I'm moving so stiffly and I'm all tensed up I guess.'

'You're right, now do you think that's an important part of your problem, or maybe you're thinking I'm missing something or should be doing something else?'

'Well, to start with I thought you were mad, but it was actually good fun and I feel a lot looser and less painful right now than I have for a long time.'

'You're making good links between tension and the pain. I want you to see that at the moment you're processing simple walking as if it were some kind of threat, which is making you tense up, be stiff and screw your face up. You're probably doing it all the time and it's now become a habit. One of my first goals is for you to practice getting the tension down while you move and that includes your face. So right now, after doing all that relaxed flopping about movement you not only feel less pain, you also feel more relaxed and, less anxious too?'

'Yes, I quite enjoyed it actually, you've made me realise I haven't moved properly for a long time now.'

'So, do you know what I mean when I talk about being tense? I want to make sure you know what I want you to get rid of!'

'Well I didn't before, but now you've pointed it out to me I understand what you mean. It's easier to know I'm tense by thinking about my face than my body I think.'

'Right, that's good. The other thing is that people are often tense when they're fearful or anxious. So my question is: are you fearful when you walk?'

'Well, I never really thought about it but maybe I am... I guess I'm frightened to make the pain worse so that makes me careful... I've been protecting it for a long time.'

'When you were walking well just now, when I had you swinging your arms and walking with a nice free waist, did you feel scared then?'

'Well, no I didn't did I?'

'Some patients have found that if they rhythmically repeat this little saying when they're moving it helps, it doesn't matter how you say it, but it's this: 'trust my body and let it relax... trust my body and let it relax... and so on... Another one that people find helpful is to breathe in for a count of 1, 2 and 3 then out for 1, 2 and 3 as they walk and swing their arms. You can try those if they help, but the main one to start is to just let your face relax, if your face is all wound up and tense, your body is and then the whole problem is being processed in your 'threat' centres. I'm going to write those down in a minute to remind you. The more you practice the easier it gets.'

She nods, and I go on....

'After a while you can run a tension check up... You have to ask yourself if any tension is there, do a scan round your body and your face and then see if you can change it. Use the silly faces and do a few swinging movements to check and then change it.'

When I wrote it all down I included this...

'Goal for next time if you can, I want you to show me a relaxed face and relaxed walking and It doesn't matter how slow you go – so long as it's free and floppy!'

This all looks like a bit of fun and certainly not what most would call standard musculoskeletal physiotherapy! But I hope that you can see how important it can be in the context presented here. It's seemingly small, but it can be a massive kick-start to getting a patient into more adaptive and less threat-processing way of moving. As here, the newfound ability to relax with movement can even generalise to their feelings, like Jude's anxiety and her pain. The use of movement to change mood and feeling states, not only beautifully embraces Damasio's somatic marker hypothesis, but also the embodied consciousness perspective that I discussed in chapter 16.1. Therapeutically let us look at it as more than just a zany treatment embellishment, but a very important part of the toolkit that we have at our disposal.

When patients like Jude improve, they often report afterwards that what helped them most was something like, 'Letting the pain go.' Or, 'It was when you showed me how tense I'd become and I started working on it.' Or, 'The best thing was when you told me to stop processing it like I'd just come across a Tiger'... Or, 'Going slowly and relaxing, then bit by bit building my confidence back up with you were the main things.'

In the above example, I've illustrated how repeated 'high-road' inputs help, in other words our 'top-down' input i.e. to get the patient thinking: why fear walking? 'I can go slow, feel safe, relax, smile, enjoy'. This can be combined at the same time with bottom-up inputs from the body i.e. reduce/trick out the tension with 'happy' movements, like swinging the arms and changing the face. Happy movements aren't processed in threat centres and along with the 'positive' 'high-road' or 'top-down' stuff are all about getting the various linked circuits/cell assemblies/pain related memories to, 'wire-apart'!

I hope the reader can now appreciate in a little more detail, the notion of 'top-down, before bottom-up?' Importantly though, the reality is that it's much better if it's on-going i.e. top-down 'during' bottom-up! Treatment and self-management activities need to be engaged, at the same time as the thinking and perceiving individual with the problem. The high-road, to consciously and regularly work on and modulate the low-road, which in turn, gets it to engage and process the pain/threat in much more adaptive ways.

Practice makes plasticity perfect... is a neat way of thinking about it!

To review: get the high road, our thinking and consciousness to shift to less threatening perspectives, so as to influence and calm the rather belligerent and stubborn 'low-road' reflex threat processing responses, at the same time, if at all possible, work with 'bottom-up' processing. That means doing something physical, that has habitually been processed as a threat and getting it to be processed as less threatening or not threatening.

In the example above, I've used relaxed and spontaneous normal movement and facial expression and instructed the patient to practice at home. If appropriate I could have used manual therapy inputs, though I rarely find I need to or want to these days. This is a far cry from doing a technique and continually asking about the pain response. It's more getting the patient to engage with an input that has the potential to be threatening but starts as easy and non-threatening and works to gradually more threatening levels as success is achieved. Tension with movement, or that produced with touch, pressure or any kind of manual therapy can be adjusted, done in a different starting position or scaled down to get relaxation and focus on letting go, then later maybe letting go with a little pain. As the patient settles and gets used to it the operator may be able to devise ways of taking it further and further. It's 'desensitisation' with a 'tension' focus or spin on it. One word about manual therapy though, is that it's often quite difficult to translate into home practice and it's rarely functional. In the more complex pain patients I tend to steer well clear if at all possible and these days even in the more straightforward, I find I'd much rather use appropriate patient-orientated movements, exercises and activities to address this aspect of their problem.

One important message is, that there's a shift of focus from pain and tension to smooth, relaxed and carefree movement. Thoughtless-Fearless-Movement! I will pick up on this again in the Graded Exposure sections later.

Using a scan to show the effects of attention and expectation on pain

A little review of some clinically important 'brain' related issues...

1. If you're fearful of something it drags your attention to it, you can't keep your mind off it.

2. Give something your attention and it intensifies.
3. Keep giving something your attention and you're likely to memorise it and it can get to you, like an annoying tune does.
4. If, because of concern or fear of pain, you stop doing a lot of the things you'd normally do and end up doing virtually nothing... and, if you're anything like most other people with on-going pain doing nothing... you get bored, you may find that your attention starts to get in the habit of spending a great deal of time listening to and looking out for any pain, that just might be there somewhere.
5. You may get into the habit of constantly scanning your body to see what's going on. As I've already discussed you can become 'preoccupied' with pain just like I can get preoccupied with learning to catch sand-rag.
6. So, if you spend time focusing on your body you'll find all sorts of 'music' playing that you weren't aware of before. Constant body monitoring and scanning for sensations and symptoms is called 'somatising'. It can become problematic and psychologists sometimes use a tool called the 'modified somatic perception questionnaire' (MSPQ) to assess this (see chapter GE 3.2)
7. If you're surrounded by folk who almost continuously keep asking about your suffering and your pain, like those close to you at home but may well include the therapist you go to, one suggestion is to move away from them, or tell them to shut up!

In my second year after qualifying, I worked with a young physiotherapist who suffered a relatively small accident but ended up with on-going and awful neck pain, headaches, shoulder pain and pain down both arms. Just about everyone in the department tried to help her using various forms of manual therapy. She eventually went off sick and she didn't return for over a year. I remember asking what helped the most in her recovery and she said: 'Getting away from all the physios who kept asking me about the pain.' I recall being shocked, almost taken aback at the time, but it stuck in my memory. It now makes perfect sense.

As you will see later, one important 'yellow flag' question is to ask 'How is your family responding to your pain?' The answer is often along these sorts of lines...

'Oh, they've been really good, my wife is always fussing over me, doesn't let me even draw the curtains now and if I do anything all of them are reminding me to be careful of my pain...'

There have been many occasions over the years that after explaining the effects of attention on pain to patients, their efforts to overcome the 'preoccupation' has been stymied by the family who keep asking about it. The only way to deal with this is to involve them, but even then it's a natural human reaction, to ask about and react to pain and pain behaviour.

Some of the ways out are easy to write down, but can be very hard to do... here are a few...

- occupy your mind as much as possible, see Glen above, who's pain behaviour settled with football, smoking and when his mates were round
- get more active, especially enjoyable activities
- use relaxation
- get reassured and get onto the activity hierarchy of recovery (see Graded Exposure section)
- start to try and process your problem away from the threat centres of your brain; try and make friends with the pain, find out that it won't be a disaster (see case history, 'Kate' that follows)
- ... and so on.

With some patients, where they report giving a great deal of attention to their pain, it can be helpful to explain to them and show them the following scans.

Figure 17.1: the picture on the left is an fMRI 'slice' through the brain of an individual receiving painful 'heat impulses' through their skin and where they're being asked to count the number of impulses received. In other words their attention is being manipulated towards the painful stimulus. Note that, extensive areas of the brain that are active and the scan highlights the bright central areas of the right and left anterior cingulate cortex (ACC), the thalamus and the insula cortex. These areas are often involved when individuals feel pain and thought to be important in the processing of nociception (see section 18).

The next two slices show the subject receiving **exactly the same heat pulses** but they're now distracted while receiving them. Researchers 'manipulate' attention, for example, they might be asked to continuously count from 1 to 10, do mental arithmetic (adds a tad of stress!), or simply listen to music. The reduction in activity in all of the areas parallels the report of a decrease in pain intensity. It usefully provides proof that if we can shift attention away from pain, the brain activity,

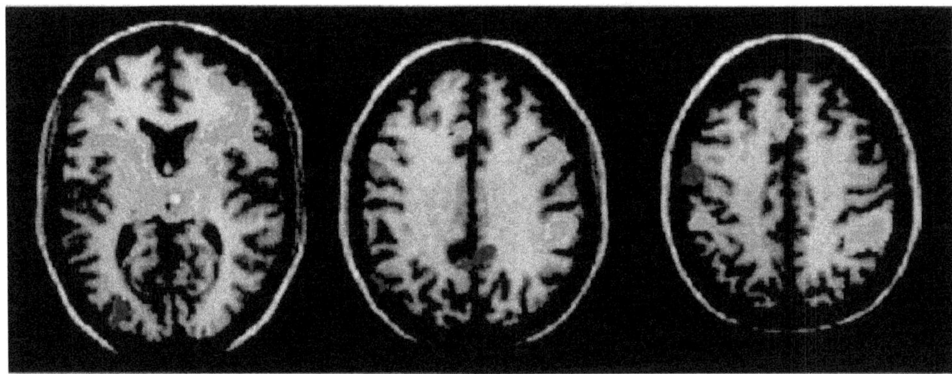

Figure 17.1 fMRI scan through brain. See text for details.

and hence the 'cell assemblies' related to the pain can reduce their activity very significantly.

'So, what you're saying Louis is that diverting attention is a good painkiller?'

'Well, yes and the more life threatening or exciting the thing you're giving attention to, the more effective the attention painkiller seems to be...'

'Can you give me that prescription for that sky-diving lesson then?'... 'Er, no, but I can give you a shot of morphine!'

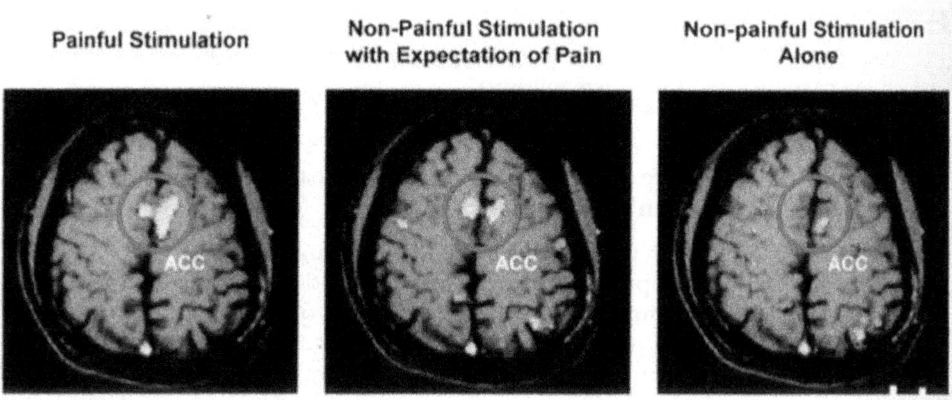

Figure 17.2 fMRI scan through brain. See text for details.

Now, figure 17.2. This one highlights activity in the anterior cingulate cortex (ACC). On the left, the subject receives a painful laser stimulation (feeling of nasty heat on the skin). On the right, the subject receives stimulation to exactly the same place but this time it's non-painful. Then the subject is told that the next stimulation will be painful, even though it's the same non-painful one that's already given. That's the middle scan picture and it shows almost as much brain activity in the ACC as the truly painful stimulus. Brilliant, it shows you what top-down beliefs, or 'expectation' can do to what we feel. The 'truth' has clearly been manipulated.

Here's another interesting study (Koyama and Coghill et al 2005) on the influence of 'expectation'.

These researchers took ten 'normals' and stuck them in a fMRI scanner to monitor their brains while giving them a heat stimulus to their lower leg. The first 'training' session involved three levels of stimulus at timed intervals. No one said anything as far as I can tell, but the subjects learned by experience that a 7 second interval signalled a mild pain heat stimulus; a 15 second interval signalled 'moderate' and a 30 second interval was 'severe' (122 degrees!). The heat stimuli were given for 20 seconds. So the longer the subjects waited the more they knew that something not very nice was going to happen! The experiment was all about manipulating expectations.

A couple of days after this training participants underwent thirty different heat trials, all monitored with the fMRI and asked to rate their discomfort using simple numerical rating scales. The key thing was that the researchers mixed the signals about one third of the time, so participants were expecting one temperature, but actually received either higher or lower temperatures. When subjects were expecting moderate pain, but were actually exposed to severe heat, their ratings of pain were 28% lower than on the training sessions earlier.

So, when a human is expecting a lower amount of pain than they expect – it is lower! As these workers pointed out, not only were the reports of pain less, so were the levels of relevant brain activation.

'28% reduction in pain just like that! Wow, isn't that as good as a shot of morphine Louis?'

Sometimes it can be helpful to discuss and explain the fMRI attention experiments and the expectation experiments with patients. I've had a great many patients make huge shifts in the right direction following discussions about what their 'brains' are doing with the situation they're in.

The key clinical thing to get over to the patient is, that if you expect something to hurt, you're going to inadvertently turn your amplifier on and wind up whatever sensation you should be getting to more than it need to have been! If you've already explained how focusing and worrying about pain draws attention to the pain and amplifies it, these pictures offer some supportive evidence. Also, you may have explained to the patient that the more you concentrate on something, the more likely you are going to learn it and put it into the memory filing system. The more activity in the brain relevant to the pain, the more learning takes place and if you really learn something well, it can be very hard to get rid of. Again, show and explain these scan pictures.

The practical positive message can be, where appropriate, to get the patient to check what their attention is doing from time to time. Here are some tips for the patient, remember though, words are not enough, instruction and practice are vital:

a) Calm down and relax about it, try not to get wound up, even, 'make friends with the pain, try not to keep processing it as a threat.' (See the next case history 'Kate')

b) Do something practical to get an attention shift. For example, exercise, read, music, walk, get on with a hobby, talk to someone, ring them up, do suduko, put on a TENS (more later!) and do something, cook a meal, plan a holiday... ANYTHING! Get the patient to find what's best and become inventive if they can. Success here can be so rewarding. Don't forget the importance of novelty.

c) Try to get the patient to avoid being frustrated if they have little success. Circuits take a long time to get into the system and become a 'habit'. They therefore can take a long time to 'undo', disconnect and change. Use fingernail-biting habit as an example and note how hard it is to stop doing...

Message? Lots of practice and be patient!) Get the patients to occasionally monitor their attention.

e) 'Behavioural experiments' can be very helpful when dealing with 'expecting' to hurt with a given activity and then finding that it wasn't so bad after all! More in the Graded Exposure section!

Chapter 17.2
Explaining pain to a patient: Introduction and thoughts

Let's look at an example of maladaptive pain in-depth with a real patient. The aim here is for you to see how knowledge of pain and the brain can be used.

I would also like to issue a warning though: that this type of patient interaction and outcome is actually rare! Why? Because in most on-going pain patients there's actually much more to it than a lengthy discourse on their pain, followed by an instant adjustment of their beliefs about pain. The patient who learned from the pain-explaining therapist that their pain didn't mean anything, who suddenly got out of the chair, went home and went riding on their bike for the first time in five years, and they were never seen again... just doesn't really exist. Don't believe what some lecturers on the circuit bullshit you about. Cure-all, miracle-type case histories and the like are, for the most part un-witnessed, un-recorded and most often exist to try and get you to buy into the lecturer's wares, fairs and affairs I'm cynically afraid to say. A great many of these therapists, who tell you what you should do, haven't seen a patient in many years I strongly suspect. Be suspicious, ask questions is my advice.

Frankly I, along with many others from the original UK Physiotherapy Pain Association hierarchy, am a bit concerned about the recent wave of 'explain pain' and the rather uni-dimensional way it seems to be delivered. The worry is that core cognitive behavioural awareness and skills have been passed by.

Having said that, explaining pain to patients was how I started my own voyage into doing better with chronic pain. Back in the mid 1990's, when David Butler and I taught our five day course 'The Dynamic Nervous System' together, I used to see real patients in front of the course participants. During the five days I actually used to see three patients out at the front, one to the whole group and then one each to the two halves of the group. The patients inevitably had tricky on-going pain problems, but mostly were nice people, whose therapist was desperate to try and help and so picked them to be plied by the forthcoming lecturers wisdom!

I had over an hour and half with the patients, often running into the lunch break and saw them three times during the course. I spent a great deal of time listening to their stories and clarifying a great deal of things, rather outside the usual manual therapy 'tick boxes'. We often went to places that therapists on the course wouldn't have dreamt finding out about, or even seen as relevant. However, and powerfully and usefully, the material, the narratives and the difficulties these patients volunteered to the group and me, fitted with the pain material that we were teaching on the course like a dream. Listening to information is one thing, but seeing it for real is another. I am very grateful to all those early patients for simply providing the group and me with the reality of 'how it is to have chronic pain'. The stories were often very, very moving.

I have to say though that it's worth getting the early few courses in context, because I felt there was an uneasy imbalance in the material. This was a course, with me teaching about maladaptive and useless pain, pain as a memory, meaningless pain and all the pain mechanisms, explaining spreading pain, chronic pain and pain super-sensitivity. All this was right in the middle of David Butler's almost world-wide tidal wave of excitement about yet even newer nervous system mobilising techniques. At this time, 'neurodynamics' was 'viral'! Adelaide physiotherapist, Michael Shacklock was an important figure here too. He convened the 'Moving in on Pain' conference in Adelaide in 1995 and was a colleague of David Butlers (see Shacklock 2005). So, all sorts of new neurodynamic tests were appearing at the time. Some used two or even three therapists to do the techniques to the patient. For example, 'doing upper limb tension test 1' while the patient was in full slump... or, 'in double straight leg raise, do bilateral upper limb tension test 2a'. Not only that, these guys had devised the most bizarre ways of doing it all: we had 'sliders' and 'tensioners' for example and I hear it still goes on in many parts of the world.

Let's say you have a patient who has bilateral upper limb pain. One technique that might be deemed appropriate to this patient, using the new neurodynamic approach would be 'doing bilateral upper-limb tension' test type mobilising in either a 'tensioner' or a 'slider' way. To do a 'tensioner' both operators would time the maximum extent of the test to coincide, for a 'slider' they would alternate. I have to say, while I quietly accepted what David was doing I hugely struggled with it and I never used it on patients. It just didn't fit, it was almost mad and do you remember that '3-of-us-holding -down-a-patient-doing-a-slump' technique I did back in St Stephen's Hospital? (Trevor's slump, chapter 2.3) but it was worse than even that to me.

At the time of the Dynamic Nervous System course I was in a far different place. I was seeing the sorts of patients, that David and Michael were doing all these fancy weird tests and techniques on and seeing that these patients had a 'processing' problem, dominated by widespread secondary hyperalgesia, not a neural or neurodynamic one. There were far better reasons for their pain 'state' than this, there had to be. Those guys just weren't getting what I was on about at that time. The very first Dynamic Nervous System course in Abergavenny, South Wales and many after too, attracted physios, who understandably wanted the 'latest neurodynamic material' from Australia and David Butler. What they got from me was pain mechanisms and a plea to see pain, especially complex pain, as a processing problem and see it from the thinking processing brain's perspective too. I taught my 'annoying tune' explanation and my 'keyboard' explanation to the real patients and the participants all witnessed some quite remarkable changes in the patients with regards their pain, their therapy and their future. I heard from many of them afterwards, often through their therapist who'd been on the course and they nearly all reported that my short time with them had changed their lives because they had understood their relationship to their chronic pain. Some of those patients had had pain for a great many years and were stuck in the system, stuck in the drugs they were on and stuck in never ending cycles of therapy referral. I remained in contact with several of them and I remember regularly keeping three of them on track for over a year after the course. Thankfully they all did well. I don't mean to puff my chest up, but at that time if I'd got nowhere, I would have left physiotherapy burnt out. I would have easily concluded that for pain, physiotherapy had nothing to offer apart from a bit of physical fiddling in a rather gloomy moment of time. However, these good early patient 'changes', especially those on the course, helped it all fit into place and make it worthwhile. It spurred me on to keep learning, to expand my thinking even further and to embrace the need for multidimensional reasoning and management approaches.

Don't get me wrong, I didn't do well with everyone I had failures, but rarely was it to the point of embarrassment on the course! In fact over the 4-5 years we did the course only one patient kind of 'spoilt it' for me and he was a patient on the Adelaide course, who'd been sent by some physio all the way from Canberra! In retrospect, he was a complex chronic pain patient who really needed to have been on a pain management programme and have all the support of the whole team. The most glaring thing was that he could hardly move or respond to any of the 'activity' sessions I tried; there was lots of maladaptive pain behaviour, with moaning, complaining and grasping and gripping, holding breath, gasping. After he left the last session we all thanked him for coming, I said I'd write to his therapist and we then gave him a hearty applause. He left and the whole class went to the window to look down on him as he walked across the concourse below and out of the college where we were. He was carrying two large cases and walking with gusto! Everyone sniggered and made derogatory comments. At the time I remember being quite annoyed by this guy from the start and what made it even worse was that one of the course participants had actually spotted him moving quite normally in the street after the first day we saw him. So we were all 'in on it,' and sadly he wasn't a useful patient to learn from. He was a good example of what I call 'the patient in front of you', meaning whatever the presentation a patient comes with, whatever you think about it, that is what you have to deal with. For this patient the bigger issues were beyond a course looking at pain processing and showing an early taste for a biopsychosocial approach. The wider issues here were important, such as the reasons why this guy was behaving in this way, his situation, his finances, his relationship with work, his relationship with himself and his life and what he was wanting out of it.

Anyway, it served a purpose and because he was so 'difficult', it stuck in my memory! The irony was that I had come full circle all the way back to Adelaide, a place where I seemed to attract a great many of these complex and hard to help type of customers (see the pain behaviour section, chapter GE 3.2 later!).

I hope you're thinking that results of interactions 'on stage' are massively influenced by the stage context. These patients become centre of attention; they're often pleased to be telling a group of 'experts' about their problem. They are almost forced to listen and attend to what you say, do and ask. If they get on with you they want to be successful for you. That's why celebrity TV shows getting people to change or improve work so well. Put a camera on anyone and tell them they'll be live on TV and they'll up the ante and perform for you. If they don't and some surely don't, they get cut out of the final presentation! I'm thinking Paul McKenna, celebrity hypnotist and self help guru of all things modern like phobias and fat. Several years ago he published a brilliant book (I think it was anyway, but, hey, I'm thin!). It's called 'I Can Make You Thin'. Well, he had a TV show in the UK but also in the USA. You can see bits of it on YouTube. The whole audience were overweight and he introduced all the techniques to them. They were all weighed at the start they were given a bit of the approach and then off they went for a week. Every week he introduced a new way of thinking about eating and eating behaviour and he backed it up with a new technique for the audience to go away and practice. Off they all went again. Well, low and behold, come the end of the programme after a few months, the results were very impressive. The fact that the individuals were being focused on, filmed and exposed was a brilliant additional motivation to succeed. There was never a one year follow up though, so we could all really see if matey had given them the tools to be 'Thin forever' or just a month or two. I doubt it somehow.

Anyway, I was always fully aware that this stage and audience thing helped me to help those patients back then.

Now, our course participants had the problem of, on the one hand hearing about all the pain mechanisms material from me, followed by witnessing a frozen moment of a real patients' pain-life over the five days they attended; but on the other hand they had to deal with the contradiction of this pain theory versus all the neurodynamic manual therapy stuff that David was teaching. Some course participants afterwards revealed that at the start of the course they were quite angry that they were not getting the 'full neurodynamics'. However, thanks to the patient demonstrations, I believe they could see that there was far more to pain than nerve mobilising and standard manual therapy. I was quite vocal at the time about my own 'recovery' from the 'conditioning' of manual therapy! As is typical of anyone young and enthusiastic, I had this big 'mission' to lead manual therapy and physiotherapy out of the passive therapy wilderness to seek and see a better place! They were good times, but I might have been a bit of a pain in the arse for a while.

What was also good was that after a few of the Dynamic Nervous System courses David could see that the neurodynamic component of the course and the manual therapy approach had to change and his own shift began. The material soon faded from the course. I don't know what David would say now, but my recollection was that just like the course participants it was seeing the real patients and the changes they made that helped fire the shift in his own thinking. David went on to research and lecture on the 'outcome' prediction research and all the psychosocial material that was available at the time. This seemed to be well before all the 'yellow-flag' material got any attention. For me his lecture on our course called 'Pain Art and Politics' will always stand out as one of the best lectures I have ever heard.

Soon after, David was brave enough to stand on stage at international physiotherapy conferences and admit that he 'was wrong'. He actually criticised the treatment aspects in his own 'Mobilisation of the Nervous System' book and, that he'd had to shift, to a new multidimensional way of thinking that embraced the new buzz word 'biopsychosocial'. He has since been an international ambassador for promoting this perspective for physiotherapy.

My big message for what follows is that information for a willing patient can sometimes make a massive difference, but for the great majority it needs to be made much simpler and far, far shorter; with masterfully contrived, easy to understand, bite size chunks of information that contain clear RELEVANT messages, if at all possible. I deal with this in the patient examples at the end of the last book.

One last criticism here is that information giving is yet another form of 'passive' therapy, at some point the patient and their brain and body have to be engaged *together*. As per the last chapter, top-down during bottom-up is a good way to go!

But it also means active graded movement, in the context of good behavioural and cognitive techniques, for patients who are chronic or anywhere near the sniff of chronicity that is so common in physiotherapy clinics and our hospital out-patient departments. Even the acute and sub-acute benefit far more from interactions that are patient-centred (meaning the patient does more of the thinking, talking and reasoning and the therapist acts to guide and encourage). So, let's at least start to consider that all interactions wherever possible, need to be laced with behavioural and cognitive skills and methods and simply, doing.

The case history of 'Kate' that follows should act as an example of how detailed some patients can go with information and questioning and also act as a nice clinical revision of why I've been subjecting you all to brain stuff in the last few chapters.

Here we go!

Chapter 17.3
Explaining, listening and interacting with a patient: Kate-part 1

Recall the super touchy, flinchy, jumpy, untouchable patient I mentioned in secton 16 when discussing temperament?

Let's consider this type of presentation, but in a pretty similar way to Jude in chapter 17.1. Kate has had her back pain for about a year and is significantly debilitated by it still. Like Jude, Kate's movements are extremely tense and careful and her back is virtually untouchable. If I go back to early manual therapy and 'Maitland' days, the interpretation of such an untouchable and immovable patient would have been that they're high in 'SIN'! Meaning high Severity, Irritability and Nature, rather than being in the grip of the Devil! High in 'SIN' for Maitland manual therapists guides the therapist to go carefully and do a very gentle grade of mobilisation. If you recall from my very early chapters, this means doing a technique while almost continually keeping up a running dialogue with the patient, asking them about the pain and backing-off or stopping should things get worse. Think about this and it's hardly a decent way to engage the high-road in modulating the low-road! If anything it's feeding more into the negative aspects of low-road processing, focusing on pain far too much, at the same time as doing bottom-up stuff that reinforces it.

Now, given a more flexible and reasoned understanding of the maladaptive nature of pain, the approach can be quite different and a great deal more productive. The following elements of importance are typical of what arises with this type of presentation:

1. A good assessment and examination to reassure me that there are no red flags and the tissues are quite capable of being progressively loaded. A key question for the therapist to ask themselves: 'Is the pain out of all proportion to any damage done or any tissue vulnerability?' I am trying to get the clinician to wonder if the pain might be said to be 'lying' or 'over-egging' it about the state of the tissues that are being reported on! If this is the case, it turns the situation into a 'positive' view of the tissue viability and that this needs to be communicated somehow to the patient. As already discussed, one important aim is to change the high-road so that it can modulate the bad habits of the low-road.

2. When tissues haven't done much for a long time they weaken, waste and lose viability. What's now wrong with the tissues can best be regarded in terms of a 'disuse', 'deconditioning' or 'tissue vulnerability' state or syndrome. The CNS will sample and hence 'know' about tissue health and the overall relative fitness status and hence may want to maintain levels of sensitivity and reactivity as a result. There is nothing actually 'wrong', it's just that the tissues maybe deconditioned and the sensory system picks up on it. This may need explaining too at some point. (Remember the numskulls?).

3. The apparent domination of a low-road 'threat' response i.e. the pain and the pain situation being interpreted as a significant threat/stressor giving rise to significant negative emotions (fear/anxiety/concern), which is in turn accompanied by associated bodily responses, hypersensitivity, high tension, antalgic postures and very guarded and tense movements, heightened cardio-vascular, respiratory (at an extreme, hyperventilation) and other more

subtle autonomic responses (sweating, gut problems, bladder, swelling, skin discoloration...). All responses which rightfully may be considered maladaptive given the lack of frank 'damage' or 'true' threat.

4. A high-road that agrees with and hence collaborates with the low-road. Hence, conscious (cognitive) interpretations are in favour of the threat perspective, like fear and concern about pain, warnings from others to be careful and that something serious may be going on, learnt coping mechanisms that are shifted towards things like helplessness, being passive, giving-up, avoidance and relying on others, hoping and praying, a temperament that is shifted to the flighty Springbok end of the continuum and so forth.

Top-down before bottom-up management dictates that the approach should start by looking at the high-road status and influences and seeing if more adaptive or productive ways of thinking and dealing with the situation are possible. If I can change the 'high-road', the thinking, believing, understanding, attributing, the cognitive-about-the-problem 'bit', I may also be able to influence what I like to call the ongoing 'high-road' noise or 'chatter', the, 'I better not do that, I better not do this, I better be careful here and there and now that's not good either'... the ongoing thinking chatter...

In order to help the reader follow what I'm trying to put over, I begin with a rather extended way of 'how it can be done'. I am going to expand on the above four points and finally deal with how manual therapy/hands on techniques can be positively engaged.

Background

Kate hobbled in;she moved tensely and didn't look happy. Her history and symptom picture took me about thirty minutes to gather. The essence of her story revolved around an awkward lift, giving her modest pain for a month or two that was followed by a slip and fall on the bottom step of her stairs. She fell on her backside and was in immediate, excruciating low back pain. It was now a year since the problem started.

She was treated with standard analgesia and had x-rays and eventually scanned. The results revealed, L4/5 disc bulging, early degenerative changes at L5/S1 and no radicular (nerve root) impingement. She was 48 years old and had only odd previous back and neck pains that usually recovered within a week or two if she was careful. She was intelligent and articulate. The current pain was right across her back, high in intensity, constant and not spreading beyond the buttocks. There was no leg pain, paraesthesia or numbness.

At first she was told she had torn muscles in her back, but after the x-rays and scans the 'degeneration' was blamed. She'd been back and forth to the Drs and seen several consultants. Rest and tablets were advised, but when no progress was made she received hospital physiotherapy for six weeks which was exercise orientated and although she tried hard it all made her a lot worse. She felt that they'd all 'given-up' with her.

I will discuss 'psycho-social' yellow flags in detail later but briefly, here they are for Kate:

- very high levels of very distressing pain... for a year… which is a long time
- lots of tablet taking and activity avoidance. Before the back pain she was a regular walker and went to dance classes once a week. She said she could barely be on her feet for more than ten minutes now and that the slightest bump in the car was agony. She had stopped dancing
- deteriorating home life, 'lack of understanding and concern' summed it up (she was also being constantly told not to bend or do anything remotely strenuous by her partner)
- diagnostic understanding was of a worn and 'degenerate' back that was highly inflamed

  (she had a strong notion that even though she had had scans and x-rays something serious might have been missed)
- lost her job as a school secretary
- low mood, wound-up, frustrated, unable to relax and admitted to feeling very depressed with the situation and negative about the future or getting better
- poor sleep
- report of high intensity of constant pain.

(If you haven't come across the term 'psycho-social yellow flags' before – know for now that if you want to predict whether or not a low back pain sufferer is going to go on to become chronically disabled by their problem, the best predictors of this are determined far more by psycho-social features than any physical or 'biomedical' findings. For example, high levels of distress and pain at onset, ongoing high levels of pain report, significant withdrawal from activity and normal functioning and being off work, are better at predicting a poor outcome than any CT scan, x-ray or finding on a physical examination.

To me it shows the importance of the impact of the problem on the 'high-road' and why 'top-down' before and during 'bottom-up, if at all possible, is such wise action. It also says that sometimes we need the help of psychologists trained in Congnitive Behavioural Therapy (CBT).

We get to the stage where I feel we're getting along.

She makes the common statement... 'In this whole year, you're the first person to take time to listen to me properly.' ...and I respond...

'I'm lucky in my situation I've got time and because no one's been helping you, I'm interested!'

Now it sounds a bit cynical but often patients like Kate are big talkers about themselves, their situation and their problem, but poor listeners. To keep us sane Philippa and I often call them 'me, me, me, it's all about me' patients, but note though that most of us, if we've been a bit ill, will gleefully give every last detail of our problem to those who care to listen, or make the mistake of asking in the first place! If patient's are poor listeners it is really important that we learn to get very good at giving very small 'bites' of information and then get on with physically doing and experiencing. The key is making the information relevant to what we plan to do.

Sometimes though, there's absolutely no point in talking!

Luckily, Kate wanted a better understanding, it turned out that she had a really keen thirst for knowledge. As an aside here, it's my experience that patients who are in constant pain, who are very flinchy when touched or when sudden jolts or movements occur, are frequently poor at listening and concentrating. As a clinician it is important to make sure you are aware of the patient's level of concentration, glazed eyes and sighs mean you are likely to be wasting your time! Try to be aware of your own communication style? Do you talk too much and not let the patient get a word in edge ways? Ah, you've a lot of re-learning to do I suspect!

Physical examination

I continued...

'I've heard your story and I've had a good look at your x-rays and scans and now it would be good to have a look at your back to see what's going on and how it's moving, do you feel happy to take some things off so I can see your back and legs?'

She immediately looked concerned and it turns out that every time someone examines her she suffers for days afterwards. I'm pleased she feels comfortable enough with me to say this by the way.

'Right, you're in total control Kate, I'll show you the movements we're going to try and you talk to me all the way, you can do as much or as little as you like, you can stop when you like, you don't have to force or overdo anything. Just say if you don't want to do the movement... OK?

'Yes, the worst thing is being touched on my back...'

'I've got that, you tell me! With everything we do, I'll tell you about it and we can go very slowly or stop or not even do it if you don't want too.'

She undressed very stiffly and slowly, but she could get her shoes and tights off by bending forward sitting. She actually sat quite slumped. I could already see that her lumbar flexion intervertebral movement was pretty full.

To see her walk was just like Jude above, tension in the face and tension in the body! A similar approach to Jude right now was totally inappropriate there was a lot to go through. She struggled to even lift her leg to do a step-up and balance on either leg was hopeless. She could just about walk on tip-toes. Walking backwards and sideways was very difficult and tense. The muscles were there but the level of coordination and tension were remarkably poor.

(Is this presentation familiar to you? It's what medicine sometimes likes to call 'the Heart-Sink patient' because this type of presentation makes you inwardly cringe and shrink and your heart sink! They're a challenge though, and I've learnt to take the pressure off myself and enjoy them! Having time is very important.).

'You don't look as if you've moved freely and normally for a long time.' I said in a sympathetic tone.

She nodded in glum agreement. I now looked at her standard standing low back movements.

'I'll show you a movement and you tell me how you feel about doing it using one of these answers I've got on the whiteboard.

Here they are, I read them out...

- 'Happy'
- 'Confident'
- 'Not sure'
- 'A bit anxious'
- 'Not keen at all'
- 'No way, get lost!'

This is a very simple 'fear' hierarchy for use with patients who have high levels of pain combined with significant fear, tension and anxiety about movement and provoking pain. I discuss the fear-avoidance model in the 'Graded exposure' section of the book (chapter GE 2.4).

I bent forward and touched my toes and came up again with a smile...

'What do you think?'

'That's a 'no way, get lost one.'

'Right watch again...'

I bend forward running my hands down my thighs so they reach to just below half way – about six inches above my knee caps.

'I'm not sure,' came her reply.

'Show me what you're 'happy' to try?'

She stiffly stooped forward a very little with a very straight back.

All her other lumbar movements were similarly feared, locked-in, tense and hugely limited. Her face was tense throughout and she held her breath and grunted even with the very small movements she did. She was almost as limited as Vivien in the Volvo from chapter 1.2, but this was in the context of over a year, Vivien was like this for only a few hours! Can you see how Kate is maladaptively stuck in this acute/early pain phase?

Now, it would be very easy to disbelieve Kate, I'd already seen her bend and get her tights and shoes off, I'd seen her sitting slumped with full back intervertebral flexion... I knew her back could bend from what I'd seen. I could have used this to accuse her of fabricating her problem but, that's what an idiot would do I now think. If you're going to help a patient like this, my top tip is accept what you see and that what you see is what you have to try and help. Accept it, see it as unhelpful or maladaptive, but try and interact with the patient to improve matters.

Now, the interpretation of all her movement restrictions and the inconsistencies is to view them as a pretty marked example of several possible things:

1. Loss of willingness to move. This suggests a conscious decision which may or may not be the case... I know that when I've injured myself I've made conscious decisions not to move or to move very carefully. It quickly becomes instinctive to protect.

2. It's become a habitual protective movement pattern, maladaptively remaining from the acute episode (on-going habitual protective patterns are likely to become subconscious, think of them as a nicely set up neural assembly)

3. Fear/anxiety about flexion and all the other movements too.

4. Also fear of the pain, that it may cause and/or fear of doing further damage (this is very common and often supported/advised by many clinicians)

5. An expression of distress and hopelessness. Think like an observing predator! Awkward and pain expressing movement signals that you are incapacitated and are going to be easy to catch. Now think like a close friend or family. This type of movement has the intrinsic message of 'help me/look after me' and also 'be careful of me'. Think now like a Dr or consultant, who's been trained to be cynical and mistrusting: 'It's a pretty weak attempt to show how bad it all is. The patient is merely trying to provide proof of disability that's needed to be maintained until compensation 'settlement' day.' Think like a psychologist perhaps: 'High levels of distress are often closely linked to high levels of pain behaviour.'

6. That there could still be something significant wrong with the tissues, that the pain is relevant to the tissue vulnerability and wisely restricting movement like this is the only way to stop the pain/structure/injury/pathology getting worse! That something is wrong? Remember, severe and serious pathology can have exactly the same type of presentation.

With all these in mind, my first goal was to hopefully reassure myself (and then her) that the tissue status was in the 'safe to start loading' category. I'd already noted that her lumbar spine could flex. Could her spine move more in different positions? I also needed to do a good neurological examination – reflexes, sensation and muscle power. The first two are easy to achieve, but muscle power can be very difficult with this jumpy, untouchable and severely restricted state.

Chapter 17.4
Explaining, listening and interacting with a patient: Kate – part 2

'Kate, has anyone spent time and done a thorough examination and explained all the findings to you?'

'No, not at all, they look at my movements, they usually sigh, they tap my knees with the hammer and they babble on and on but as far as I can see it amounts to 'Kate, there's nothing wrong'. At first they said take tablets and rest, later on they said I needed to move and get going, that's when they sent me to physio for exercises. Neither work, it's so frustrating.'

'Right, well so far, I can see a back that doesn't want to move at all – pretty obvious eh?'

'Hopeless case me, I'm not very hopeful anymore.' (Good, she's comfortable enough with me to come forward with some issues relating to how she's feeling).

'Well, we need to look a little more. One thing's for sure, it's all horribly tense in your back right now. I'm collecting your problems, can you see? First up: back won't move. Second: back's tense. I've put them in my 'Shopping Basket' of things that need addressing!'

She looks slightly puzzled and I think whoops, not quite appropriate going to that yet. I go on...

'I want to check to see if the nerves that come out of the bottom of your back and go down your legs are working, if that's OK. One of the big things, is that when something goes wrong in your low back, the nerves that run down your legs can get injured and then don't work properly.'

We sit down and I get out the articulated spine, show her where the nerves go, where the spinal cord ends up at L1/2 and reassure her that her spinal cord is well above the area of the problem and that it's therefore safe. I also show her the discs and how the nerves can get pressed on by them and I tell her how the nerves are labelled S1, L5 etc. I show her the ones that are relevant to her pain distribution. She stops me.

'No one explained to me that my spinal cord stopped way up there. In my head I've been thinking that this disc bulging is going to press on my spinal cord any moment and that'll be it.'

'So, how are you thinking now?'

'Pleased to be listening to what you're telling me!'

I nodded to communicate 'good'. I got the first hint of a smile and a strong sense of her enthusiasm for more knowledge.

'What's good, is that it's easy to test the nerves and make sense of the tests. If they're OK, it makes me feel a bit more confident about your problem. I'll explain as we go along.'

'Right there are three things to test, your muscle power because nerves make your muscles work, so if a nerve's been badly injured the muscles can get very weak. Then your reflexes, which I think you said you've had done many times before and lastly, your skin sensation. If a nerve is injured you can lose your reflexes and sensation, it goes numb, just like you get at the dentist when they inject you to do a filling. Now, you said you've not got any numbness or pins and needles so that's a good start, but I'll test skin sensation anyway in a moment.'

'Let's stand again and check a few muscles.'

Because her balance was so poor I got her to stand at the end of the treatment couch and hold on. I demonstrated a movement/test and asked her to have a go, using the same fear-hierarchy as before. Walking on tip toes on the spot holding on, was no problem. I noted and nodded encouragement at the fact that she was doing it well. I then got her to go up and down on both tip toes together and also go up and transfer weight from one to the other. She did well here too. I then got her to stand and walk on the spot on her heels to quickly test dorsiflexion power. She found it a bit awkward and painful, but she managed it.

Note, that during all physical activity, including standard physical testing as demonstrated here, there's always an opportunity to use behavioural/reinforcement techniques. For example, simple encouragement via eye contact, nodding and appropriate words like 'good, you're looking relaxed', 'nice' and so forth. Extinguishing unhelpful pain behaviours involves, ignoring, subtle body language, silence and words like 'just do what you feel you can'. The worst thing to do is to start empathising, asking about pain and looking fearful yourself. With Kate, I was encouraged and she was looking a bit more relaxed.

'The muscles you just worked are good, which means that the sacral 1 and lumbar 5 nerves, the two main nerves at the base of your spine I showed you just now are working OK. I appreciate that the tests bring on a bit of hurt but if we can, let's do a few more. We'll do them sitting and I can also check your sensation and reflexes too.'

She sat on the treatment couch with legs dangling and I knelt down and did her quads and calf reflexes and also light touch. It was all fine, reflexes were really brisk, not only did the reflexes go off quickly but her whole body jerked too and sensation was quite normal. Doing sensory testing by light touching her skin with my hands (quick test really) was the first time I touched her and I notice that she jumped a little here too.

'Did that hurt or are you just jumpy?'

'I'm sorry, Louis, my whole body seems to want to jump away whenever anyone comes near me...'

'Have you always been like this or is it just since the pain problem?'

'Well, I guess I've always been a little jumpy but nothing like as bad as this.'

I also wanted to quickly test the Babinski sign and proprioception. I explain what the tests are for and how I'm going to do them, demonstrating on my own foot for Babinski sign. With Kate, it causes a whole leg withdrawal the first time, but after a couple more gentle strokes I get the normal toe curl-down. Proprioception was normal as you might expect for someone with 'just' low back pain. I wanted to be thorough because it was important for reassurance.

Seeing that her reflexes were so brisk I quickly test calf clonus, I tell her what I'm going to do as clonus testing involves a quick jerk of the foot into dorsiflexion. The test was actually 'positive', in that there was a cog-wheel or jerky type muscle contraction, followed by the well-known beating as I dorsiflexed the foot. Be aware though, that to be positive for upper motor neurone pathology (think stroke/spinal cord damage/multiple sclerosis) at least five ongoing beats are required. Anyone who has worked with neurologically damaged patients will know what abnormal clonus is. In my experience, whenever there are very brisk calf reflexes and a heightened physical 'tension' in patients, a bit of clonus can be elicited normally with foot dorsiflexion. Always be careful to not be too dismissive of it, but here I was inclined to think on edge, flighty, 'springbok', heightened stress type of state, rather than anything nasty! These are the folk who jump to the ceiling when any sudden or unexpected thing happens and Kate was certainly one of these.

She now looked confused and concerned.

'I'll explain it all in a moment, but can I test a few more muscles first?'

She agrees and I proceed to get her to resist knee flexion and extension. I can't get a normal build up of power, I'm getting the classic chronic pain 'cog-wheel' jerky on/off muscle contractions, that most medics dismiss as proving the patient is less than straight forward and mentally and behaviourally flawed.

That's fine with me, interpret it as you like, but it's such a common 'chronic pain disabled' patient finding that whatever it means I take it on board as just that – a 'finding'. To me it's an expression of a functionally but not pathologically impaired system. Trying to explain it in a reductionist neurological way may be of value. All I can say is that it can disappear and become normal when normal movement, functional confidence, a lowering of tension and stress and normal strength and coordination returns. The key thing is that this response is not at all what you get when there is a peripheral neuropathy and 'true' motor weakness. Here, however hard the patient tries to perform a resisted contraction there is a sustained and smooth giving or breaking of it. It's not jerky. To reassure yourself that this finding is 'invalid' in terms of pathology, watch what happens when the tested muscle is used with functional and coordinated movement. For instance, Kate walked in, she could get out of a chair and with a bit of assistance could go up a step. Yet, the jerky quads contraction assessed on its own, in terms of raw strength, would suggest these movements to be impossible. Consider the 'context' too – function is processed by the brain a whole lot differently to an isolated muscle contraction done while the patient is sitting and concentrating. Could it be a processing block associated with high levels of tension and fear? I've never seen this type of response in anything but chronic maladaptive pain presentations and it is very common. As an aside for those who feel it's a 'made-up' type of phenomenon, you can't imagine that all these chronic pain patients ring each other up and agree to produce this jerky sign when tested? Further, a great many haven't met others like themselves, so there's no chance for learning off others either. So to me, it's not a learnt response but a response that naturally occurs in association with high levels of distress and poor pain coping. I tend to see it as an expression of loss of confidence on the one hand and on the other, an exasperated effort or attempt to provide some evidence that something hurts or is wrong. Sadly, over time, it can become a very deeply conditioned habit and one that usually doesn't bode that well for the future recovery of the sufferer.

I now lower the plinth so Kate is sitting with both feet on the floor.

'More strength testing for a minute, are you happy to stand up and sit down from here two or three times? Go as slowly as you want.'

She uses her hands a bit to push off but stands rather tensely but perfectly well in terms of leg strength. I put the plinth up a bit and get her to stand, take her weight over to her left and sit trying to bias the weight to the left and then up again on both and the same over to the right. We go back to the step-ups and with support for balance she steps up well enough for me to assume her quads are strong enough, or at least non-pathological, but they have to be terribly deconditioned if she's been moving like this for a year.

I get her to sit again with the plinth back up and feet dangling. I now check foot eversion. I get her to keep both heels in contact with either side of my knee and take both feet into eversion. (I usually kneel in front of the patient to do this). I then ask her to hold the position and resist my pressure into inversion. It's all a struggle and there's more of the jerky cog-wheel stuff. I reduce the pressure until there's a nice sustained contraction and I start talking to her about her general health.

'I didn't ask you just now, but how's your general health?'

'It's fine as far as I know...'

'How's it been throughout your life, any problems, operations, hospitalisations and so forth...?'

'Let me think, I broke my collar bone when I was fifteen and had some problems with ear infections about ten years ago...'

She tells me and I get a bit more information, all the while I very gradually increase the pressure and find that I'm getting a reasonably good strong contraction.

'Now focus on this a minute' I interject.

'You've managed to let your muscle stop being so jerky, can you see?'

'Oh, I... was miles away, you're right.'

'Try and be relaxed now and let's do it again, this time concentrating rather than thinking of other things.'

I go back to the very slight pressure.

'Feel the steady resistance? Now, you try and push my hands away and I'll resist.'

She goes too quickly and it starts to jerk.

'Go back, less, less, now build up more slowly...'

I spend three or four minutes doing this with her. It's good, because she's learning a more normal contraction and I can use this to show her that change is possible, given the right way of doing things.

I finish the neurological examination by doing static holding to all her hip muscle groups i.e. pressing knees together and apart, pushing up through the heel and getting her to pull her knee up into my hands to resist hip flexion. As an aside doing 'statics' is only one aspect of muscle contraction. If you're on 'remote thinking' here, as in 'I'm testing muscle strength because I have to for motor nerve function,' or even worse, this 'I'm testing muscle function because this is what I was taught and it's part of my routine', you're missing a big chance to check muscle through range capability, confidence to contract, fear and anxiety about moving under load and so on.

In case you're wondering I am now over an hour into the exam. I have an hour and a half slot booked for her. If you're going to help these sorts of patients you need time. Any patient who I know has an on-going problem I like to book a double appointment with. If that's not possible I stop after forty-five minutes and get them to come in later that day or the next day to continue. I never rush. In this first stage of management it is vital that enough time is given to setting the scene and building rapport, it's one of the most important parts of the whole process.

A big thing that pisses me off is getting referrals from 'healthcare providers' – the middle men in the chain. Companies asking for a thirty minute assessment, a form filled in, the patient given advice and a recommendation as to whether any further physiotherapy is appropriate! In that amount of time, even an acute whiplash couldn't have a fair hearing, examination, appraisal and advice. What hope is there for some of these complicated patients when treatments have become so commercialised? What hope is there for the therapist who is trying to really understand and help these patients in three sessions of thirty minutes? It is nuts. I'm afraid I ignore the commercial demands and give the patients what they need, which is time!

'Kate, that's the end of the nerve-checking part of the examination, let's discuss what I've found so far.'

'I'm wondering what you are thinking!'

'That was thorough and I'm pleased you've been explaining it to me, but I'm not sure whether what you've found is good or bad?'

'Right, as you've seen, your reflexes are very good, in fact they are what we call 'brisk', meaning they jump quickly. When a nerve has been injured in your back you can sometimes lose your reflex, meaning nothing happens when I tap the tendon. Quite often when people lose a reflex they also lose sensation in the part of the leg that the nerve goes to or supplies. Remember I showed you the S1 nerve on the skeleton just now, well that nerve feeds the skin and muscles down the back of the thigh and then into the calf down to the outside of the foot and the little toe, if it's been upset you get numbness or maybe pins and needles over that area. The other thing that can be lost is power in some of the muscles. For the S1 nerve the most common muscle to go weak is the calf muscle, which means you can't go up on tip toes, when it's L5 it's difficult to walk on your heels and turning your foot out. Holding it like you did, involves both the nerves. The next one up, the L4 nerve, goes to your thigh muscle and if that was weak you'd have difficulty getting up out of a chair or going up and down stairs.'

Kate then complains that she does have difficulty doing these things, I point out that it's not because of any nerve injury but more to do with the pain stopping the muscles working as hard as they need to. I also mention that the muscles haven't been doing much for a long time and are likely to be pretty weak and deconditioned. (It's good to get that word in – deconditioned, because the only way to 'recondition' it is for the patient to get to work using it!).

'Now, to summarise where we've got to, from what I've seen so far your back and general movements are very limited and there's a great deal of tension in all of them. I need to look at your movements further, with you lying down and maybe in some other positions too, to see whether taking weight off allows things to be freer or move a bit better.

On the big positive side, the nerves that relate to your back are all fine, as we've found out reflexes and sensation are fine and your muscles, though weak, are not weak because of any nerve injury. The jerkiness you get when trying to make them work and resist is very common with patients who have long term pain, we don't fully understand what causes it but what I can tell you is that in others like you, it goes as you gradually improve. What was good just now was that, with a bit of fiddling about and you helping, we managed to stop it in your foot. Practice should improve that and I can show you what to do with all the other muscles too, if it's necessary.' (In reality I'll avoid it and only come back to testing it when she's more active and confident.)

'Now, I want to tell you where I'm coming from and what I'm thinking with what I have found so far. Do you want to ask anything or point anything out before I do?'

She shook her head thoughtfully, slowly and deliberately.

'I had a look at the x-rays and scans just now and I read the reports, remember the reports are written by experts in looking for serious disease, as well as any abnormalities and they've found evidence of quite normal age-related changes, involving the joints and discs at the base of your back. There're no fractures, no nasty diseases, no pinched or squashed nerves.'

She's nodding and almost transfixed.

'If I took thirty normal and fit people off the street that were your age and build, then scanned and x-rayed them, I can promise you that they would have similar findings to those you have. Many of those people will be highly active, putting their backs through physical stress with their work and lifestyle day in and day out. They move normally and enjoy a pain free life most of the time. Just about everyone gets back pain from time to time and most recover fine, it's a normal part of life, just like having the occasional cold or flu is. Right, can you see what I'm saying? It's that there's nothing nasty to worry about. The main thing, from my perspective is your reduced movement, and that's what we need to look at more right now.'

'Big question Kate, I'm wondering what you're thinking with what I'm saying... be honest and tell me, anything?' I smile and she slowly looks at me.

It would be wonderful if she had looked relieved, but as I've come to accept and expect many patients tend to feel uncomfortable and confused at this sort of juncture.

Kate could have said...

'I'm confused and slightly annoyed. I really don't know what to think... I feel like screaming or crying... You're saying there's nothing wrong, yet I've had pain for a year. You're saying everyone else has a back like mine and they don't hurt, but I do, so why's that then? What have I done to deserve this? I'm wondering if I'm making this up and wondering if you're thinking I'm making this up?'

But I knew she wouldn't say this – why? Because when you're explaining to patients and they're interested, they're attentive. As I said earlier, beware the glazed-over look, it usually means the patient has lost you and is getting wound-up because you're waffling on and not doing anything to 'fix' them! Kate was surprisingly attentive for someone so wound-up and jumpy – so I knew she was following me. She said...

'I'm following you but I'm puzzled as to what would cause my problem. I'm a bit confused because the two consultants blamed the degenerative changes and inflammation from the scans. I'm feeling like I should believe them because they're the experts, but on the other hand they didn't spend more than three or four minutes examining me, hardly asked any questions about the pain and spent most of the time looking at the x-rays and scans. Like I said to you earlier, I'm pretty convinced something's been missed and it's serious, you hear about Drs missing something serious all the time.'

Now, this is one of the most difficult times for the 'lowly' physiotherapist. Who does the patient believe? Little physio you, the Dr, the big consultant...? The scan..? What the neighbour said..? What your best friend Doreen told you that her reflexologist told her to tell you..? What the chiropractor told you about your leg length and pelvis being out of alignment..?

If our job isn't hard enough without this 'expert' hierarchy! This is a huge gremlin for us, as it often stymies the highly knowledgeable and skilled physios attempts to give the patient a much more credible and useful understanding of their pain problem. What's the answer? How do we deal with it?

Well, you could try to raise your own status, 'I'm a 'Highly Specialist Pain Therapist', I know far more about pain than any Dr or Consultant... I've got letters after my name to prove it.' You may need a white coat, a dickie-bow and half moon glasses! Some people like to inflate themselves in order to have control and status over their patients. I don't. I like to be sincere and honest. That stuff makes me shudder, particularly coming from therapists with a relatively few years experience and even then it's seems pretty arrogant to me. The wiser you get the more humble you become, surely?

I prefer this for Kate...

'I'm a physiotherapist with a special interest in managing and treating pain problems that come from your bones, joints, nerves and muscles. Some family doctors have special interests but mostly they're experts in over-viewing all health issues, knowing about diseases and using medicines to treat them. Some difficult problems and diseases require a more specialised physician or consultant and it's the Dr's job to refer you to the right one. The problem with medicine and specialist training is that with pain from joints, muscles, nerves and bones, especially on-going pain, there is no medical speciality. Surprisingly, Dr's only learn the very basics about pain, so I suggest you see them as experts at diseases and injuries, but not pain. When Drs want to become specialists they focus on narrow bands of diseases or on surgery. For example, a 'rheumatologist' is an expert physician in joint, muscle and 'soft-tissue' diseases – like rheumatoid and osteoarthritis. Your Dr referred you to three orthopaedic surgeons. Orthopaedic[1] surgeons are trained in surgery of bones and joints, so they're good at putting broken bones back together, mending torn tendons and replacing arthritic joints. Now the first two he sent you too are specialised in joint replacement, the first one does knees and hips and the second, does hips and knees! The third one was nearer the mark, he does spinal surgery, but his big thing is straightening out badly curved spines and putting big rods in and he occasionally does operations for back pain. Operations like discectomies, where they remove a bit of the disc that's pressing on a nerve, or facetectomies, that cut away bits of the little joints in your back if they're pressing on your nerves and giving you pain, remember the little joints I showed you earlier?'

Kate follows, nodding. I go on...

'They know from looking at your scans and x-rays and doing a few of the basic tests that I did, like checking your muscles and your reflexes. All specialists and Drs are mostly very good at looking for and identifying serious diseases. Unfortunately they are not as good at reassuring the patient that no serious disease is present. They tend to always want to tell you what's wrong as opposed to what's right! So, because they

1 - *Orthopaedic actually means 'straightening children!!' 'Ortho' is from the Greek 'orthos' – meaning 'correct' or 'straight.' 'Paedic obviously refers to children, as in paediatrician. Anyway, it's a throwback from when correction of spinal and bony deformity in children was the meat and potatoes of orthopaedic practice.*

can't see any disc or facet joint pinching your nerves, they're blaming the only thing they can see on your scans, the 'degenerative' or age related changes or they may say it's 'wear and tear'. And because they don't yet do 'back replacements' like they do 'hip' or 'knee' replacements, they've nothing much to offer you. One thing's for sure though, that because you've seen three highly skilled surgeons and clinicians in their fields they will all have ruled out any serious disease causing your pain.'

You may need to add this as well if necessary:

'So, if you want help with on-going pain, there are a few physiotherapists who are trained like me and more and more hospitals now have 'Pain Clinics' and 'Pain Management Units' which are for patients where there's no evidence of any serious disease that can be treated. Pain clinics generally help patients control pain with drugs, but also sometimes use acupuncture and TENS machines; Pain management units don't use medicines, but concentrate on helping people with long-term pain deal better with their problem, change their lifestyles and get fitter and they're often very successful.'

I pause for a second to let Kate come in...

'There's a lot we patients don't know isn't there...?' She pondered.

I agreed and said...

'I want to convince you a bit further. In the last ten years there have been clear guidelines for the diagnosis and management of common back pain. Most physios here in the UK are trained in looking for things that you tell us and that we find with our physical examination that indicate something is seriously wrong, they're called 'Red flags'. If I find a 'Red flag' I refer the patient back to the Dr for further investigations, things like bone fractures and nasty diseases like rheumatism of the spine and cancer. If you want I can show you the list of Red flags, but for now be reassured that none have cropped up, if one does I promise I'll let you know! Remember what I said just now – those consultants are experts in looking for serious disease.

(Note the only possible red flag with Kate so far relates to, 'persistent and severe restriction of lumbar flexion'. Severe loss of lumbar flexion is associated with lumbar pathology – think bone metastases, disc infection and fracture. Recall though that Kate had revealed normal lumbar flexion in sitting and undressing that I'm going to investigate further.)

Kate's eyebrows are raised and I say.

'It's time to look at your movements a bit further, I'll come back to any of this stuff later or next time when you've had a chance to think about it. If you're confused, ask? And if anyone at home gets confused when you try to explain all this, bring them in too! I'll give you a hand out overview of what I've said at the end though.'

'That'd be great'

An aside here, is that while patients may hear and get the gist of what you say, they still don't necessarily believe it, but if it's written down – it's far more likely to be believed. Don't forget to sign the material off with all the letters after your name! Kidding!

Chapter 17.5
Explaining, listening and interacting with a patient: Kate – part 3

Because Kate's standing movements were so limited by pain and tension I decided that the physical examination should follow a 'fire-apart-depart' approach, meaning get the best possible movements with the least amount of pain or no pain/low pain. I couple it again quite simply with the 'fear' hierarchy introduced earlier, whereby I demonstrate a movement and then give the patient the option to have a go and see what they can do.

Recall the hierarchy up on my whiteboard:

- 'Happy'
- 'Confident'
- 'Not sure'
- 'A bit anxious'
- 'Not keen at all'
- 'No way, get lost!'

Because Kate was so dreadfully tense and fearful moving I decide to show her all the starting positions I could use to do movements in. This is how it went:

'I'm going to demonstrate to you some different movements in various starting positions that you may be able to feel you can do, I want you to tell me which position you'd prefer to start with.'

I showed and talked through the following. Note that I did the full movement, but also emphasised and demonstrated how I could do a much smaller and slower movement of each one:

- supine lying: head end of couch up with pillows under head, crook lying – to do crook rotation, easy grab-a-knee, grab-both-knees, pelvic rock, bridge, hip hitching, legs out straight

- all fours: arch and hollow, flex knee/leg towards chin, curl-up (into 'mecca' position!) and slowly go forward and let hips go down towards 'cobra' position (i.e. extension)

- side lying: curled up, straighten up and extend, then curl up a bit again and grab top knee/leg to flex

- finally sitting: flex forward with chest to knees, but with hands on knees to control the movement, up tall, easy twist and easy side flexion.

'Any look any good to you?'

'I'm happy to have a go at the sitting and the all fours movements...'

With that, we went ahead with the clear instruction...

'If you can, try to be as relaxed with the movement as you can be, most people find they do best if they go really slowly, so that it's easier to stop and feel in control.'

'Tell me about it, two of those orthopaedic guys actually pushed me further than I wanted to go, one got hold of my leg and suddenly lifted it up without telling me, I screamed and it took days to settle down, in fact I think it never really settled after that...'

We then looked at what she could do slowly in these positions and pleasingly, she could still bend quite well sitting! But not as well as she did when she was taking her socks and shoes off! Why? Malingering... or how about 'different context', sitting putting on socks and shoes is a habitual goal-orientated movement? It's in the 'thoughtless-fearless-movement' processing category and not associated with bending in quite the same way as say standing and bending forward is, during a physical examination. Also, the same sitting movement in the context of 'examination' and 'pain', changes the processing and brings in the 'threat' component and therefore the 'low-road'. It not only produces an increase in pain, but also an increase in all the other outputs with it, think at one end of the scale, 'fear' feelings and at the other, autonomic/ HPA (adrenaline/cortisol, heart rate, blood pressure) and somatic motor (increased protective tension – antalgic movements etc.).

After showing me a very slow forward bend in sitting, I then demonstrated flexing my leg up to my chest saying, 'What about hugging your leg?' She tried it and was happy to do the full movement. I didn't jump up and down with glee, I just said a fairly neutral 'good' and moved on to the other leg. But here was near full hip flexion and near as damn-it full back flexion, as a result. I'd just like to note that this type of finding is just as common in acute low back pain as in chronic back pain. Sitting-grab-a-knee style flexion is often a very good way to 're-examine' evidence of poor flexion in other movements, like in standing. It can be good in lying too.

Sitting up tall was more problematic, but twisting while sitting produced a reasonably good half to two thirds range. Side bending was poor, but made easier with the presence of a low stool next to her as a stop and somewhere to reach to. Appreciate that reaching over to the side while sitting can feel like you're going to 'topple-off'. It also requires some good muscle control and a bit of good basic balance coordination. The low stool can make that 'unease' lessen right off and very often better quality movement appears spontaneously. See that I'm trying to use 'all the tricks of the trade' to facilitate good relaxed quality movement. (Tip: think and work like a neuro physio would!)

We went to all fours (yes, I crawl around on the floor with my patients... don't you?).

Here, Kate demonstrated that she actually liked curling up into the full, knee, hip and back flexed position. Again, this is massively common in all back pains, acute or chronic. It also usefully shifts any flexion loss/pathological restriction, red flag thinking, into a much more 'downgraded' reasoning corner; it increases your confidence that the spine will move, does move and that given a better experience with movement for the patient, can hugely help them get going again.

(This situation of 'can't bend in standing' but likes curled up is very common,

especially in acute low back pain. Recall that it may be that pain problems get 'stuck' in a specific 'phase' of recovery and don't move onto the next, as here, in the early-tense-don't-move-it phase, but also in the inability to bend under load, but likes curled up flexion.).

'I often do this to get relief and stretch it out' she said.

'I'm pleased with what I'm seeing!' I returned. But I knew she didn't really see any big deal, it was something she'd been doing many times a day for the last year!

Arch and relax (arch and hollow) were very jerky and poorly controlled – which is also common. She was very unwilling to go anywhere near the cobra position. The cobra position is like extension in lying, but approaching from the all fours position with straight arms allows the patient to drop the hips and pelvis very slowly, to whatever position they feel comfortable with. It's a good way of doing it for patients who are poor at lying flat and are likely to struggle with doing the standard 'lazy press-ups'. Try the going-from-all-fours method yourself and note the feeling of forces that come into your back and whole waist area. I find I become very aware of the back coming into full 'jamming' extension. Knowing the anatomy, it's a facet-end-range-bone-on-bone feeling, rather like I get when I fully extend my elbow and let it relax. As I go further, I get a gentle but increasing pulling feeling through my anterior abdominals.

I would urge every therapist to open the 'gates' to consciousness and make a mental note on all movements and exercises that you do and give to patients and also, get a pile of normal friends to do them and ask them what they feel. It's what I call NORMAL KNOWLEDGE, no one teaches it you, no one thinks about it and no one has written it down. The point is how can you be expected to 'normalise' something with a patient when you've no real idea what normal is yourself? My suggestion is to start with your own body and every single exercise you can think of, but don't assume everyone feels it like you do!

Tip: before doing all fours-extension towards the cobra position, I always get the patient to shift their hands forward about a foot from the standard all fours position.

During this type of examination, if a patient is not keen or very unwilling to do a movement, like Kate was here, show them it in an easier way, this usually means going very slowly into only the first small part of the movement and then quickly and easily back-off again for example.

When I showed Kate the first, very simple, part of the cobra she tried and found she actually could do it a very little. This time when I looked at her with quizzical eye brows raised, she nodded with a more pleased expression.

I now showed her all fours hip waggling (in neutral all fours) which she managed to do very slowly and showed that some side flexion was quite possible.

(Note that most people find this hard to co-ordinate, even some physios, but it doesn't take a minute to teach. I find touching the iliac crest and then the lower ribs at the same time as the instruction –'pull your hip bone here... up towards your ribs, here..' seems to work fine... followed by the word 'banana!' Big blokes and the

elderly are often too stiff to get much lumbar side flexion, though it's worth a try. Also, make sure you get the patient to try in different positions of flexion/arch and extension/hollow to get the best biggest, easiest movement possible!).

'How are you doing?'

'A bit more sore but not bad... I wish I could move more easily...'

We now had tears for a few minutes and I gave her a hug – but don't do this if it's not 'you'. I do what comes naturally, tears with patients is common and no problem for me or Philippa (my partner and colleague). We definitely don't get all soppy with patients, that wouldn't be a helpful strategy at all. It's best to just hand the tissues over, quietly wait and then ask what they want to do. The great majority, if you're being trusted by them, will want to carry on.

When things had settled a bit I said:

(Note, no pain talk, no, how's the pain, has the pain gone down, where's the pain at the moment, what's the pain on a 1-10 scale? Absolutely, none of that)

'Kate, I've seen enough of your spine movements to know that it can move and I believe if we get going in the right way your movements can get better and then later a lot stronger. Have you any comments or anything you want to bring up here?'

You might expect her to start going on about how sore she was now but this is what she said.

'As I've been doing these movements with you and watching and listening about all those nerve tests you did, it's really hit me how incapable I've become and I guess I'm a bit annoyed.'

She wipes a tear.

'Yes' I simply respond.

'I've got pain fighting me to go one way and I've got me giving up and letting it win. I feel so weak, almost pathetic with it.'

'If you want to stop now and call it a day, we can? But you're telling me the exact same thing that others in the same situation do. It's fine, and it's normal.'

'I want to carry on, even though I feel shit, there's another side of me going, stay with this Kate, at last you may be getting somewhere, but I know it'll be shit later and I'll get mad with it.'

'Big rule comes up now Kate, it's try not to overdo stuff and then crash-out after as a result, we call it 'pacing'. That means it's best to do little bits and build up. For the great majority that's by far the best way. So, stopping is a positive tactic, it's not a giving up thing, is that OK?'

'You've hit another nail-on-the-head, that is me to a tee.'

'So, how about we stop for today and you come in again tomorrow or when ever is most convenient?'

She agreed.

'Right, for now I want you to go away with these messages.'

As we discussed, there's nothing seriously wrong in your back, meaning broken bones, massive discs 'out' pressing on nerves, serious arthritis, cancer or serious diseases of your nervous system like MS or Parkinson's. I'll give you the handout on pain and medicine I promised.

I'm going to explain why you hurt so much next time. For now, understand that sometimes the circuits and nerves in our spinal cord and brain can keep processing normal and very light 'inputs', like light touch and ordinary movements, as pain when they shouldn't do. It's as if the messages coming in are being posted to the wrong address. Instead of going to the areas of the brain that process light touch and gentle movements, they're going to a 'make-pain' destination!

The best example to help understand, 'pain with gentle light touch', like you mentioned you have, is the horrid skin sensitivity that people sometimes get after having shingles. You may have heard of it? Shingles is caused by a close ally of the chicken pox virus, a great many of us have the virus in our nerves but mostly it lies dormant and does nothing at all. Occasionally it becomes active. If it does, it goes down the nerve to the skin and causes chicken pox-like skin eruptions, which can be very sore. After a week or two the eruptions disappear but in a few people with it the horrid skin soreness remains and gets worse, it becomes supersensitive, even though the skin now looks completely normal. The condition is now called 'post herpetic neuralgia' – neuralgia means pain from a nerve. People who have it say that the skin is almost unbearably sore, they find that they are unable to touch it, that the slightest touch makes horrid pain and even gently blowing on can really stir it up. It seems that the virus leaves the nerve supersensitive, long after the skin has healed.

The key thing is that there is nothing wrong where the soreness and pain are, it's all healed up and yet the sensitivity remains... Can you see that we know the mechanism by which pain can remain after healing has taken place? I will give you a handout to read on this too.

That's an example of skin sensitivity to touch but a similar mechanism can occur for the muscles and joints to, making the slightest movement insanely painful.

If you can understand what I'm getting at and follow along with me, I can see no reason why you cannot move better and be less sensitive in the back. The way we improve things is by starting very slowly and gently and gradually building up. A major thing, is that I can show you how to start and progress, but it's you who decides what you do, how much you do, how quickly you progress and how you get going generally. I'm never going to force you or insist that you do something that you don't want to.

(Note my handouts are basically what's written here – the pain expert stuff, the red flag, reassurance stuff and this on shingles and pain being related to upset processing etc. The important thing about handouts is that the material in them fits with what's been said.

I actually really like to personalise the handout and write up a summary of what I've said and discussed and then email it to the patient. Standardised handouts that aren't personalised are rarely read – think of those handouts you get given at the Drs. I did a personalised information sheet for Kate and she got the material early that evening. I started it with a note saying read and make a list of questions for me if you have some. If you've no questions then I'll be giving you a test on the important points! (I mean it and I do give them a test)).

I now finished off...

'Your homework for next time is to read the handouts and discuss them with your partner. Then come back to me with anything you want to bring up. Some people come back and are cross and mention things like, 'You're telling me that it's all in my head, that I'm making it up, that it's all psychological. Or, 'Why wasn't I told all this before?'... Or, 'If there's nothing wrong, it's all healed. Why does it still hurt?'... Or, 'You're suggesting I get going, I've tried to get going and every time I do it just gets worse and worse...' Or, 'My chiropractor says that it won't get better until my spine is fully corrected...'

She nodded her understanding, we stop there; she's 'done-in' with all the concentration and I can see she can't take anymore.

Chapter 17.6
Explaining, listening and interacting with a patient: Kate – second session 1

Kate came back the following day. I'd booked her in at the end of my day, so as to have as long as needed. She walked in a little looser I felt. I didn't say anything but used eye contact and facial expression to show I was subtly pleased. Her first words were...

'I didn't sleep much last night, so I'm really tired today.'

'Tell me about that?'

'Well, I was going through everything we did, everything you told me. I'd had a long chat about it all with Greg my partner, he gave me the 'how can he say all that, he's only a physiotherapist' type stuff and I got a bit upset and found it hard to explain. I ended up making him read the handout you gave me on pain expertise and Drs and medicine. We both calmed down after that. I went to bed feeling quite calm but I was actually quite excited about finding out more today. I'm daft because I kept coming back to that jerking you got out of my foot and how I couldn't make my muscles go hard when you pushed against me. I was thinking that maybe I've got MS or something like that.

(Note that this is probably my fault – if you mention something bad to a worrier they'll easily engage with it and start to cogitate on it! I mentioned red flags, serious neurological diseases, sciatic pain and symptoms down the leg etc. – at the time I knew it could be a problem, but on the other hand Kate was intelligent and I felt I could easily deal with it at an appropriate time. It's certainly something to be aware of, but for me, the dishonesty of the past, the 'we don't want to worry the patient unnecessarily' often leads to more problems, uncertainty and worry.)

'The good thing in all that is that you wanted to chat to Greg and it sounds as if he may have come on side a bit with it all. You also mentioned looking forward to coming again today.'

'Yes, but what about MS, what about that?'

'Well, you tell me with all we did yesterday, what do you think I'm going to tell you?'

'That I'm a daft-bat probably!' She smiled and shook her head at the same time... She had an 'I'm hopeless aren't I', type expression about her.

I nodded strongly and we both smiled.

'It's all in the email you sent me, I know...'

'Good!'

Note that I didn't boringly go back over all the old stuff from yesterday. One of the big problems with some chronic pain patients is that they get in the habit of wanting constant reassurance. I didn't need to tell her again, she'd listened well yesterday; I'd emailed her the hand outs, she'd seen three different consultants and a whole pile of Drs. The idea of MS popping into the picture is all part of how negative emotions about something drag in negative and fragmented knowledge from the 'medial temporal lobe memory systems' (whoops, brain-centric!). My main goal is to get on with the practical, more positive side of things and build positive associations bit by bit. Circuits that fire-apart, depart. Don't dwell on them and re-visit them!

So, get the patient to learn to work out the answers for themselves from what's gone before.

Another note here. I did as full a neurological physical examination as I could yesterday with her. Think about it and you might be thinking that it could have easily have been left out? Not for the standard reason that she's only got pain in her back without leg referral and really not because I needed to reassure myself, I didn't. Perhaps all her awkward movements and the poor balance should have alerted you to some more sinister nervous system disorder? The thing is, it's probably always best to err on the side of caution. BUT ...

The reason that it could easily have been omitted is that she'd seen three consultants and many Drs, had a pile of tests and, that'll do! Even if she has MS, she's still a chronic pain disabled patient and needs to get going again. My thoughts are: an experienced clinician will know the difference between a chronic pain disability presentation and an MS or any other neurological disease presentation, BUT, will never be so arrogant as to not always have the need to test further in the back of their mind. I worry that newly qualified physiotherapists are trying to specialise too soon into musculoskeletal pain treatment and management, without having regularly seen, assessed and handled the vast array of diseases that humans suffer and which they will experience only on general hospital rotations. ***My advice is experience at least three years on general rotations before specialising***. One of the most important of many clinical rotations that I ever did was to work with neurologically diseased and injured patients. Those skills apply hugely to chronic pain management. Major and fundamental skills of rehabilitation are only gained through experience in this area and in general orthopaedics.

The reason I did the neurological examination here was that it was important for me to add a 'reassurance' input in the form of 'laced expertise' if you like. I ended up doing tests that none of the others had done, that she now had had explained and that were all fine, or at least 'normal' for her 'state'. If I want her to listen and believe what I may explain to her later, I want her to feel that I know what I'm talking about and it's worth listening to and if at all possible, worth thinking about believing. But, I certainly didn't want to be that 'impressive-I'm-better-than-all-the-others-because-they-missed-all-these-important-tests-kind-of-expert'. That's a 'dick-head' in my book.

I learnt a hugely valuable thing teaching and working with colleague and friend Suzanne Brook many years ago. She was Suzanne Shorland back then and Suzanne is a cognitive behavioural therapy trained physio. She worked in St Thomas' Hospital INPUT pain management unit in London and more recently at the London Hospital for Neurology and Neurosurgery, continuing her work with chronic pain disabled patients in the pain management facility. If Suzanne got a patient like Kate, she would assess her, but very soon she would get almost straight on with 'doing' and at the same time using behavioural techniques. The patient change that she could get without any of the trappings of biomedicine and manual therapy testing and analysing were, frankly, amazing. The big lesson is that when a patient has had a pain problem for a long time, they've usually been checked out by a great many others, from top to toe if you like. Suzanne had no issues with any of the nitty-gritty manual therapy stuff, she didn't need it and didn't like it for these patients and she was the first to admit that she didn't know it at all well either. The basic red flag stuff, fine. When you witness patients make good changes in a single session, it is very persuasive that better models of management for the on-going pain disabled patient are essential to our profession. This is a personal big thank you to Suzanne, I loved teaching with you those few times, you are one of the most amazing therapists I have ever met, so thanks.

Read her very clinical material and hugely relevant material in Topical Issues in Pain 1 (chapters 8 and 9 where she's Shorland); Topical Issues in Pain 2 (Chapter 8 with Toby, where she's now married and 'Brook') and Topical Issues in Pain 3 (Chapters 6 and 7, also Brook).

Let's get back to me and Kate. Where to go now!

'Are you ready to carry on?'

Tired though she said she was, she looked eager and responded positively.

'Yesterday you told me that you were really fearful of your back being touched?'

'It's a big problem, because every time someone goes to touch or pat or hold me on my back and you know we do that stuff all the time without realising it, it makes me jump and frankly, I can't stand anyone near me in case they do that. I'm frigid-rigid Kate' she quipped rather sadly but with a wry smile.

'That's fine, so my next thought is, can **you** touch it at all? For example when you're in the shower or even lying on it in bed?'

'Well, yes I can if I go carefully... but it feels like I've burnt the skin.'

'Can you show me what you can do...?'

She slowly got up and quite gently pressed over her back and upper buttock areas, she was relaxed and didn't flinch.

'What you are showing me are the 'no-go' areas for anyone other than you!'

She smiled and nodded...

'I'm with you and I don't want you thinking I'm going to go touching and pushing on your back in a minute, is that OK.'

'That's a massive relief, I was dreading the bit where I have to take things off and my back gets pushed on. The Dr's all did that and I basically froze. I was so frightened and like that Dr who lifted my leg suddenly, it stirs it up so badly.'

I nodded and then said that the session could go two ways, a bit more of a talk or a bit more moving or if there was time, a bit of both!

'I need more information' she responded. 'I think I'm going to find out more as to why it hurts and what can be done to help, that intrigues me.' She paused. 'Those handouts you sent me were so useful for me and Greg to discuss.'

'OK, there will be more handouts. My aim is to help you understand how we all feel pain and why your pain has gone on so long... and what we can do to try and help.'

Lesson: normal pain, injury pain, healing pain... (see section 13)

I produce a safety pin.

'Pin-prick', I smile, 'I'll do it gently to you and tell me what you feel.'

I prod her gently on the forearm.

'Sharp or blunt or in between?'

'In between!'

I repeat in two more places, first in the middle of the palm of her hand, then on the hypothenar eminence – where the skin is usually thicker and then on the skin on the dorsum of her forefinger just proximal to the nail bed, where the skin is usually really sensitive to pin prick. I make sure I do it with roughly the same force in each area, I then move between the three areas, tapping and moving...

'Compare them all... as I move round...'

'They're all different!'

'Roughly the same pressure though, surprising isn't it?'

'Now what's the reason for the pain and what's the reason for the pain being different in the different areas? How do we get pain?'

'I presume it's because nerves tell us...' she said...

'Where's us?'

'Up here!' She smiles and points at her head.

'Correct! Inside your skull is a brain that processes the information that gets there via nerves from your body and it all works together to give you the different sensations.'

'Next question... Is there anything that can be done so that you stop feeling what I'm doing?'

She looks lost for a moment... so I add this...

'Anything that would make it – I could even cut your skin without you feeling anything?'

'Ah, anaesthetic, is that what you're after?'

'Exactly! Think dental injection for teeth and surgeons anaesthetics in hospitals for operations that go through the skin. The dentist uses the anaesthetic to deaden nerves, in particular the nerves that send information into us about damage. The surgeon uses a 'general anaesthetic' that knocks you out, so you don't feel anything... the obstetrician can give you an epidural to deaden the nerves below your waist so there's no pain with giving birth. So, how do they all work?

Kate looked puzzled.

'Anaesthetics are chemicals that stop nerves from working, it's as simple as that!'

'Right, back to the pin-prick – I've shown you how it can vary and you're like me in that it's more sensitive on the skin by the nail. Can you think what it would be like if I used the pin on two or three day old skin wound?

'Ow!'

'Exactly, again and what makes the cut more sensitive? It's the same nerves but somehow they react to the pin-prick far more. The reason is that the healing chemicals, the chemicals from the inflammation, make the nerves more reactive, they send far more and stronger electrical messages than when it's normal.'

'So, we have the basics, there are special nerve fibres in your body that respond to injury or physical threats, like my pin... these nerves send their messages into your spinal cord... (I start making a drawing and build it up as I speak) and then on up to be processed in your brain.'

'You usually feel pain... unless you're under anaesthetic or your nerves have been deadened. Now, another question, can you think of some kind of injury or threat where there's no feeling of pain, and when you haven't been given an anaesthetic, when you're perfectly conscious? Has that ever happened to you, or can you think of examples of this?'

'I'm remembering one of those TV hypnotists who put a girl under the spell and then put a large needle through the loose skin on the back of her hand, she didn't flinch, she was wide awake and she said she felt nothing.'

'Good answer, so how about the opposite, can you think of a situation you've seen where there's no injury or only very slight one and where there's a massive amount of pain...?'

'Yes, my neighbour's eight year old daughter, she cries and screams at the slightest knock or scratch... she drives us mad when they come round.'

'And I bet you know of kids who can take all manner of knocks and bangs without getting too bothered?'

She nods, 'That'll be my nephew Jamie, he's always covered in bruises and you know when he cries there really is something up.'

I nod.

'Summary: normal pain is caused by injury or physical threats to the body, messages go in special nerves to the spinal cord and up to the brain. Somewhere on the way the message can be dampened down, so we might feel less pain and sometimes it gets amplified, or turned up, so we feel alot of pain.'

'We all have a volume control system that can turn what we feel up or down, it depends on what we're doing and we note that some people seem to hurt more easily than others. We really do have a 'pain-on' system and a 'pain-off' system and researchers now understand a great deal about them both. Here's an example, you're running for your life and you trip and fall bruising and cutting your knee, you know you're injured but you get right back up and keep running. The knee doesn't bother you at all. Ten minutes later you're safe and the knee starts killing you and you roll your trousers up to see what's happened.'

'I want you to remember that we've all got a pain-on and a pain-off system and you might be starting to see that you need your pain-off system to work better and your pain-on system to calm down a bit!'

I go on...

'Interrupt me if you don't agree or don't get what I'm on about?'

I pause, she's listening and I go on, 'Soon after an injury everything hurts – think of the bruised knee, it's a horrid ache, it soon stiffens up and small movements give you horrid sharp pain that stops you using it and makes you limp or walk stiffly. Yes? Maybe? No?'

'Yes...'

'I call that the 'STOP MOVING ME' phase of recovery and healing! It's usually the same for back strains, or for that matter any other tissue strain. Patients say their back 'went' and they froze, being unable to move.'

'Now, usually, within a few days, it all starts to get a bit more comfortable, sometimes it's within a few minutes or hours, mostly it's a few days. The ache lessens a bit and you can find positions where there's no pain. It still hurts to touch and move, but there's a bit more movement before the sharpness. This is the phase when you start to move a bit more normally but still cautiously. Sometimes when you're resting a stiff ache builds up and it actually makes you move which though uncomfortable at first, soon relieves it. You also find that if you go slowly pushing into the sharper pain it actually feels good and frees it a bit more too. Sometimes if you overdo it – it makes you take it easy again.'

'I call this the start to GET ME MOVING phase!'

'After a few more days, you're starting to forget it and getting back to some normal activities again, though a little cautiously with anything a bit extreme. A month or so on from there and it's largely forgotten about. Does that sound generally about right to you..?

'It does, but I wish it had been like that with this!'

'OK, skin is pretty quick to reach normal function again, even though we know that its healing process actually goes on for nearly a year... which surprises most people and er, even Drs are unaware of this, they'll tell you it's a few weeks usually! The important thing is that skin is safe to start loading or moving again even while it is healing and that as healing goes on it actually needs to be loaded for the best result and the same goes for all other tissues of the body too – especially muscles, tendons, ligaments, bones and even nerves. They all reach a stage after a few weeks where healing requires movement for the strongest outcome.'

'You're now making me feel bad Louis.'

'Don't. You're the reason why I'm here, what's happened to you happens to a great many people, my job is to help people find ways of getting moving and getting their tissues stronger, when their pain seems to be stopping them doing just that. In some people and we don't understand quite why, their pain doesn't move from the 'stop' phase to the 'go and get me carefully moving' phase and finally to the 'forget about me I'm fine' phase. Yours is still very much locked into the 'stop' phase!'

'Now, if you can take a little more… we're getting there... the next thing is the brain's 'threat control centre'. I'm going to build a diagram up. But if that sounds too complicated, or something for another time, we can get going doing something.'

'I want to hear more!'

Lesson: the threat control centre...

Note: Figure 17.3 shows a possible first diagram that deals with some kind of physical threat from the environment, but it goes on from there as you'll see.

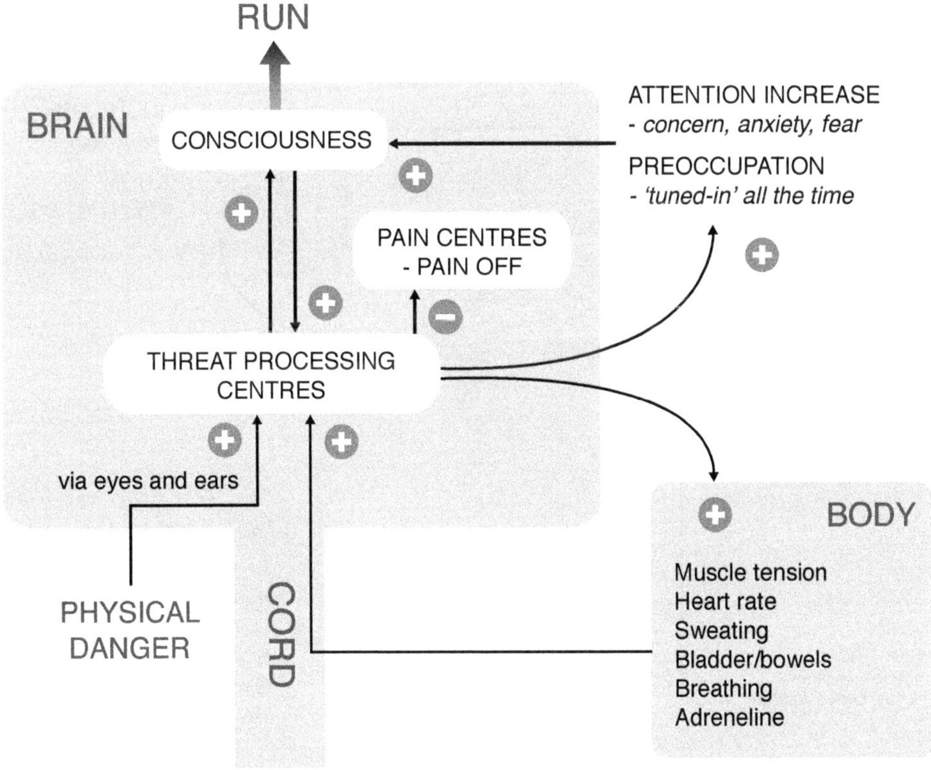

Figure 17.3 A 'build-up' diagram – basic material for explaining 'threat' processing centres in the brain and what happens when we're under threat.

When I'm explaining this material to my patients I tend to 'build diagrams up' on a piece of paper and 'ad-lib' what's put on, depending on the patient's problem and what crops up as we chat along (hence what I call 'build-up' diagrams, figure 17.4 and 17.5 are also a 'build-up' diagrams). You very much need to know what you're talking about and have all the material at your finger-tips. Stumbling along is not a good place to be and handouts that don't fit with what you've been saying aren't helpful either. Take your time if you can and try to tailor everything to the patient wherever possible. Learn and rehearse – do it as a presentation to your fellow therapists, it'll make them think and should create good discussions!

I talk and slowly build up the first diagram as I do so. (If you are good at power point, this slide can be 'animated', so as to add small bits with every click of the mouse or forward button and then you can email it to the patient).

'Right, the next thing I want to get over to you is a bit about how the brain processes a threatening situation and then look at the threat an injury provides, you'll see why I'm doing this when we start to discuss how to tackle your problem.'

I now draw the basic cord and brain boxes and put the words 'Physical Danger' on, (bottom left of 17.3).

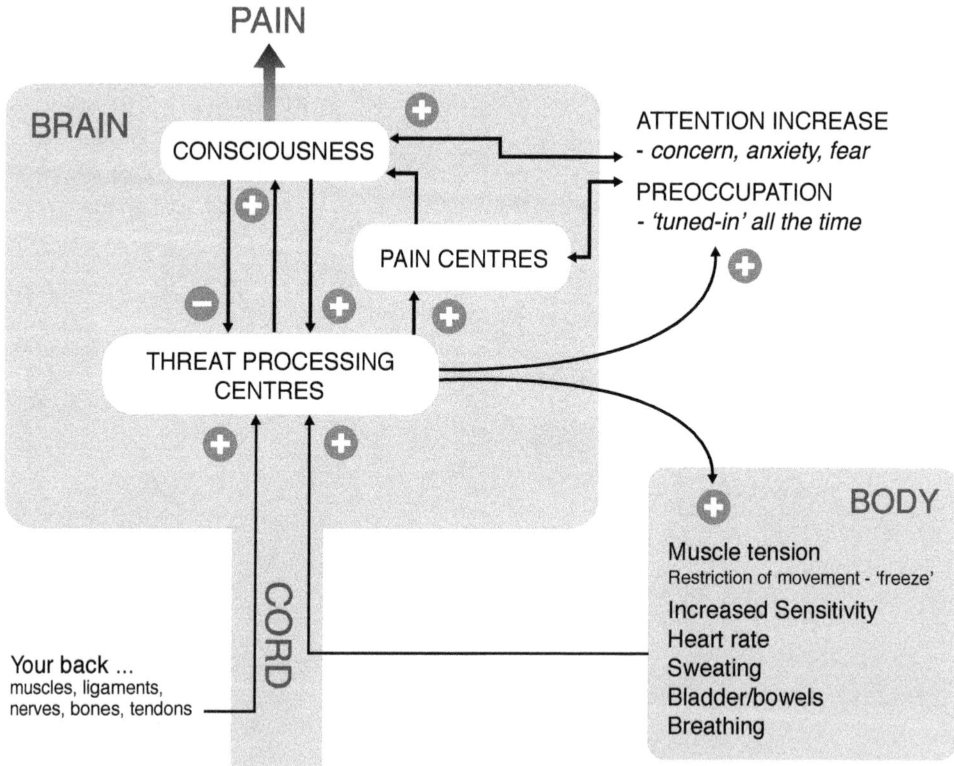

Figure 17.4 Another 'build-up' diagram – basic material for explaining pain being processed as a 'threat' by the brain and what can be done about it.

'Imagine you're being confronted by someone who's very threatening, not nice I know, but you take in the situation via eyes and ears, messages go into your brain and straight to an area of the brain that processes 'threat' (draw threat processing centre on it). One of the main areas involved is called the amygdala if you're interested! Anyway, this area is really subconscious and reacts very quickly to get you ready to save yourself, up goes your heart rate, your blood pressure, your breathing rate and your tension, (see bottom right). Alongside this you become very aware of what's going on (draw the vertical line up to conscious 'you') and the threat processing centre makes 'conscious you' give full attention to what's going on and you're mind doesn't wander one bit – it fixes you on what's going on. Also, you feel tense, anxious or fearful. Conscious 'you' then decides what to do and you make a fast dash for it. Run! You may have heard of 'fight or flight' and the hormone adrenaline. Well, it's this part of the brain that organises all this. Follow so far?'

'Yes, it's just what happens to me at night when I think I hear an odd noise... my heart's beating and I feel tight in the chest.'

'Very good! You've got the idea... When you're in possible danger like this, the threat processing centres also send very strong messages to the areas of the brain that process pain and actually stop them from working, so it doesn't allow you to feel any pain while you're escaping! It's the pain-off system at its best! So a big fear of something can often make any pain that you may have, go. It allows you to be a super-hero, even when there's quite serious injury.' (Draw on the arrow with the negative sign going to the 'pain centres').

'Wasn't there someone recently who finished a race and afterwards they found they'd got a broken bone in their foot?'

'That's it, it's the same system that's operating there too.'

'Now let's do another diagram that's similar but put on your back injury and see what happens. (This builds up to something like Figure 17.4). When you lifted, or when you fell on your back down the stair all those months ago, I want you to see it's very similar to our 'fight or flight' example, as far as the brain is concerned. Any injury is a threat to our health and up it goes into the threat processing centre, where it produces similar effects out in the body as before... draw on the big circle and add, the tension, heart racing, breathing rate goes up and sweating if the pain is really bad... plus a huge protective 'locking-up' of movements of the back. Nasty, sudden pain stops you moving, as we've discussed. In many injuries there's often a widespread increase in sensitivity, it becomes incredibly sore to touch over a large area (can you see, this is normalising her spread of sensitivity and jumpiness). All this then feeds back into the threat processing centres and it maintains the situation.' (Follow the arrows and plus signs – from the body-spinal-cord-to threat processing centres.).

'The other thing that happens is that sudden pain takes your attention away from what you're doing and puts it to work on itself! I'll draw an arrow up from the threat processing centres via the pain centres to conscious 'you' and then another arrow to show the pain emerging at the top! In our first example with the threatening person, the conscious 'you' said, 'Run', forget any pain. Now, when there's injury to the body it says, 'Pain, stop, focus on me (I'm the threat), look after me, don't move' and so forth. I'll put this stuff over here on the right of the diagram. Look, attention increased to focus on pain, there's concern, anxiety, frustration and even fear about the pain. Plus the brain gets quickly 'tuned-in' to the pain problem and can become 'preoccupied' with it. The nastier the pain the more these things kick in.'

'Are you still with me..?'

'I'm seeing what you're getting at. I'll need your diagram though.'

'No problems, I think you're seeing that what I'm putting on the sketch are a great many of your current symptoms, it seems that you might be stuck in this early 'STOP' don't move phase of healing and haven't moved on to the 'get me moving' phase. I'll come back to this in a minute. What I also want to put on the diagram is an arrow from conscious 'you' down to the threat processing centre. If conscious 'you' is highly concerned about the pain and what it means, if it's super-concerned that if you move you'll make the pain worse or injure yourself further, or maybe if it's concerned that something is badly wrong, then you send messages to the threat processing centres – which keep them going. Hence it all keeps up the anxiety, concern and tension, as well as the lack of movement and so forth. It's a vicious circle and it's why I'm spending a bit of time in trying to get you to see a different perspective on the problem.'

I now draw a downward arrow with a big negative sign, it goes from the 'conscious 'you' brain box down to the 'threat processing centres' box below.

'What we have to do, is to try to stop all your inputs being processed in the threat centre and this requires the thinking 'you' (I point to it on the figure) helping, while we do things! For example, we want normal touch and normal movement processed into 'normal touch and normal movement' processing centres and not by your 'threat' processing centres, we want it diverted away from the 'danger' processing to the 'it's nice/non-threatening' processing centres and I'm going to help you try and do that. If successful you'll be shifting into the 'get me moving' phase of recovery!'

I pause and give Kate a chance to comment or query...

'This looks hard, my brain is constantly drifting to my back pain all the time, it makes me tense, I've a constant dry mouth, I can't think straight and I'm feeling like nothing's going to improve it. Wouldn't it be so good if you could just fix the back and this whole thing would slip back to normal?'

'Yes it would, but with a bit of practice and a little success, even the tiniest amount of success, will help you to see that it can improve and you'll start to feel better with yourself. Ideally, for the next three to four weeks, I want you to be entirely selfish if you can, because there's going to be a lot of little practices to do through the days if you can fit them in.'

(Note that my sketches are clear when they start, but as they're built up by the end they're a bit of a mess, what I do is give the patient copies of figures 17.3 and 17.4 to take home with them, or email it to them if they have the right programme).

Chapter 17.7

Explaining, listening and interacting with a patient: Kate – second session continued

Lesson: the recovery graph...

(Again, as in the last chapter, I start with a fresh piece of paper and I build the graph up as I go through things. I'd also like the reader to appreciate that there was far more of a two-way conversation going on, with Kate asking questions and me answering or drawing the answers out of her, where appropriate. What follows is the essence of the material and conversation we had.)

'Here's another diagram to show you where patients similar to you can go. I call it the 'recovery graph' and on it is a list of important things that other patients just like you and many far worse, have found useful in their recovery.' (see fig 17.5)

'I'm assuming you're comfortable with graphs? The vertical axis here is all about health and well-being, as it goes up, so pain usually goes down but we're careful to make no firm promises here. Along the bottom axis is time, as time goes on there's a progression steadily upwards, which I often divide into two phases: the first phase may be a week or two or many months, there's huge variability and it's very hard to predict how fast people will move along here. The key thing is 'start-easy-build-slowly', doing too much too soon, getting over ambitious or over enthusiastic

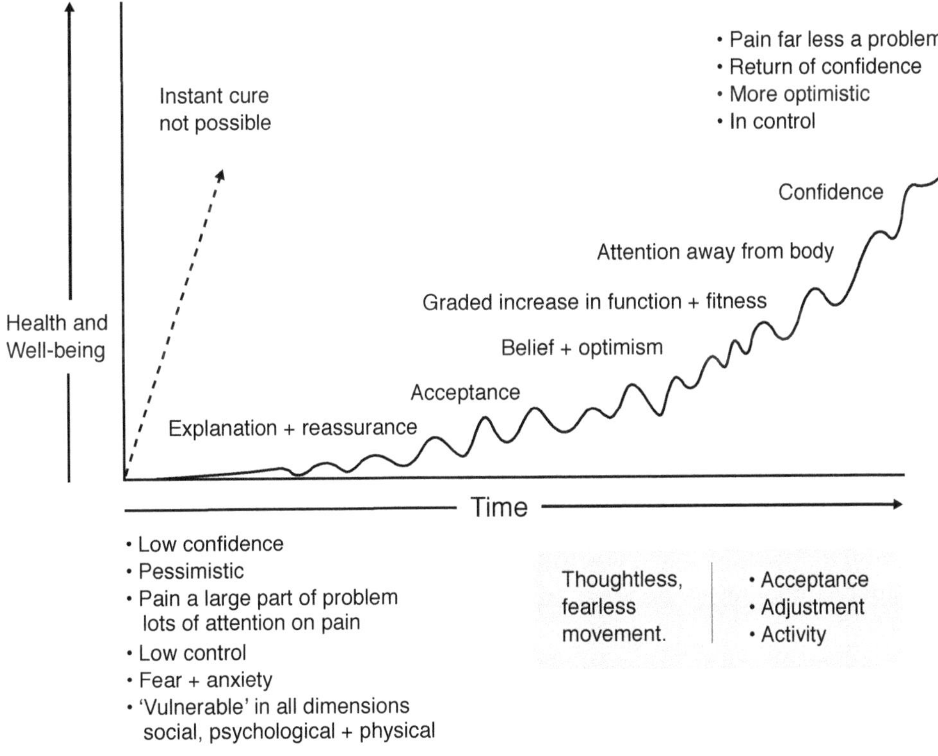

Figure 17.5 The Recovery Graph – another 'build-up' diagram.

often leads to big flare-ups and then you're put-off doing anything and you give up. We also add the simple phrase 'succeed-not-fail', to remind you to go easy and not overdo it. Sometimes patients get over enthusiastic or even frustrated with not doing enough, they then do too much, the pain flares up and they end up not wanting to do it again. They fail, they get frustrated and the door which was slightly open to them closes. The 'threat' centres fire up again. 'Succeed not fail' means go gradually and succeed rather than go like a bull-at-a-gate and end up failing because of the pain flare. In order to do this you need to learn how to pace activity and any exercises that we might try.'

'I'll keep reminding you of these two phrases of ours as we go along. What we are going to do is take very small steps with movement and touch, taking great care at the start and to get the most comfortable and most relaxed situation we can. We're going to try to 'trick' your system into processing in the 'nice', 'neutral, or 'couldn't care less' centres in your system, rather than the threat and nasty centres and then it's practice, practice, practice! When you get good at that we move on to slightly harder levels.'

'Let's just finish what's on the graph. Note that I've put a line going vertically up that says 'Instant cure not possible'! That's definitely what most patients don't want to hear but I hope you're starting to see that...

a) The Dr's and consultant specialists you've seen haven't got one...

b) The physio hadn't; but...

c) You may have heard of people who've had miraculous cures, from all sorts of alternative therapists and want to try them. You can go off and do that if you want, or you can come along with me now, or, if you do go want to go away and try other therapies and don't get anywhere – you are welcome to come back later on and we'll carry on! The big thing is, that the reason I've drawn that line is because with problems like yours, 'instant cures' are actually very rare, even though many alternative practitioners would have you believe otherwise.

She took a deep breath...

'I've actually got something to admit and thought it best not to tell you, but I have been to quite a few therapists already, most of them have promised a lot, helped a bit for a while but overall it's no better and they've been very confusing... the worst was the one who told me to lighten-up and that it was my fault that her therapy wasn't able to work. Overall, I think they've made me emotionally worse because I've started to get cross with myself over it. It's so hard when your friends say things like 'Well they helped me, it was brilliant' and I can't agree with them. It makes me feel guilty for failing all the time.'

'You're not the only one out there. All I can tell you is that I've been working with problems like yours throughout my career and I hear these stories over and over again. Don't feel bad about it and don't get mad, because when normal ways of getting better don't work, it's quite natural to seek other forms of help. You sound like you're happy to keep going with this?'

'Indeed, it's easy but sort of complicated, but it's making sense. I know I need to think about a great deal you've told me and somehow I'm feeling better in myself, just because at last someone has given me a way of looking at it that fits with how I feel.'

'Stuck in the 'STOP' phase of injury!' I say quietly. I smile and she agrees.

I'm getting somewhere!

'Back to the graph now!'

(Note that, as here, it's quite nice to use the 'third person' to bring issues up that you may feel a little awkward or sensitive to ask about. The 'third- person' nicely detaches the clinician from any personal relationship with the material being put across. It certainly helped me in my early communications with patients on this sort of level)

This is what I said, 'Down here, is where a great many patients like you start.' I point to where the X and Y axes meet.

'I'm going to make a little list of some of the things that many patients say about how they feel when I first see them, some of which you may feel are familiar and apply to your situation. So:

- they're low in confidence – that's physically but also generally, social, work, home etc.

- a great many report that they were once happy and positive but have become 'half-empty' – they're pessimistic about themselves, about what they can do and importantly about their own future

- they've lost control in their lives because they're doing so little and have become dependent on their family doing a lot for them

- they find they're giving on-going and high levels of attention to the pain and the problem Some say they become almost preoccupied with it, or that it's overwhelming their normal ability to concentrate, their mind keeps wandering off looking for pain or concentrating on the pain that's there and analysing it

- they find themselves talking about it all the time and trying to make sense of its behaviour

- many have lots of worries, fears and anxieties about the pain and their situation

- a great many feel that the word 'vulnerable' sums it all up and it's not just physically, it's socially and psychologically too

- a great many feel physically out of sorts, their fitness, their weight, their appearance and this all dents their normal confidence. Many would rather stay in and not meet anybody.

Kate had been nodding all the way through, she agreed.

I knew I was comfortable enough with her to not need to go into great detail of any of the issues then and there, but it was good for her to realise that I 'understood' what she was going through in terms of not just the pain, but also in terms of 'life' and general mental and physical well-being.

'I'll just carry on, stop me, comment anything you like...'

I knew that this could easily have been a little 'breakdown' point, which would have been fine, but rather than pause and let it happen I took her attention back to the graph. I wanted to shift the thinking to seeing what could be done and what we could do together.

'Now look what I'm writing along the graph line...'

> **'Explanation and reassurance** – I think we've done a fair whack here and I feel I may be able to see a spark of a new perspective and maybe slightly more confidence, but some of this stuff can be quite confusing? You must let me know if there's something bubbling in your head that's upsetting you...'
>
> 'Louis, I've been listening and all the time my feeling that I'm going to be helped is growing, it makes sense, but I need to review it at home too with Greg. What's actually happening is I'm popping up questions in my head, but then I'm getting the answers from what you are saying a few minutes later.'
>
> I now wrote **Acceptance!** 'This is a big one that helps to reduce the activity of the "Threat Processing Centre." This is what I mean: a great many people in your situation keep harking back to what they used to be able to do and that they can't do it now. If I can get them to come to terms with their current situation and accept where they're at right now, it helps hugely. A problem is that early on we're aiming for goals that may seem pathetic, compared to what they used to be able to do, but if patients can accept the situation and start to recognise small goal achievements, then they usually do very well. There's a lot of research that shows that when patients accept their situation, even accept and make friends with their pain, they also do very well and the pain get's less! It kind of means you stop fighting the pain, you stop processing it in the 'threat control centres.'
>
> I pull out the two diagrams from the day before (17.3, 17.4) and point to the Threat Control Centres on them.
>
> 'I fully realise that someone telling you to 'make friends with your pain' could make you scream, but in the context of getting things processed away from the threat centres, it makes sense. A big thing is that some levels of pain are so nasty that this is impossible, but lower levels can be accepted sometimes and this helps.'
>
> 'Some patients have found that thinking of their current pain as a pet dog is useful: it's a 'Great Dane' to start with and gradually and eventually morphs into a 'Chihuahua'! The Great Dane is massive but get to know it

and it's friendly. The Chihuahua is tiny and friendly. *(You may think I'm going crazy here – but 'Top-Down DURING bottom-up' requires mental images that trigger positive processing and this is just one way of getting it. Later Kate may be doing an activity of exercise and I'll want her to be engaging helpful 'top-down' processing, having an easy image, or a repetitive phrase to say as the activity/exercise is preformed is designed to trigger this i.e. Chihuahua, Chihuahua...!)*

I write **'Belief and Optimism'**. 'When you start to achieve a little success, which means reaching a few easy goals, I want you to be able to reflect on what you've done in a positive way. If you can achieve a basic goal, you can then go on and achieve a slightly harder one and so forth. Success breeds success and gives you BO! We call it 'BO' for short, not 'body-odour' but 'Belief and Optimism!'

Now, **'Graded increase in function and fitness'**. Big one here: generally, the majority of fit people and I mean all round well-being here too, are happier, healthier and feel good with themselves. Their bodies are less painful and if they injure they heal quickly. Their 'pain-off' systems, that we discussed earlier work really well, they're efficient.'

'Now, fitness is a massive issue for anyone who has had a pain problem like yours for a long time. It's mostly because pain stops you moving normally, you do far less than normal and you become generally unfit. The muscles and joints of your back become weak and stiff and as a result become more vulnerable and hence will become more sensitive. The problem is that while moving them helps to get them fitter – it hurts and flares up! The good news is that if we look at your movements in a bit more detail, we should be able to find a great many that are easy to do and are either comfortable or you feel happy to start doing, this process is 'graded' – meaning gradual.'

'Attention away from body – Most people move their bodies without giving them a thought, they move around, pick things up, do their work by moving on automatic. This is a great goal to achieve when you've been super-cautious for a long time. I note with many successful patients, that when they are really getting somewhere, they start telling me they're doing activities without thinking about their pain area. This usually happens spontaneously as they improve, but it's good to give yourself a little star for realising you did stuff without thinking about it.'

'Confidence, I always write four points at the top of the curve here. They are the four things, in this approach to problems like yours we can almost guarantee, if you stick with it. Here they are:

1. When you're further up the curve here, back comes the feeling of being in control.
2. Patients almost always say that pain is far less of a problem than

it was. BUT! I like to say to the patient, try not to let the pain level and its behaviour be the only thing by which you judge progress, I know that is hard.

3. There's a return of confidence and the outlook becomes positive and more optimistic.

4. The big goal in all my patients is 'Thoughtless fearless movement' and I write this at the top. It's hopefully self explanatory.

(Note that this phrase can be used as a 'Top-down during bottom up' trigger to say when appropriate. For example, a patient may have a specific exercise to do and while doing it I will get them to specifically shift their thinking away from the movement/symptoms etc. if I can. I often get patients to sing, listen to music, radio, TV, talk to friends, fiddle with their phones or ipads... think nice thoughts about the movement. Repeat phrases like 'GreatDaneChihuahua'! I'm afraid with a patient like Kate, or for that matter any patient if I really think about it, I am not at all keen on the muscle imbalance therapies that get patients to focus on muscles and movement and that it has to be 'correct' in some way. To me if a movement is thoughtless and fearless it's just fine. The notion of 'bad' movement patterns is a danger to the spontaneity of our existence. Save it for the obsessive sports stars... not here! Read Eyal Lederman's papers to get a realistic perspective).

That just about completes the session, but with a few patients I finish off with the story of the Australian surgeon who wrote a book called 'Cry of the Damaged Man'.

The book is summarised thus: while driving to work in 1984, Dr Tony Moore was hit by a thirty tonne truck, crushing him and his car and changing his life forever. A well-known surgeon and rehabilitation specialist, he tells his story of recovery from a patient's point of view, but with a doctor's knowledge and experience. Temporarily disabled and emotionally devastated, Tony Moore records how, from the depths of despair and isolation, he emerged as a more perceptive doctor and changed individual.

At the point in the book when he started to really recover he realised that there were three really important things that helped. They were very simple:

- **Acceptance**
- **Adjustment** (to the current state of health and function)
- **Activity** (getting active and fit again was centre to his recovery, despite the pain)

In the next session we started the get-going process.

Chapter 17.8
Kate – early physical management

Cargoes

Quinquireme of Nineveh from distant Ophir,
Rowing home to haven in sunny Palestine,
With a cargo of ivory,
And apes and peacocks,
Sandalwood, cedarwood, and sweet white wine.

Stately Spanish galleon coming from the Isthmus,
Dipping through the Tropics by the palm-green shores,
With a cargo of diamonds,
Emeralds, amythysts,
Topazes, and cinnamon, and gold moidores.

Dirty British coaster with a salt-caked smoke stack,
Butting through the Channel in the mad March days,
With a cargo of Tyne coal,
Road-rails, pig-lead,
Firewood, iron-ware, and cheap tin trays.

John Masefield

I actually started Kate with some easy movements using the 'wire-apart-depart' principles discussed earlier. I will deal with how this is achieved in a practical way in later chapters. What we actually did physically, was very simple.

Kate had got going with:

1. A graded walking programme – I did some movement things with her similar to Jude, but not quite so tongue in cheek to start with, as her personality didn't allow it. The main thing was that I taught her to how to use top-down during bottom up i.e. consciously letting go in her face and trunk as much as possible while walking, using loose waist and swinging arms. After that, she agreed to a graded walking programme doing two walks a day to start with, we started with just two minutes outside, weather permitting and incremented by thirty seconds every two days, with an emphasis on quality not quantity to start with. She used a 'floppy-let-it-go' mantra for the top-down during bottom-up part of walking and walked as slowly as she had to, in order to get the quality of movement. She also agreed to practice the 'relaxed walking' at any time for a few paces throughout the day.

2. She charted her walking progress.

3. Similar techniques were used for back exercises that were essentially the same as the ones she'd chosen during the earlier examination. She agreed to find time to do these three times a day starting with 5-10 repetitions (our classic ridiculous amount!), depending on the movement and gradually building to 10-15. The exercises she felt confident about were the all four's ones and those done in sitting.

4. I was keen for her to tackle her concentration. So she agreed to start to read a book she'd been thinking about and then make a few notes on each chapter to show me (she actually volunteered to do this). The idea was to get her to start practicing concentration again and also see if what she could manage, for how long and how easily. It was a simple 'base-line' finding exercise, with a strong emphasis on the principles of 'start easy build slowly' and 'succeed not fail'. She agreed to try to be satisfied (rather than get mad) with only a paragraph or two, if that was all she could manage. If you think about it, this is just applying the make-it-easy and start-easy-build-slowly principles of 'graded exposure' and by doing this and being successful, she would hopefully learn to apply this to many other situations too.

5. With her agreement and understanding why, I referred her to a reliable non-whacky relaxation therapist who works hugely out-of-the-box with patients like Kate. I think these types of therapists are rare.

Most tense and wound-up patients like Kate, are hopeless at relaxation and just can't get the concentration or stillness required. As a generalisation, the very people who are likely to benefit from relaxation are the most difficult to train. They're the: 'I've never been able to sit still for five minutes, the idea of relaxing or anything like that, just isn't me,' type of people. But note, Kate was one of these, yet she was very able to be with me and concentrate for long periods, as the last few chapters have illustrated. Sometimes our brain 'compartments' just don't see the discrepancies!

'I can't sit still for more than five minutes.'

'Hang on, you just sat there listening and discussing with me for over an hour?'

Tip: don't do it like this! It's confrontation and challenging!

It's only me being mischievous. The point is, I know she can do it.

The relaxation therapist, strangely called 'Blame', reported that he was initially able to get her to be calm for about five minutes by using a short, one minute session of counting breathing out-loud, followed by reading short poems for a few minutes. As things progressed, he started repeating the little sessions, giving her mini standing and moving breaks in between, which was cool in itself – to use movement and changes in posture!

By the end of the third session (after two weeks) she was able to repeat the five minute cycles three times with no problems. 'Blame' told me that he'd recorded the poems and she practiced at home twice a day – with the instruction to use them at anytime, if it helped how she felt. He had focused on using poetry because she'd said she really enjoyed it at school. Most of the poems chosen were those she knew well and had grown up with. 'Cargoes' by John Masefield was one of them.

Interestingly, as time went on he started bringing in more rhythmical nonsense type poems, as well as reciting words from some of her favourite songs. The idea was to get a mix of emotions, from neutral, through story-telling, to amusing, to calm and peaceful scenes and on to more complex passages. Eventually she was able to relax well for around twenty minutes using a tape.

Within the three weeks that followed the first two 'ground-work' sessions I've described in detail, I saw Kate twice more, to instigate all the above. I then let her get going for ten days before following up again.

She walked in for this fifth session smoothly and with a smile. This was exceptional I thought.

'I'm walking occasionally without having to do my 'top-down' phrases and I think I'm doing better.'

We discussed the positive aspects of progress – nice! In the old days it would have been all pain talk and misery talk. There was still a lot to be done and a great many possible directions to go in, more exercise, new starting positions, start adding a little resistance, start getting into stretching, do more functional patterns like sit-stand, steps, balance, physio-balls, even light gym work, even hands-on!

I asked her about any difficulties and things not going so well – sleep was still a big issue. She tired easily, she'd had some terrible days, she accepted but hated the pain killers, she wished she could control the pain better and she was still really jumpy and sore in her back. She had days when she was low but was doing her best to keep on track with the relaxation (liked it!) and the programme.

Hands on...

'Is there any particular thing that you'd like me to deal with or look at today?' I openly asked...

'I'm dreading it, but you mentioned touch and this tension and flinching in my back, if we can do anything there I'm sure it'd help my overall pain too...'

'Great, so if we're going to get anywhere I need to know more about your back sensitivity and I would like to start by trying to find something positive. One positive thing is that when I first saw you – you showed me that you could touch yourself quite happily.

'Just remind me, what's it like washing yourself and drying yourself after a shower?'

'I tend to dab it with the towel, but I can just towel down OK and washing seems fine.'

'No flinching... it doesn't make you jump when you touch yourself...?

'No, it doesn't seem to.'

'You're looking concerned, as if I've just found you out! I haven't, because what you're describing is typical of people with super-sensitivity, they find that they can touch it and feel OK, probably because there isn't the prospect of anything sudden or surprising. When you touch it yourself, you're in control, someone else touching you is a potential threat, off it goes to the threat processing and up to the pain processing centres and, bang, Ow!'

'I'll tell you a story that may help set the scene. When I first trained I worked with patients who'd had severe burns, when skin recovers from a burn, as you probably know there's lots of scar tissue and scar tissue tends to tighten up and contract. If it isn't kept moving from the early healing days the patients end up with very restricted joint movements, because of the scarring. Burnt hands were particularly problematic. The other thing was that if the injured tissues weren't moved, touched and handled – they ended up supersensitive. So, even though it hurt at the time, early movement and lots of handling and touch helped to prevent the contractures but also eventually helped reduce the sensitivity. The patients who got used to it quickly and accepted the pain, usually did the best *(don't say this if it's going to make the patient feel guilty or bad that they haven't got used to it)*. So, some patients coped a great deal better than others, but the ones who made the biggest effort and started touching and moving it for themselves and were also happy to let us therapists do it – did the best. What always happened though, was that we started out light and gently but soon did more and more, this way the pain system and the patient got used to it and found that slowly the sensitivity got less and less.'

'You can see what I'm saying? We have to somehow start a touching programme and you have to be involved too – it's exactly the same process as doing your movements, the more you practice the more you get used to it and the more you can do.'

Kate got it and we started by seeing if we could find inputs to her back that she could do at home that were either neutral or even pleasant. *(This is the fire-apart-*

depart thing and I could have explained that to her here.). I got her to do the towel rubbing through her clothes. Sure, she'd done it before but this needed to be done in a conscious way, so she realised that the tissues could be pressed on and at the same time, joining up the two contradictory 'compartments' (one is the: 'I can't be touched on my back it's so sensitive' compartment, the other is the: 'I wash myself and towel it down every day without thinking about it.' Therefore it can be touched, it depends on the context etc.). I wanted her to engage top-down in a 'preparatory' sort of way.

Once she had got the idea with the towel, I now got her to do a similar rubbing movement across her back with her hands. I got her to do it low over her buttocks as well as higher above the pain area. I then took the towel, with her agreement of course and repeated in the two areas above and below... and then asked how she felt about the same thing across the back.

'If you keep it the same pressure...' came the rather tentative reply.

I started the see-sawing movement over her low thoracic area, kept it constant and slowly let the towel descend over the low back.

I said we could call this 'the new towel therapy!'

Within five minutes or so she allowed me to rub her back in the same way.

She now had tears in her eyes.

'This is the first time anyone's touched my back without me being in agony and jumping a mile since the problem started...'

And so the graded progression from touch to massage, to mobilisation went on over the next 1-2 months. By the end of the second month I was able to do what I would call normal 'posterio-anterio' ('pa') type pressures for about ten minutes. That was fine for me, but for real-life 'pa' pressures are largely irrelevant. She needed to be desensitised to the normal hustle, bump and bustle of life. To this end I did lots of balance type pushing her around in various starting positions – all fours, standing, sitting on a 'physio-ball' etc... We even tried a pillow fight, did forward rolls and a 'jarring your body' programme – sitting down with a bump,– starting on a physio ball and progressing to a chair with pillows then reducing them and so forth. This is a cynical ex-manual therapist purist (long-ago mind), acting and thinking much more like a neuro-physio! FUNCTION AND REAL LIFE!

A few important things from this touch/desensitising input:

1. Top-down during bottom-up – was occasionally required, but the key thing she told me was when she realised that her own touch was for the most part OK. She realised that all she had to do was overcome her fear of being touched and the best way to do that was to practice and slowly get used to it. Pleasingly, she eventually trusted her partner to be involved and like many others found that firm touch was better than light touch.

2. She practiced a great deal and it took her a long time and a lot of work before her flinching reactions diminished. She trusted me, then her partner but the

wider community was more problematic for quite a long time (another year).

3. Initial manual type input, using top-down 'during' bottom-up almost always requires it to be done while constantly directing the thinking of the patient. For example, in prone lying doing gentle soft tissue work to the low back, the patient often flinches and jumps, or the muscle goes rigid and solid, not uncommonly more on one side than the other.

What follows is a likely running conversation. But first, think about lying prone, think what the patient's feelings might be. They can't see a thing, lying prone for many isn't the most comfortable, they've little idea where you are, have no feedback of your body language or facial expression and most of all, they've no idea what you're going to do. I wouldn't put a patient like Kate prone, I'd always have her in side lying so she can be comfortable, see me and we can make eye contact and communicate easily.

Here's the conversation and details:

'I want you to feel what I'm feeling in your back at this point here (soft and relaxed), compared to what I feel here,' (firm and tense, no give...). I go slowly forward and back from one place to the other...

'Try and let go in the muscle so that it softens, softer, like here. See if you can feel the difference that I'm feeling?'

She lets go for a second or two and then it comes tense again. I keep going giving occasional feedback about the tension and their success. 'Can you feel what I feel? Try to soften, let that tension go. Maybe try sending it to our 'friendly' it's OK processing place if you can.'

If there's a bit of success, it's often good to then do a few movements, for example up into all four's to do easy arch and hollow – flexion into extension.

'Floppy, smooth and relaxed, try not to be jerky... slow it down a bit, smooth, smooth, keep the smooth little movements going... trust your back to relax with the movement... now increase the movement a little, keep it smooth... trust your back...'

'Now Kate, I'll keep going and how about you tell me what's happening?' She's getting it and letting go and telling me too. She's soon getting it right all the time. It's simple 'learning', she's learning the skill of monitoring tension in her back, in this context, with me. It might be helpful, but it might be a waste of time. The big deal is transferring it to real life movement and function; if it doesn't, I think, forget it. However, patients often get up and move better and feel better. The more they experience what a relaxed back feels like the easier it is to get there again and again later.

I hope I've given you a few thoughts and ideas. I could have recited 'Cargoes' with her as we did the touch or the movement...!

There are a great many patients like Kate, some are very difficult to shift or change and some respond well like she did. The amount of information given was relatively massive, because she required it and could concentrate enough to take it. With others, I'd have watered it down a lot and most likely just got straight on with simple relaxed movements, at the same time chatted about processing, or not at all. Of which, more later!

What's the brain got to do with pain?

Here's one way of summarising some of what's cropped up in this section:

- *Top-down before bottom-up: i.e. prepare to change the 'background' cognitive influence on the maladaptive pain and movement 'noise' that's being amplified by the current beliefs and attributions.*
- *The unhelpful 'bottom-up' and low-road processing needs modulating by any reasonable means possible.*
- *High-Road – Listen and physically examine and then explain/ reassure/ change beliefs/thinking/attribution – the introduction of a less threatening perspective/view is sometimes valuable but not always possible. You can spend a long time here, but ultimately it may not be that productive. Getting on with 'doing and proving' can be more efficient, but a balance is always needed.*
- *High-road issue: tissues not being pathological – 'deconditioned' is the best perspective.*
- *High-road issue: the concept of maladaptive pain and 'threat' processing may help.*
- *High-road issue: concept of maladaptive hypersensitivity and desensitising process may be helpful.*
- *Review of bottom-up issues that can be addressed (RELEVANT physical findings in the shopping basket – try to err more to the 'functional/ activity restriction' compartment than the traditional manual therapy love: the 'Impairment' compartment.)*
- *Start Bottom-up DURING top-down! Example here using exercise, normal movement, gym and fitness work, pain modalities, manual therapy!*

Section 17
Read what I've read

Damasio A.R. (1995) Descartes' Error: Emotion, reason and the human brain. Picador. London.

Damasio A.R. (2000) The feeling of what happens. Body, emotion and the making of consciousness. Vintage. London.

Damasio A.R. (2003) Looking for Spinoza. Joy, sorrow and the feeling brain. William Heinemann. London.

Koyama T, McHaffie JG, Laurienti PJ, Coghill RC. (2005) The subjective experience of pain: where expectations become reality. Proc Natl Acad Sci; 102(36):12950-5.

Lederman E. (2010) The myth of core stability Journal of Bodywork & Movement Therapies 14, 84-98.

Moore T. (1992) Cry of the Damaged Man: A Personal Journey of Recovery. Pan Books.

Section 18

THE MATURE ORGANISM MODEL AND THE BRAIN

Chapter 18.1
The Mature Organism Model (MOM): feelings and homeostasis

You're Gonna Make Me Lonesome When You Go

I've seen love go by my door
It's never been this close before
Never been so easy or so slow
I've been shooting in the dark too long
When something not right it's wrong
Yer gonna make me lonesome when you go.

Dragon clouds so high above
I've only known careless love
It's always hit me from below
This time around it's more correct
Right on target so direct
Yer gonna make me lonesome when you go.

Purple clover Queen Anne lace
Crimson hair across your face
You could make me cry if you don't know
Can't remember what I was thinking of
You might be spoiling me too much love
Yer gonna make me lonesome when you go.

Flowers on the hillside blooming crazy
Crickets talking back and forth in rhyme
Blue river running slow and lazy
I could stay with you forever
And never realize the time.

Situations have ended sad
Relationship have all been bad
Mine've been like Verlaine's and Rimbaud
But there's no way I can compare
All those scenes to this affair
Yer gonna make me lonesome when you go.

Yer gonna make me wonder what I'm doing
Staying far behind without you
Yer gonna make me wonder what I'm saying
Yer gonna make me give myself a good talking to.

I'll look for you in old Honolulu
San Francisco, Ashtabula
Yer gonna have to leave me now I know
But I'll see you in the sky above
In the tall grass in the ones I love
Yer gonna make me lonesome when you go.

Bob Dylan – from the Album: Blood on the Tracks 1975

As I've already discussed in section 11, if you read the pain literature you'll find that the small unmyelinated C fibres and the myelinated A delta fibres are mostly referred to as nociceptors – or even more frequently as pain fibres. In that chapter, I reviewed Schiable and Schmidt's work showing that linking these fibres solely to 'pain' and 'high threshold' only activity, isn't the situation at all and that they may be best considered as 'tissue sampling' (and supporting) fibres. In this chapter I look at their broader and more biological role in relation to body or 'homeostatic' sampling and reflect on the brain and central processing of it in relation to feelings that include pain.

What I also want to try and do here is reinforce the notion of a continuous 'sample-scrutinise-respond' process in biology – that occurs at all levels, from the lowly tissues to the supporting nerves, up into the spinal cord and finally through to all the various levels of the brain and back out again. At each level some kind of scrutiny occurs that gives rise to the possibility of an appropriate response.

A brief thought about the word 'scrutinise' though, because it tends to make one feel that some kind of complex thinking and decision-making is going on. In a sense, that is true, decision-making is going on, but at lower levels it usually boils down to a simple choice – like switch on? Or, switch off? We therefore have: sample-scrutinise (Turn on? Or off? Or allow/prevent)-respond. At higher levels it may not be as simple because there is likely to be competition between networks of on and off cell assemblies, all vying to produce one or other response. Think of it as a democracy, a voting system whereby the majority win out. This democratic system allows for a 'spectrum' of response strengths. For example, a strong vote in favour (really go for it), or against (stop it right away) a given response, gives instant and unhindered facilitation or inhibition. At the other end of the spectrum, where the gap between those in favour and those against may be very narrow – the response that emerges is likely to be somewhat weaker. A go nowhere 'hung' vote may even be a possibility. Nerve cell assemblies can be envisaged as competing with each other over a given decision or response with the strongest, fittest and most robust winning the day. Think 'dithering' for a close vote and think a landslide 'go for it' or 'don't go for it' where there's a big majority!

At a rather reductionist level of reasoning, nervous system scrutinising decisions are made at the level of the synapse and are also related to the strength or 'efficacy' of the synapses involved (remember Shane and Claudia?). Right now, it's all about synaptic democracy!

The 'interoceptive' cortex

I am now going to lean heavily on Bud Craig's (Craig 2003, 2010) notion of an 'interoceptive' system – because it fits nicely with the Mature Organism Model (MOM) and my easy sample-scrutinise-respond way of viewing things. As an aside here, one thing not hugely in Craig's favour, is that he is the epitome of a 'brain-centric' pain researcher, he seems very determined that one day he is likely to be able to describe the actual 'pain network' and all the various zones, areas and organs of the brain responsible.

Anyway let's pick on what's useful. Craig's research has led him to the conclusion that we have specialised neural networks, assemblies and brain nuclei[1] that are dedicated to checking and managing the body's health and physiological status. He refers to the network as the homeostatic or 'interoceptive' component of the nervous system and brain. In the original MOM I described the brain as 'sampling its own body' i.e. 'interoception' and that this occurred alongside 'sampling the environment' i.e. 'exteroception' but also, and finally, the brain 'sampling itself'. Meaning sampling the individuals' memory libraries and networks for any useful information or experiences it may have from the past, which could have some relevance and use to the current situation (see section 16 chapters).

It looks as if the 'interoceptive' cortical areas are where key body sampling information goes to seek a hearing and receive some kind of scrutiny. Section 16 mentioned this and also the visual, gustatory, olfactory and somatosensory cortices too. There will be more discussion of the somatosensory cortices in section 19 because they seem to be 'trending' in physiotherapy treatments for chronic pain. To me, they're collaring a bit too much attention over other sampling, scrutinising and responding areas, who, by the way, are feeling somewhat left out; I've interviewed them, if you're wondering how I knew that!

1 - The term 'nuclei' when used in the brain refers to a compact cluster of neurons. In sections of the brain nuclei show up as regions of grey matter. The medulla and pons contain numerous small nuclei with a wide variety of sensory, motor, and regulatory functions. The thalamus and hypothalamus are made of numerous interconnected nuclei.

Let's get on, sorry it's a little heavy on brain bits and pieces for a couple of paragraphs but bear with me and keep the figure in mind (18.1) if it helps?

In the brain, Craig is particularly fond of a cortical area called the 'insula'. It's best visualised from a coronal slice through about the middle of your brain (figure 18.1). In the figure it's called the 'Interoceptive cortex'. Note that it's deep in the fold of the cortex that separates the lobe above, the parietal lobe, from that below, the temporal lobe.

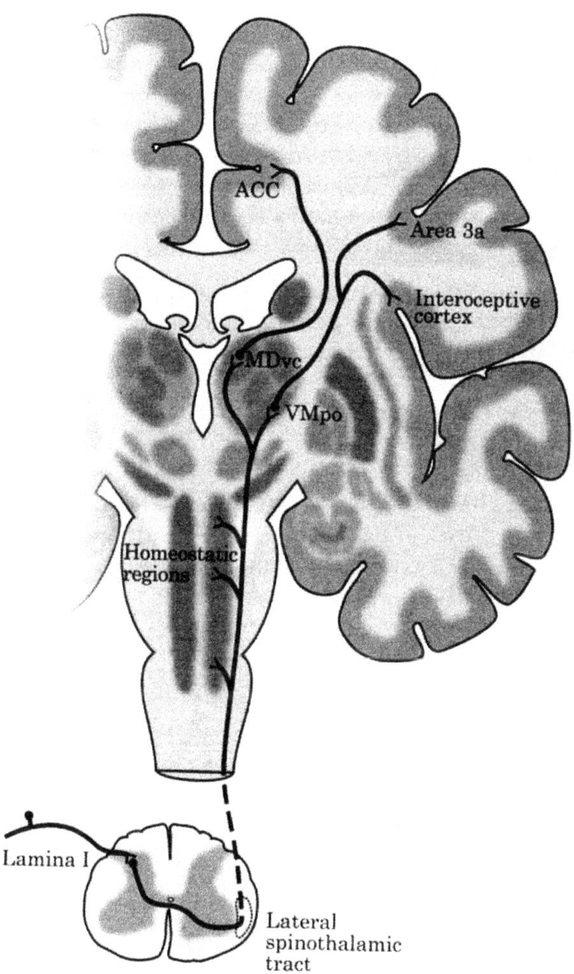

Figure 18.1 A cortical area called the 'insula'. It's best visualised from a coronal slice through about the middle of your brain. In the figure it's called the 'Interoceptive cortex'. Note that it's deep in the fold of the cortex that separates the lobe above, the parietal lobe, from that below, the temporal lobe. Also on the figure is a schematic of an ascending tract (that's many millions of nerve fibres but where only one is shown!)

Also on the figure is a schematic of an ascending tract (that's many millions of nerve fibres but where only one is shown!), whose origins are from our small afferent 'sampling' fibres (Aδ and C fibres). These fibres synapse in the outermost layer of the cord dorsal horn grey matter (lamina 1), then project across the cord and on up in the lateral spinothalamic tract to the brain – the classic (Cartesian) 'pain pathway', which more correctly should be termed a 'nociceptive pathway'. The diagram unfortunately omits important projections from lamina 1 to the autonomic systems, whose columns and synapses lie in the lateral horn area of the cord. In other words, C and Aδ fibres project via an interneuron (or two, or three) directly to the sympathetic and parasympathetic systems, which then loop back to the tissues, in order to make any adjustments that might help the situation. Brilliant, there's a quick route into the cord and straight back out again, just like the simple motor spinal loop we all observe when testing reflexes. More on this soon, but at this level it's all about quickly reacting and controlling, followed by a smidgen of a moment later a bit of 'context related' adjusting, thanks to 'scrutinising' and 'controlling' higher level processing... 'Oh, sorry, we can't help you out right now he's busy winning Wimbledon – you'll have to wait until later.'

In the brain stem you can see branches from the spinothalamic tract to 'homeostatic' regions there. For example, the periaqueductal grey (PAG) and the rostroventral medulla (RVM), which we've already met in relation to the pain-on and off systems and also another little area of processing importance, the parabrachial nucleus (PN). Above this the tract reaches the thalamus where further 'processing' and synapsing takes place. The two areas shown are the VMpo (posterior part of the ventral medial nucleus of the thalamus) and the MDvc (ventral caudal part of the medial dorsal nucleus). From the thalamus, the tracts' destinations of interest to this discussion are Craig's 'Interoceptive cortex' (part of the 'Insula') and the ACC – the anterior cingulate cortex that's in the medial forebrain that we've already come across... and probably a whole host of other destinations and processing regions too.

These basic one-wire type wiring diagrams are useful for us to visualise, but a problem in that they miss a massive mass of 'other' connections. For example, as you might imagine, this ascending system must reach and have potential impact on all the key stress or threat processing centres. It's best to go back and review the 'low, quick and dirty' and the 'high, slow and accurate' roads to see what I mean. So, think: amygdala, hypothalamus, all the sensory cortices, the medial temporal lobe memory system, the forebrain working memory areas and so forth.

Bud Craig feels that the interoceptive cortex is vital to the conscious formation of bodily sensations including pain, well he would, he's got a reputation for being rather 'reductionist' and rather 'line-labelled too.

My advice is, see the notion of an interoceptive cortex as interesting – but realise it's unlikely to be just the insula and far more likely to be a massively dispersed system.

Homeostasis and feelings

Let's think about homeostasis for a minute, because what I think is really being presented by Bud Craig is an extension of the well known sub-conscious homeostatic control goings-on in the brain stem to include, or add on, new knowledge of conscious awareness processing of that very same information. Craig is trying to put the 'brain-centric' – 'I found the areas where it becomes conscious' hat on the subject unfortunately.

I'll try and explain from my grounded and 'loopy' perspective. This is much lighter.

The homeostatic/interoceptive sampling systems of the body give the brain information about important physiological needs, for example:

- blood sugar levels – hence hypoglycaemia when they're low
- blood fluid levels – blood osmolarity
- blood oxygen levels – e.g, hypoxia
- body temperature
- bladder fullness
- bowel fullness
- gut/stomach fullness
- the presence of poisons and toxins – gut, skin, etc.
- food or fluid in the mouth
- physical damage
- healing
- pathology and disease
- needs of musculoskeletal system – muscle metabolite levels
- skin 'threats'

The list may be longer of course.

In normal humans all the above are associated with some form of feeling, or sensation that motivates appropriate behaviour to 'go-sort-it-out!' These feelings can be weak or strong or anywhere between on the spectrum. So, let's now consider a few of the common sensations we get and what they mean:

1. Low sugar levels – produces hunger, which motivates food seeking behaviour ('go sort out my low sugar levels') When sugar levels are high, the feeling disappears and if combined with stomach fullness sensations – there's a satiated feeling (which is supposed to be a 'stop' message!). When I've done marathons I've noticed that I get very strong cravings for fruit. It seems likely that the CNS/brain is capable of giving a specific food message to meet a specific requirement. Call it a craving perhaps, but see it as a smartly evolved module that registers what's needed and directs our behaviour to seek it. Hence, hungry for a specific food item, like fruit or meat.

2. Low fluid levels – thirst... fluid seeking behaviour.

3. Low oxygen levels – desire to breathe more... or if local hypoxia the behaviour is often to move, rub, shake – remember botty-rot!

4. Body temperature – too hot or cold feelings, cooling/warming behaviour.

5. Bladder fullness – desire to pee, toilet, or ideal pee-spot seeking behaviour.

6. Bowel fullness – desire to poo, toilet or poo spot seeking behaviour.

7. Gut fullness – bloated stomach, full up feeling, stops feeding behaviour.

8. Gut, feeling of nausea – stop feeding/drinking, go and be sick, (think expel toxins, as in Friday-night-too-much-alcohol-and-curry-for-body-detoxification-systems-to-cope-with, get rid of what you can, be sick in the street, lie down and go to sleep) The numskulls must be going nuts with his excessive behaviour!

9. Food/fluid in mouth – taste, good/bad? Swallow or spit out.

10. Sudden physical injury – injury pain, leads to reflex avoidance behaviour, then orientation, assessment and self help or help seeking behaviour.

11. Wound vulnerable and healing – healing pain/vulnerability awareness/ discomfort, gives rise to vigilance and care while using and moving. Later aids in getting slowly moving/recovery behaviour etc. as already discussed. (Also see chapter GE 3.1)

12. General malaise – likely to relate to infection but also pathology and disease. Hence feeling poorly, having a temperature, the full sickness response and the result, 'sickness behaviour'. It allows and motivates the system to slow down, find safety and focus resources on countering the threat (see chapter GE 2.3)

13. Toxins or infection – often produce headache, which may be a part of the sickness response. To me, a headaches' 'adaptive' purpose, is to bring about resting behaviour to allow focus of resources on dealing with toxins/ infections. Think of the post binge drinking headache. The body wants a rest and time and resources to deal with it all, at least the liver does.

14. The needs of a musculoskeletal system that's been working hard: we get muscle cramp and that heavy leaden muscle ache feeling that pleads for rest, or at least a slower pace, to allow some recovery time or more careful use of dwindling resources.

15. Skin threats – a remarkable variety of sensations – think varieties of pain, but itch too (makes you scratch and hence ***remove the threat!).***

Note how incredibly precise some of these sensations can be. Note also, that a great many of those sensations, that are not considered to be 'pain', actually do become painful when at their extremes. For example, a very full bladder, or extreme hunger make any sensation more intense and it enters the realm of the words 'unpleasant' and then 'pain'.

What I have just done is give a list of sensations and feelings that bring conscious attention to the body's needs and in so doing provide the motivation to do something about it.

The rest of this chapter and the two that follow, look at what we know about processing pathways and regions of the brain that are concerned with these homeostatic sensations, well, mainly peeing and pain!

From the bottom up!

Bud Craig emphasises that the C and Aδ fibres are more or less ubiquitous – being found in not only all of the musculoskeletal system but all the viscera too (reviewed in Gifford and Thacker 2013 p 43). Note that visceral C and Aδ afferents project to the spinal cord in parasympathetic and sympathetic nerve trunks going ***in the opposite direction*** to the much better publicised 'efferent' outflow, that was discussed earlier in section 12. The majority of these gut afferents travel in the sympathetic 'splanchnic' nerves and amount to only 1.5-2.0% of all spinal afferents that have their cell bodies in the dorsal root ganglion. Compared to the skin which has an understandably massive somatic sensory afferent contribution, the viscera seems to be poorly represented. Well yes, but visceral afferents also reach the CNS via several cranial nerves, the vagus being the largest and most far reaching. The vagus is the tenth (X) cranial nerve and considered a major nerve of the parasympathetic system. Hear this though, a massive 80-85% of the vagal nerve fibres ***are visceral afferents*** and they all terminate in the 'Nucleus of the Solitary Tract' or NST, in the brain stem. This is where a mass of information comes in about our *physiological or homeostatic* status along the lines listed above. Hence afferent traffic with 'physiological' information from the trachea and lungs, heart, stomach, pancreas, spleen, liver, gallbladder, blood vessels and so forth.

It's thanks to the wonderful vagus nerve that the brains of those with para or quadriplegia still have contact with the viscera and are able to maintain a degree of controlled function there.

As an aside, note that I used italics for the words 'physiological and 'homeostatic' above. I've done this because, unlike much of the sensory information from our skin, joints, limbs and trunk – which gives us an awareness of our body and its position and posture, the viscera doesn't have this, we have no specific 'awareness' of deep visceral organs and tissues in the way we do from our musculoskeletal system. It's a proprioceptive deficit if you like. To test this think first 'elbow' and you instantly know where your elbow is, now think gall bladder or liver or adrenal gland or small intestine and you haven't a clue. There are simply no sensory maps in the brain for our deeper structures like the viscera. I'd like the reader to also think of deeper structures that we more commonly have to deal with, like discs, bodies of vertebrae, bones, deep muscles and so forth. The more you start thinking about it, the vaguer our bodies seem to be. There are massive voids of awareness, because there are simply, no maps but, given the right opportunity, which is usually when there's been some injury, infection or pathology, it may just be possible for the brain to make new maps. Think bladder infection for example!

Unsurprisingly, you don't have to look too far to find that some people can be trained to be more aware of their internal organs and their activity, or they can be trained to be!

Back to Bud...

'Line labelling' – can we trust what we feel?

Bud Craig is at pains to point out that all fine homeostatic afferents (visceral and somatic) coming into lamina I of the spinal cord, are 'modality specific' – meaning they accurately carry and report specific information derived from their tissue origins to their targets in the CNS and brain where they then produce a feeling appropriate to the stimulus given. This stance is what neurologists call 'Line labelled' – meaning a single 'line' or nerve pathway is dedicated to specific sensation. Part and parcel of a 'Line-labelling' stance is that the degree of activity in any given pathway produces a sensation that accurately reflects the physiological status in the tissues that the pathway is given over to. It's the way most people would reason our sensory system work. It's called 'specificity' – a specific stimulus travels in specific neurones via specific pathways to specific regions of the brain to produce a specific sensation.

When Pat Wall was alive he constantly struggled to get medicine to overcome the 'dualistic' reasoning associated with pure line-labelling and 'specificity.' In fact, it made him very angry that his colleagues couldn't see that while individual sensory fibres and their sensory endings could be very, specialised to particular types and ranges of stimuli – what happened to that information within the nervous system and brain didn't guarantee a specific sensation. The nervous system 'modulated' – meaning varied and manipulated, the sensory information it received, so that the end result might range from absolutely nothing at one end of a spectrum, to a very intense sensation at the other.

Specialisation accepts specialised inputs but doesn't guarantee an exact replication of that input as a conscious output. At this moment in time you may have many hundreds of thousands of specialised 'itch' fibres firing but you are totally unaware of any need to 'itch.'

Specificity accepts specialised inputs and guarantees an exact replication of that input in consciousness. At this moment in time you may have many hundreds of thousands of specialised 'itch' fibres firing and you are overwhelmed by the need to 'itch'.

Clinically, specificity boils down to an unbridled belief in what might be called 'sensation honesty' and accuracy! When the patient reports bad pain there must be plenty of neural sensory activity, sensory processing and appropriate tissue disruption to reflect it. If clinical examination and investigations are unable to corroborate this – this drives the assumption that the patient must be fabricating or consciously over-egging their symptoms for some kind of gain. Pat pleaded that before assuming an unsympathetic psychiatric/malingering and patient-blaming diagnosis Drs searched for other alternative explanations first. Thankfully his early research work with Ronald Melzack in the 1960's and the massive amount that followed from it, has enabled a much better and more balanced understanding of what can happen. As we've seen (Dorsal horn chapters) and will see more of in the nerve root section of the book, there are plenty of mechanisms that can explain why symptoms can be out of all proportion to the degree of tissue abnormality. Unfortunately, a great many Drs and clinicians still haven't embraced Pat Walls' sentiments, even though they think they have!

In discussing pain, Pat Wall would not have got on with Rene Descartes but Bud Craig would have!

So, is the notion of 'line-labelling' and specificity OK or not? ... Well clearly it is not. The wording has to be changed from 'Specificity' to 'Specialised' which allows a system to have the potential to be very precise but where the conscious output isn't written in stone. In other words, it is open to being modulated and changed and that depends on a whole pile of intervening variables that can be neatly whittled down to issues relating to 'context'.

'Did you smell those hyacinths just now? Wow, it was overwhelming.'

'You know I didn't, I was thinking of buying some fresh bread and some Gorgonzola on the way home...'

Let me make a short list of some homeostatic inaccuracies that have come into my head right now:

- feeling of hunger/wanting to eat when blood sugar levels are fine...
- same for thirst
- hyperventilating
- being desperate to pee and nothing happening or only a dribble
- something tasting disgusting when there's nothing wrong with it at all
- physical pain when there's no injury or excessive pain when there's a minor injury – massive injury or pathology and little or no pain
- chronic headache when there's no sign of a toxin
- itchy scratchy skin when there's nothing irritating it.

Thanks to the fact of evolving on the already evolved, the notion of scrutinising an incoming report from the tissues or the viscera and dealing with it, just isn't as simple as gathering it all at a specific place, doing the processing and then activating an appropriate response. As I've said a few times, for things to get more complicated than they already are (or were), evolution has to try and come up with something that can still work alongside what's already there.

So, being saddled with pre-existing 'Sample-Scrutinise-Respond' modules means that evolution of greater sophistication and complexity has to accept and adapt to those modules already working quite happily and already securely in place. That means, if evolution is true to form we should find module on module on module!

The next chapter looks at this in more detail.

Chapter 18.2
Sample-scrutinise-respond modules and peeing

'My eyes have made a pact with my ears against my vulgar senses: urination is a holiday on the edge of a soothing lemonade waterfall.'

Bauvard, Some Inspiration for the Overenthusiastic

Let's now take a look at a very basic processing level or module. I'll call it sample-scrutinise-respond (SSR) level I 'module'. It's the spinal cord. And a good example to illustrate how things work is peeing. The urge to pee as we all know can shift from the moderately nagging into the realms of extreme pain. Not peeing is dangerous – so a very, very full bladder is a significant threat to homeostasis. This painful urge to pee is fundamental to survival! Back to this shortly, but for a moment, maybe you can see that pain is just the end of the spectrum of any given homeostatic stressor or threat? So you can have hunger pain, full bladder and bowel pain, the pain of extreme heat or cold and so on. In this sense, pain is just an expression of the urgent need to correct something that's in a physiologically bad place.

Here at peeing level I SSR, all the components required are in place to allow bladder filling and voiding. The young baby, or 'naive' organism, pees when its bladder is full, with not a care in the world and quite unaware of it most probably – just like that new puppy doing it all over the best carpet in the lounge! There's no need for a brain at this basic level and this is confirmed when the spinal cord is damaged; paraplegics do not pee all the time, their bladders fill and when they're full, they void. Some paraplegics find that they can condition the void reflex to switch on by stimulating the skin on their legs. The point is that it all works without descending control mechanisms – in the baby they are yet to develop and in the paraplegic they have been destroyed.

The bladder is a muscle bag that continuously fills with urine produced by the kidneys. The smooth detrusor muscle of the bladder walls receives its nerve supply from branches of the lumbar sympathetic and sacral parasympathetic nervous systems. In order for the bladder to fill the detrusor muscles must remain relaxed. Its contraction is held in check by the inhibitory activity of the sympathetic supply.

Urine is prevented from leaking out of the bladder by two sphincter muscles: the 'internal' urethral sphincter lies either side of the urethra, right where it leaves the bladder and its contraction pinches the urethra tight blocking any fluid exit. This smooth muscle is held in contraction by its sympathetic supply. In sum, the sympathetic system as described so far is all about, 'no peeing' and 'don't-pee'.

There is also an 'external' urethral sphincter that consists of skeletal muscle and is supplied by the pudendal nerve – a branch of the sacral plexus (originating in the cord from levels S2-4). The external sphincter muscle actually runs the length of the urethra, therefore produces its control over a wider surface area than the internal sphincter. It's this sphincter that we have direct voluntary control over and the one that's exercised with 'mid-flow' stopping and starting. So, we use it to stop flow mid-stream and of course, we have to 'let-go' when want to pass water.

As the bladder fills, afferent sensory traffic relays the 'stretch' or filling status of the bladder to the spinal cord. The 'spinal cord bladder scrutinising centre' therefore receives continual input about the state of the bladder and in turn, organises the sympathetic vs parasympathetic balance of activity. During bladder filling the sympathetic system predominates, keeping the internal sphincter closed and the detrusor muscle relaxed. As the bladder gets nearer to being full there is a significant rise in afferent firing activity (a gathering and strengthening vote for change emerges!). The big majority required is eventually reached; democracy reigns supreme and without further ado, the 'voiding' module is voted 'on'! This module has to do two things; inhibit the sympathetic system that is keeping the internal urethral sphincter contracted; at the same time, facilitate the parasympathetic sacral system to bring about detrusor contraction. This also means, that the sympathetic supply to the bladder detrusor muscles must be inhibited, in order to prevent it inhibiting the contraction produced by the excitation of the parasympathetic system. Confused? No you're not? It's simple 'on-off' stuff – even the spinal cord can manage it!

This is how it is for the very young, the not house-trained and paraplegics! For healthy adults we have awareness of our bladder's filling status and we can control when we wish to void. This means that there are additional SSR modules involving the brain and plenty of bottom-up and top-down influences via consciousness, which come 'on-line' in the first year or so of a child's life. So don't get cross with the baby when it 'wets' on the carpet, it can't help it.

What fascinates me here is to note that not even a simple spinal 'reflex' or 'SSR' module seems to run in isolation, there's always some 'higher' spinal or brain-stem-and-beyond involvement too. We can actually be aware of one hell of a lot!

'Oh yeah, what about iron metabolism then Louis? You don't get this thing in your head that goes, 'low on iron, go stock up now' and you certainly don't get one that goes, 'too much iron can you dump some now'. Well, yes, but maybe when iron levels are low, you get this urge to want to eat eggs and meat and when they're too high you get this overwhelming urge to go and give blood!

It's surprising how much our behaviour is actually manipulated to fulfil a great many homeostatic needs. It is certainly one of the main points made earlier and one which I think Bud Craig would agree. That homeostatic challenges and moment by moment reporting of the body's homeostatic situation, is gathered in by the brain and given an awareness value (or awareness potential) in consciousness. Even the most basic elements of life seem to have a quasi accurate niche carved for them in our consciences. Bud Craig and Antonio Damasio (see refs) are strong supporters that this homeostatic reporting and processing is important in giving 'body-image' awareness, as well as contributing to our feelings and emotional status. That consciousness is so involved, or more accurately such a big part, underlines, yet again, how important it is to move beyond the uni-dimensional consideration of just the tissues when dealing with injury and pathology.

Bladder filling eventually 'signs-in' to produce an amazingly distinct want-to-pee sensation and the more it fills the stronger the sensation becomes, until it becomes painful. But sometimes the situation demands that the sensation be switched off. Modulation!

So, my second level SSR module or loop (2) now involves the brainstem and back to the cord – hence afferent input coming up in the cord from the spinal bladder inputs of lamina I in the dorsal horn... and entering the brainstem. There are two destinations: the Periaqueductal Grey matter (PAG) and a fancy little place nearby called the Pontine Micturition Centre (PMC). These areas are just like the brainstem nociception processing points – with similar bladder filling sensation-off/pain-'off' and sensation-'on' cells and connections back down again.

Both of these brainstem areas have further SSR loops, for example there are loops to and from higher cortical centres like the hypothalamus (which in this context can be seen as an emergency action organising centre i.e. the HPA and SNS output systems); the medial frontal cortex (recall the working memory areas and especially those concerned with action decisions – like the anterior cingulate cortex, ACC) and the insula cortex. The insula cortex and ACC are what Bud Craig calls the 'Interoceptive cortex' and are undoubtedly important regions that play a part in conscious awareness of all the 'homeostatic' sensations I listed earlier – bladder filling sensation being one of them. I hope the reader can see that all these loops on loops on other loops all back and forth all the time are likely important in producing conscious awareness?

The PMC, as you might guess, also has strong connections back to our lower spinal level 1, peeing/not peeing SSR 1 module. The PMC is actually held in check by low level ascending afferent traffic, but as the 'heat' rises with bladder filling the 'majority mass vote' now swings in favour of action. All it needs is the OK from above!

'Hang on a minute I'm giving a lecture!'... or maybe it's... 'I'm hovering over the urinal now, go, go, go... ahhh..!'

The decision from cortical structures 'above' is all about situation and sensation. If the situation is not conducive to having a pee – like giving a lecture, cortical appraisal structures get in contact with the PAG module. 'He's busy right now, there's no way he can pee and I want you to stop your bloody full bladder sensation coming up here and putting him off.'

Recall that the PAG, along with the RVM are areas, which when stimulated can strongly switch pain off – they're part of 'Claudia's family' (chapter 5.3); descending down to the lamina I synapses, inhibiting the activity there and preventing the onward flow of the nociceptive message and it's the same here – peeing is right alongside pain! The strong desire to want to pee can magically disappear given, the strong gating mechanism arising from the PAG. So 'pee-off and pee-on' control is much the same, if not identical to, the SSR loop for 'pain-off or on' in all but the ultimate destination address.

Once the all clear is given (he's finished the lecture now/stress is off), the PAG lifts the inhibition, ascending impulse traffic ramps up and gets through to conscious processing and the sensation of wanting to pee returns. The working memory now fills with strong bladder full feeling and the need to 'find a friggin' toilet'. Eventually, when we're in a position to be able to pee, the PMC can go for it. Downward efferent traffic to the spinal level 1 SSR voiding circuit gives, 'on' with the parasympathetically controlled detrusor muscle, causing bladder contraction. Simultaneously, there's 'off' with the sympathetically maintained tone in the internal urethral sphincter and 'off' with the pudendal skeletal muscle circuits contracting the external urethral sphincter – tone goes down, you relax and off you flow.

So, the brainstem level 2 SSR is all about, 'If he's busy we'll stop the sensation and we'll put the voiding on hold.' Or, once it gets the OK from the level 3 or 4 or more SSR's up above, it'll send the messages down to release the voiding circuit.

As we've seen, 'level 3 SSR' involves the cortical areas of the interoceptive cortex, along with whatever else is going on in the 'high-road' processing circuitry touched on in the last chapter. To put it crudely, the 'full bladder feeling' along with the 'I want to pee' action-thought now emerge into consciousness and consciousness goes and flips on the action modules that enable one to find a toilet and do the business!

Hopefully it's not a giant leap to see that injury/pathology – nociception, pain and all the other homeostatic processing and 'sensations,' operate in a very similar manner to the peeing circuit? It's an on-going hierarchically dominated democracy! I've just started wondering if it's possible to be able to train your bladder to fill a lot further, before you start feeling you want to pee? I bet it's a part of some kind of yogic ritual, but in a sense it's exactly what we are asking patients to do with many pain states – to reset their 'it hurts' level to something more conducive to everyday life. Just keep it all away from the low road and those 'threat control centres'... is probably as good a place to start as any.

At spinal level 1 SSR for tissue injury/threat, just like in the bladder control circuits, small diameter afferents (nociceptors) bring in messages of concern about their tissues to the cord. These neurones synapse in the dorsal horn and then via segmental interneuronal circuits can output back to the tissues, in appropriate pre then postganglionic autonomic nerve fibres. In this way the damaged, healing or pathological tissues may derive some support – in the form of SNS secretions (section 12), as well as appropriate circulatory control if needed. There is also the dorsal root reflex, whereby impulses travel back down the C fibres to instigate neuropeptide release from the fibre terminals. The scrutinising, on-off element here, amounts to whether to allow the helping process to continue, i.e. inflammation and healing or, to put the healing on slow down or, 'on-hold' for resource conservation, as discussed in the healing section 13-15. As with urination and the feeling of a full bladder, descending control from SSR levels 2, 3 and more also plays a part. Notable brainstem nociception (and homeostatic) processing occurs at the parabrachial nucleus, the PAG and the Rostro-ventral medulla (RVM) for example and just like urination – there's plenty of influence from above! Flip back to a numskull type conversation can help!

Tissue processing numskulls in brain stem to Mr Ed (consciousness): 'Er, Mr Ed, could I trouble you a minute? You just stubbed your toe quite badly and it's not looking so good, in fact it could be broken, 'cos the guys from the big toe distal phalanx bone are making a riot. Er, we'd like to turn on the big toe pain quite a bit, we think it needs you to have a look?'

Slightly subconscious forebrain numskulls: 'Sorry guys, he's just about to have sex with his new girlfriend, he stubbed his toe rounding the end of the bed – suggest you keep it to yourselves and come back in about 20 minutes or so... shhhh!'

Get your priorities right, spread your genes around at every opportunity...!

Hmm, that just might be another fundamental 'rule of nature' – like 'get as much as you can for as little effort as possible!'

Chapter 18.3
The MOM: the neuromatrix and brain processing of pain

What Brain Areas?

For years researchers have been trying to understand and indentify the areas and regions of the brain involved in processing and producing pain. Medical thinking would just love to know where to target to provide the 'cure'. But unfortunately for Doctors and patients, biology and the beauty, yet complexity, of messy evolution by modules on overlapping modules; when pain evolved, it just hadn't got those 'find it and cut it out to fix it' guys in mind.

Still though, if you read about pain and the brain you'll always find a list of structures that are active, when something painful is done to a willing subject, when they're in a brain scanner. Researchers commonly use painful heat stimuli to the skin and then watch what happens.

When I ponder what the brain might do with a tissue injury, I come up with a list something like this:

- ow! that's intense... awful, sickening...
- fuck, that stings..!
- where is it..?
- shit, it's a bee on my leg...
- that's going on a bit...
- bothers me...
- a bit concerned and quite worried really
- what shall I do...?
- don't move it and be careful of it when I move
- I'm getting the hell out of here...
- could happen again better be ready
- I might just have to cancel golf tomorrow... oh, and work...

... and so on.

Pain doesn't just come into the head in an isolated sensory way. That's this, if you can imagine total neutrality:

- I have a pain.

No more, no less and in reality it doesn't exist like this at all, not even in a scanner, unless you're very, very stoned!

Pain from all homeostatic quarters has a message, it means something and it wants you to make sense of it and then get on and do something sensible about it. You may need to draw on past experience or get help from others, but it's a message that says, 'get it sorted!'

The types of issues above are often referred to as 'the pain experience'. So it's mood, it's context, it's how you're thinking and interpreting, its location, it's who you're with and what you might gain or get out of it, it's also intensity and duration and it's synapses, chemistry, nerve activity/inactivity, plasticity and much more.

Now, in the light of all that... what brain areas?!

List? Why not? Let's give it a go. It'll have to include:

1. Conscious working memory areas, along with medial temporal lobe memory system and all the relevant cortical and transitional cortical areas, which are involved in planning and executing. I've covered them. Don't forget the hippocampus, a fine word and a fine organism (Hippocampus is the Sea Horse).

2. The 'threat' centres, the stressor processing and stress response centres and modules, throw in the amygdala and the hypothalamus, driving the autonomic and neuroendocrine responses.

3. The areas of the brain that tell you about 'location'. Think sensory cortices. Then, there are all the arousal centres and attention, orientation and even vigilance processing modules.

4. Action stations: the pre-motor and motor cortices along with brainstem and cerebellar motor centres, involved in protective postures and movements. The planning parts of the brain too, the Anterior Cingulate Cortex (ACC) gets the nod.

5. Oh and in amongst all this, some regions have to be somehow, making the actual pain sensation! Easy, bang it on Bud Craig's 'interoceptive cortex' or is it all this and more?

6. Lastly, to embrace the 'whole' and Damasio's somatic marker hypothesis, we must acknowledge the important part of the efferent effects out to the body and the re-sampling back again, that results. Go beyond this again and we're all barking up the 'embodied consciousness' tree... which will never give a specific place to any of this. It's all in the circles, the multiple MOM's – the SSR modules or whatever you'd like to call them.

Could pain be all of it? (Big, YES!) ... Brain pain researchers love the terms 'diffuse' and 'dispersed', but Bud Craig feels that there are some areas that continuously crop up. He likes these:

> His 'interoceptive' cortex, in particular, the 'parieto-insular cortex (part of the insula, which is sometimes called the 'limbic sensory cortex') which receives inputs from lamina 1 dorsal horn neurones via an area of the thalamus called the VMPo, the posterior ventral medial nucleus and it's side-kick-best-mate, the VMb (the ventro medial nucleus of the thalamus). Remember, the thalamus is a key 'projection' area of the brain – moving and shuffling bottom-up messages to their appropriate destinations, but always under the heavy influence of top-down modulating.
>
> The anterior cingulate cortex (ACC) which in many brain texts, is considered to be particularly fond of making action decisions and then instigating, what's rather nerdily called, 'motivational behaviours' (he's scared, er, best ... hmmm, yeah, 'run!'). So much so, that the ACC is often referred to as, the

'limbic motor cortex'.

> According to Craig activation of the ACC correlates well with sensation unpleasantness and is accompanied by activity in our 'fear' and threat related friend, the amygdala. The trouble is that if the brain is going: 'I'm fearful about the situation, I'm in that's brought this pile of nociception on – I'm out of here', then the ACC is bound to be working and correlating with unpleasantness.

Interestingly, these areas are also active in hypnotisable folk (actually in a scanner), who can be made to feel pain without any tissue stimuli at all (Derbyshire 2004). I wonder if this can be classed as a form of hallucination? Anyway, my mate Mick Thacker tells me that he's now doing research using hypnosis to induce CRPS-like pain and symptoms in normal people. Again, scanner observations of brain activity point to the above areas as important.

What's the consensus about the pain processing areas of the brain then? Thankfully I found a readable article called, 'The cerebral signature for pain perception and its modulation' by Irene Tracey and Patrick Mantyh (2007). In their meta-analysis they found the following brain areas to be active in the acute pain 'experience':

- primary and secondary somatosensory cortices (more on this in the next section, 19)
- insular cortex
- anterior cingulate ACC and prefrontal cortices
- thalamus.

These are the commonest areas involved in all the studies analysed – utilising experimental nociceptive stimuli. Tracey and Mantyh comment that when pain is reduced in the subjects using analgesic drugs, there is a sizeable reduction of activity in these areas when rescanned.

The following areas are also included, but 'depend on the particular set of circumstances' for that individual...

- basal ganglia
- cerebellum
- amygdala
- hippocampus.

Beautiful! The first two are classically associated with movement, the third with fear and emotional stimuli and the fourth with memory formation!

So, 'Dr I want you to nobble my pain centre and cure my life ache.'

As Pat Wall so often pointed out, you can do some treacherous things to the brain (meaning surgery) and while the pain may go for a while, it eventually returns with something far worse. Or, you end up dependant and disabled like poor old H.M. did following the surgery to cure his seizures.

Could it be a case of my brain does this with pain and yours does that? Within certain limits, very much, so probably!

Ronald Melzack and his 'Neuromatrix'

I now come to Ronald Melzack, who I had the pleasure to meet and invite to speak at the Birmingham Physiotherapy Congress, in October 2002. His article that contained the 'neuromatrix' theory first caught my eye in the excellent journal of the American Pain Society: Pain Forum. That was back in 1996, when my first thoughts about on-going pain states and the biology of memory were gathering apace. After all, it was Ronald Melzack, with Joel Katz, who were using the terms 'somatosensory pain memory' and pain 'imprints' to explain phantom limb pain, knowledge of which spurred me on to thinking that the same mechanisms were likely in a whole host of on-going pain states.

It was wonderful to be able to reproduce Melzack's Pain Forum paper in full in Topical Issues in Pain 3. And I still cherish the humorous and informative communications and conversations that we were able to have. (But also see a more recent update: Melzack 2005).

Ronald Melzack had of course done a great deal of work on phantom limb sensations, as well as on phantom bodies, as applied to those with paraplegia or quadriplegia. It was from these observations that he developed his neuromatrix proposal. For my purpose, what was so beautiful about it was its simplicity and hence the ease with which it could be transferred to something useful for patients.

Here is the meat of it from my perspective:

As I sit here and write I am aware of my body, I know where it is. If I close my eyes I still know where it is. I feel it. I can cast my attention to it and move around my body. It's hard to explain what I feel, but if I concentrate more specifically, some areas are easier to be aware of than others. For example, I am well aware of my hands, but if I think about my forearms there isn't much happening. If I really concentrate I can feel a light awareness of my shirt on my forearm. I can easily feel the pressure of the chair on my backside and I have a clear notion that my legs are crossed. I'm not aware of anything in my abdominal cavity right now, no, not even my heart beating, the bladder's fine and I'm barely aware of breathing movements. I'm in balance and upright. This is my 'body-self' image right now and from a sensory analyses point of view it's proprioceptive, skin sensation, slightly deeper tissue pressure feelings in the buttock – maybe even a smidgen of low grade ischemia related nociception, that makes me shift position occasionally (mild botty-rot!). There's a small feeling of chill around the shoulders that I hadn't noticed...

Rather than piece together the activity in the various brain area body processing modules, like for example, the intricate details of what's being processed in the sensory and interoceptive cortices, then feeding into working memory/consciousness, Melzack uses the all encompassing term 'neuromatrix'. The neuromatrix is seen as a widespread network of nerve cell assemblies and interconnected loops throughout the brain. On-going and varying cyclical activity and interactions between these cell assemblies produces what Melzack calls the 'neurosignature'. It's this neurosignature that gives rise to our body awareness. Melzack describes the neurosignature as a 'continuous outflow from the body-self neuromatrix', which is then projected to 'areas in the brain' – 'the sentient neural hub', in which the stream of nerve impulses is converted into a continually changing stream of awareness.

It's pretty simple I think and avoids the bitty, 'brain-centric' reductionism that tries to divide the brain up into anatomical and functional zones and then put them all together. It kind of makes you go: 'Well who cares where it's all coming from, it just does.' 'Ah, but it's too vague, we haven't got a target, what's the target, what's the use without some target?' 'Look, it's far too easy to say that the pain's coming from a 'sentient neural hub' and then not tell us what or where that is.' 'So Melzack's neuromatrix proposal is lazy, a bit of a cop-out, is that what you're saying?' 'Well, it's a point, but ultimately it's actually very wise because let's be honest, no one has got a clue.'

To review: the brain takes in the mass of information that is arriving all the time from the body and comes up with a vague overview of what's going on in it! Simple, it's called the output of the 'body-neuromatrix' which is the neurosignature that then becomes conscious via the sentient neural hub.

In the last six years I've had two epidurals for operations below waist level. Unfortunately, at the time of the operations, they also gave me what I call a 'take you to paradise' dose of diazepam as a 'pre-med' which I wasn't going to refuse. Anyway while 'semi-out' I was determined to think about my legs and try and locate them somehow to see if my sentient neural hub was keeping operating, and of course I couldn't find them at all! With eyes closed and almost comatose, I even tried to imagine where my legs might be and hazarded a guess, then peaked a quick look. I was shocked to see they were up in stirrups and there were a pile of students gazing at my bits! Conclusion: the neuromatrix requires input from the periphery to produce its neurosignature (in me!).

Melzack also talks about an 'action neuromatrix' whose role is in organising and producing appropriate physiological and behavioural motor responses. He links the body-neuromatrix to it, in what to me looks like a 'sample-awareness-respond' kind of way.

Integrating the MOM I'd do it something like this:

- sampling of the body gives rise to the body-neurosignature produced by the 'body-neuromatrix'
- sampling of the environment gives rise to the environment-neurosignature from the 'environment-neuromatrix'
- sampling memory gives rise to a memory-neurosignature from the 'memory-neuromatrix'
- scrutinising all this means there have to be 'scrutinising-neuromatrices' , for body, environment and memory

- responding equates to the products of the 'action-neuromatrix'
- I also have a feeling that we could throw in a 'homeostatic-sample-scrutinise-respond-neuromatrix' too. A 'Homeostatic neuromatrix'.

Pleasingly, in discussing the action-neuromatrix, Melzack does seem to allude to scrutinising:

'Thus, in the action-neuromatrix, cyclical processing and synthesis produces activation of several possible patterns and their successive elimination, until one particular pattern emerges as the most appropriate for the circumstances at the moment.'

I guess I would stick this bit into a 'scrutinising-neuromatrix', because some decision or choice has to be made and then once the decision about what to do is made it would trigger one of a whole host of ready and waiting 'pre-programmed' action-neuromatrix response signatures. The chosen response would then organise and produce the desired motor output/behaviour.

It's a slight pity, in Melzack's model, that there's no mention of the part played by conscious thinking, scrutinising and then choosing of the appropriate response – via the 'high-road'.

I can also see a way of thinking that sub-categorises the neuromatrix even further, for example, the 'peeing neuromatrix' discussed earlier and so forth. In the end it probably doesn't matter, but what is for sure, the more you think about what the brain is doing, the more you realise a great deal is going on. It's little wonder that the various areas of the brain get assigned different functions depending on the discipline you are reading. For example, read the pain literature on areas of the brain, then read the fear literature, or the reward literature and you'll see what I mean. I talk about specialists getting stuck in their burrows and not coming out of them to see who lives in the burrow next door, in the Graded Exposure section of the book (chapter GE 2.7). It certainly seems to apply to those who study the brain in the context of a single phenomenon, like pain brain researchers not being hardly aware of what the guys over in the happiness, flow, reward and emotion labs are up to!

For me, as you can probably see, the only way to get a useful handle on it is to see it all in terms of sample, scrutinise and response loops or modules. Each loop influencing and regulating the activity of another and each one, being in a variable position on a complex hierarchy. Whatever the case, any 'decision' that is made ultimately may just boil down to mere 'voting power' and democracy.

At the beginning of chapter 16.1 I made the case for nervous systems' function being related to movement or behaviour. What has become clear to me the more I've thought about it, is that the greater the number of behavioural options that have evolved, the more complex the nervous system has had to become. And, that in order to make the correct (survival/most beneficial) choice, given the current situation or context, the individual has had to have some means of interpreting and understanding what is going on. This cannot be done without some form of current (working) and long-term memory. In short, this means there has been a need for some form of consciousness to bring it all together! Thus, when considering how highly developed conscious may be in a given organism, start by considering all the behavioural options the organism may have in a given situation. Remember the Cichlids in chapter 16.1? Now they looked very smart in that one situation where they had to work out which fish they were most likely to beat in their Saturday night brawl, to impress the girls. They used a bit of 'transitive inference' to work out which fish was the weakest, having sneakily observed them all fighting each other. So, from a whole pile of behavioural options they invariably picked the right one because they were smart. Ah, but only in this one situation... So the next rule in looking for highly developed consciousness is to not only look for an organism that has a large number of behavioural options it can choose from, but also has a large number of situations.

Just a thought!

The ageing body image and on-going pain

It's probably reasonable to say that a normal, healthy, young person's body-image is void of discomfort. The young body is in good confident working order, the interoceptive sampling from the body's tissues is reporting a continuous 'we're good' message and this is reflected in the vague and unobtrusive body feeling the young person has. Unfortunately, as time goes on, we accumulate the consequences of wear and tear, ageing and the legacies of old injuries. The afferent traffic surely must report a 'not quite so good' message and the body-neuromatrix has the option to add these issues to the out-going body-image neurosignature? Hence a spectrum of bodily sensations that may run from grumbly aches and pains through to full-on disabling chronic pain.

So, why don't we hurt all the time and more and more as our bodies crumble around us. In fact it's pretty amazing how little we hurt when considered like this.

Here are some thoughts:

1. We do hurt more and more, most of us just accept it and ignore it! It's simply like my tinnitus, if you take note of it, it's there, playing its annoying tune. Most humans, up to a point are quite good at getting used to things that are going on, more especially if they happen reasonably slowly. As Mick Thacker says, what anyone feels in relation to their body is a balance between 'input' and 'modulation' and that as long as the 'modulation' system remains intact then there's no need for us to have pain. Moral? Look after your modulating system!!

2. Are you rigid or are you adaptable? Good question! Do you ever get patients in their 50's or beyond, who feel that they should be feeling like they did in their 20's and 30's and because they're not, there's something wrong!

3. Is there any point in hurting? Why produce a pain in a given tissue when altering behaviour or patterns of movement are unlikely to be of any help?

Wear and tear or degeneration in discs is a good example that I'll return to later. For now, note that the biological turnover rate of disc material is in terms of years, possibly your whole life, and therefore it has a very poor healing capability. In other words, there's no logic in it 'hurting' if it's not going to mend or benefit from careful behaviour! Ignore it. Some can, some can't though. I have a feeling that a great many of our successful therapies turn on the 'ignore' it modulation switch.

On the other hand, giving you a degree of back 'vulnerability' may just make you that bit more cautious and prevent further injury or wear and tear. It might even protect the now vulnerable lumbar and sacral nerve roots as they pass through the degenerative and encroached upon area of the low back. That feeling of vulnerability might just stop you doing quite what you might have done in the past. Wise action! For example wear and tear in the knee, ankle or hip, it's not bothering you but you're just not so confident jumping down off that wall anymore. You youngsters reading this have no idea yet!

4. The tissues would like 'you' to change your behaviour for a little while, but you're just too busy doing something important to want to allow it into consciousness. Like hunter-gathering, having sex, having fun or maybe having a fight with neighbouring villagers.

5. The tissues would like a change of behaviour from you but it's not absolutely necessary. In other words, they'll get better the best they can regardless, but a bit of rest when you can spare it would be nice. It's almost as if the CNS scrutinising turns away from the tissues 'Look I can hear you but you can get on with it yourself, I've more important things to be getting on with...'

6. You've got a really well trained pain-off system. Think lots of rough and tumble as a child, plenty of falling out of trees, stinging nettles, cuts and bruises, fights with the lads next door, falling off the bike, rough manly games like rugby a life where knocks and bruises are mixed with fun, where rubbing it quickly better, sticking a plaster on it and getting back in the mêlée is where it's at.

7. You were trained by your parents not to make an unnecessary fuss and you were shown that what you were crying about wasn't much and would soon get better. Nobody panicked or made a big scene. You've got well practiced pain suppressing neural assemblies.

8. You do feel discomfort from time to time but you don't let it bother you or dwell on it too much, in other words, it's not processed in 'threat' centres because you 'accept' it. Hence, no repeated orientation towards it and little if any 'threat response'/autonomic reaction/tension/altered movement patterns/stress response etc. You get on with it or you just adapt and work round it a bit.

9. If you do hurt you seek reassurance, which you get and you don't question,

so you brush it off and get on with life.

10. The body scrutinising modules sense that 'its body' is strong and can cope. As opposed to one that is weak or vulnerable. With patients I always use the phrase: 'When you're low you hurt more easily' and I give the example of flu symptoms. Here you feel rotten, not only do you have a temperature, you also have a headache and every move you make feels sore and achy. If you knock into something by mistake it's ten times as painful as usual. When the body's in a vulnerability state its 'sensitivity' setting is increased, hence hurting more easily. The answer is to get over the flu and the sensitivity setting should return to normal, in parallel with improved health. For our patients it may be to get fit, stronger and healthier in the right context and at the right time. This is a good thing to explain to them and will be dealt with later when I discuss the 'Vulnerable Organism Model' (chapter GE 2.3)

11. There are likely to be heritable and developmental factors favouring less pain response than others.

But some people do hurt a great deal with seemingly the same ageing, degenerate or injured body status as those who don't.

Here are some thoughts on this:

1. There are a whole pile of 'pain panic' and 'pain-on' modules in your medial temporal lobe memory system – learnt responses to pain if you like. Think the more or less total opposite to the points above! In other words, if there's the slightest bit of nociception coming up, then pay attention and put it into high importance category, stop what you're doing and be careful. Top-down facilitating bottom-up. The high-road agreeing with the low-road.

2. This may be politically incorrect and a tad cynical, but to me, it's pretty straight forward to see that the culture and commercially driven times we live in are subtly shifting our understanding of the world around us, to fear and reject any semblance of dirt and pain. The sanitised, disinfected, paranoiac, obsessive-compulsive rich and spoilt westerner promotes a plastically driven cradle-to-grave shift towards all kinds of hypersensitivity. One wonders if there will be any turning back.

3. Cynical again: we live in a world where, if we're not careful, our brains will have enough time to ponder a great many of the calculated eleven million pieces of data it receives at any given moment! What I'm getting at is that having little to do, allows some of us, to give more attention than we otherwise would to incoming 'sensations' and then pondering in a negative way about what it might mean.

4. Try American TV commercials – you get the most amazing adverts that urge you to check out and 'go ask your Dr' for medications that will help, well, speed up slow peeing, lower blood pressure, better erections, lower

cholesterol, relieve back pain, stop skin irritation, sort piles, mouth bugs, gut bugs, concentration and memory problems, coughs and colds and on and on and on.

5. There may well be poisons, toxins, contaminants and pathogens in the air and the environment – but I consider this as hugely hyped-up compared to the social and cultural or psychosocial aspects. Have you noted how humans, including scientists and researchers, will do anything to blame the cause of a problem on a single, specific and concrete thing, rather than on multiple more nebulous issues that subtly conspire to work together? For example a broader consideration of factors involving mind/thinking/culture/occupation/relationships/knowledge/misinformation/nurturing and parenting is almost always required too. But note how reluctant or even insulted we all are, to even consider them as playing a part of the issue?

   'Are you intimating that my parenting skills are to blame here?'

   'Oh, no, never, not at all, but don't you think the video games your Benedict spends six hours a day on might be at the heart of the problem, I see he smashes your place up if you try to stop him, can't be very nice can it...?'

   Bang, the one-issue-instant-diagnosis-reflex just tested positive. That's just the same as the clinician concluding, 'It's obviously a disc madam'.

   Take 'Attention Deficit Hyperactivity Disorder' (ADHD), where blame has been attributed to a 'gene' or maybe eight genes and, as a result, some kind of 'brain defect'. Solution, you're stuck with it, the brains hard wired now, it can't change, you've got to take Ritalin for the rest of your life! Or, on another side of the fence: the problem is due to consumption of dangerous food additive chemicals in junk food: solution: alter the diet/take Ritalin. Both of these explanations are popular, because they downplay the societal and relational issues that are considered to be of significant importance in this ever so wonderfully heterogeneous maladaptive behavioural presentation. Is it maladaptive or is it just a throw-back from our evolutionary past that was once very useful, but now just doesn't sit well with hours of free time, disinterested parents and little purposeful or productive physical activity? As you might expect I rather like the 'hunter versus farmer' hypothesis for ADHD. Good hunters have a tendency to be more flighty and busy by nature, whereas farmers need a great deal of patience and time. Farmers are maybe better suited to boring modern life-styles than hunters – who basically go behaviourally bonkers and play up all the time.

   'Buy the little one a fishing rod and a gun, that'll sort it for him.' Trouble is, there aren't any fish anywhere in the middle of the city or, any good hunting forests, there's a good X-box game for fishing and hunting though...

There goes that reflex 'single issue' thinking thing again!

That pain patients and their Drs and therapists get sucked in to a merry go round of trying to find something 'concrete' to work on, mounts to the same sort of thing. Changing thinking, beliefs, behaviour, lifestyle, fitness as a fix is just too vague, complicated and difficult. Ah the magic bullet! It 'aint there folks – the cure is within you, but the past is impossible to change. It's far easier to learn a piano when you're young than when you're old... it's easy to learn 'sensitivity' when you're young – it's hard to unlearn it and learn anew when you're older.

6. Some of us may be genetically predisposed to hurt more than others – but genes don't work in isolation from their environment. I have a patient who has an identical twin who has rheumatoid arthritis. My patient has occasional joint aches and pains like anyone else her age. When you compare their lives, both have had some very difficult times, but the twin with the RA had a particularly rough time in the few years prior to the disease manifesting. Both may be genetically predisposed to RA, but the environmental factors and influences only impacted one of them.

On a last note, I think I've made my point about our reflex single thing thinking, my request then is to please be vigilant! When we consider pain and chronic pain especially, those who wander towards single modality approaches are not best placed to help. I worry a bit here and in the next section I take a look at one form of treatment that is currently taking the physiotherapy world by storm and which needs a little reining in I feel.

The therapy is 'graded motor imagery'. Why rein it in? Because it's seducing therapists into believing that it's simply a matter of changing our patients' sensory cortex to cure their on-going pain. I love the fact that it's getting therapists to see that the brain is important but it's missing the important multidimensionality of pain rather. I, and others in the field of physiotherapy and chronic pain, feel it's dangerously focusing, yet again, on a single issue to target, blame and treat, at the expense of the same old 'bigger picture'. Don't get me wrong, it's exciting, but it could well be giving a great many a false sense of power and hope and that criticism might be just as applicable to the therapist as the patient.

Section 18
Read what I've read

Craig A.D. (2003) Interoception: the sense of the physiological condition of the body. Current opinion in neurology. 13:500-505

Craig A.D. (2010) Interoception and Emotion: A Neuroanatomical Perspepective. In: Lewis M, Haviland-Jones JM, and Barrett LF (Eds), Handbook of Emotion, 3rd Edn.

Damasio A.R. (1995) Descartes' Error: Emotion, reason and the human brain. Picador. London.

Damasio A.R. (2000) The feeling of what happens. Body, emotion and the making of consciousness. Vintage. London.

Damasio A.R. (2003) Looking for Spinoza. Joy, sorrow and the feeling brain. William Heinemann. London.

Derbyshire, S. W. G., Whalley, M. G., Stenger, V. A., & Oakley, D. A. (2004).

Cerebral activation during hypnotically induced and imagined pain. NeuroImage, 23, 392-401.

Gifford L.S. (1998) Pain, the Tissues and the Nervous System: A conceptual model. Physiotherapy: Volume 84, Issue 1: 27–36.

Gifford L.S., Thacker M.A. (2013) A Clinical Overview of the autonomic nervous system, the supply to the gut and mind-body pathways. In Gifford L.S. (Ed) Topical Issues in Pain 3. CNS Press, Falmouth.

Melzack R. (2005) Evolution of the neuromatrix theory of pain. Pain Practice 5(2):85-94

Melzack R. (1996) Gate control theory: on the evolution of pain concepts. Pain Forum: Official Journal of the American Pain Society. 5: 128-138. (Reproduced in Topical Issues in Pain 3).

Ridley M. (2000) Genome: The Autobiography of a Species in 23 Chapters. Fourth Estate. London.

Ridley M. (2004) Nature via Nurture: Genes, experience and what makes us human. Harper Perennial. London.

Tracey I, Mantyh PW 2007 The cerebral signature for pain perception and its modulation. Neuron 55:377-391

Section 19

THE TRENDY SENSORY CORTEX AND MORE!

Chapter 19.1
How to become a chronic pain sufferer!

'Two things are infinite: the universe and human stupidity; and I'm not sure about the universe.'

Albert Einstein

If you've come along with me so far you'll realise that I'm keen on the notion of on-going pain equating to an on-going memory, it being analogous to an annoying tune like the famous brass band marching tune, 'Colonel Bogey' playing in your head continuously. But, clearly, to the sufferer pain is not in your head, when the pain tune is 'playing' the awareness is in the body, exactly where it hurts. The difference between hearing Colonel Bogey in your head and a constant pain located clearly in your body is that with the tune, you know it is not actually happening, you know it's just your memory, your imagination, your brain doing it, the brass band isn't actually there. The pain though is very real, you know its location, it may even be tender or painful to touch – that's real and that's clear evidence that it's real. To be told the pain is like an annoying tune doesn't necessarily quite hold water with the patient therefore – Colonel Bogey is obviously imagined, but the pain in the leg is very real! I'll come back to dealing with this later. There's a 'warning on the can' so to speak: that telling a patient their pain has no value whatsoever, is meaningless, that they are healed and therefore the pain is being generated wholly from within the central nervous system by 'central mechanisms' – may be unhelpful and I think needs modifying. That the CNS and brain are processing tissue weakness or deconditioned tissues in an amplified way is far better. There are many ways of explaining pain and in addition to those already given there will be more.

When I was teaching regularly I occasionally used to do this lecture called 'Chronic pain, if we know how it starts can it be stopped?' One of the key parts of my talk related to one of the 'yellow-flag' predictors of a poor outcome, which was: high intensity of **acute** pain, especially if it was associated with high levels of distress – predicts a poor outcome.

It was Dworkin (1997) who said, 'The severity of acute pain has consistently emerged as one of the most reliable predictors of chronic pain, as evidenced by research on postoperative pain, herpes zoster and low back pain.'

This makes sense when you consider that maladaptive central changes associated with chronic maladaptive pain, at the dorsal horn level of observation, relate to:

- intense afferent barrages impacting on second order cells (review Shane and Claudia from section 5): massive barrages can come from injured tissues, but also, most aggressively, from injured peripheral nerve fibres (see nerve root sections)

- poor segmental, inter-segmental and descending inhibitory control mechanisms – in other words 'pain-off' systems not working well (Claudia's family) and maybe the 'pain-on' systems working too well and encouraging things (Shane's family).

Jump now to thinking about how we engage our memory to the best of its ability:

If you really want to consciously memorise something you...

- must deem the thing you're trying to remember as important, you give it 'high value'

- you need to focus and concentrate on it, give it plenty of attention, even getting a bit obsessed and pre-occupied by it will help!
- you need to keep repeating it to yourself and come back to it often! That's daily practice...
- try and make it as pleasurable, enjoyable and as rewarding as you can!
- or... the complete opposite can work too – get really scared about it! Get someone to be prepared to wire you up to a really nasty shock, or throw you into icy water or off a cliff if you don't learn what you're supposed to – put the pressure on a bit. Fear is a motivator in some contexts.

Now, that's active memorising, as in when you're forced to recite a poem at school or you're in the school play, or having to give a lecture.

Lots of things and experiences just end up in memory without us having to really work hard to get them there. As I've just been suggesting, it's those experiences that have high emotional content that get most easily memorised, 'learned' or 'imprinted'. So, translating this into the clinic: pain that's given high 'threat' value, a high focus of attention and a source of anxiety and worry is likely to have a high 'synaptic-impact' and hence get imprinted! This is supported by the well known brain and pain researcher, Herta Flor (e.g. Flor and Birbaumer 2000) who states that the key emotions for imprinting are a high degree of fear and anxiety.

In the earlier brain chapters I discussed at length how fear and anxiety focus the brain on the object creating the fear and anxiety, which in turn intensifies the stimulus and also its potential to be remembered.

I like what's shown in figure 19.1 (from Posner and Raichle 1997). It's a recording of the activity of a single neuron from the sensory cortex of the brain of a monkey in two different conditions – 'attended' and 'unattended', as you can see. The neuron being recorded responds to a given stimulus let's say a simple light touch on the hand. On the left, the monkey's hand is stimulated while being distracted elsewhere. The neuron responds a little. Now, on the right the monkey's attention is drawn to the hand while it's being touched and as you can see the neuron responds far more. The results of the same experiment on humans are shown in the bottom pair of graphs, here the recordings aren't quite as accurate being taken via scalp electrodes – but the effect of attention is marked.

I've already discussed, that the greater the activity, the greater the likelihood of an increased relationship between firing neurons. It's Hebb's, 'cells that fire together wire together' of course! If you want to make better connections in your brain, you have to give that 'something' your attention and by doing that, the activity which occurs gets amplified and facilitated. Add a bit of motivation to the mix and the product is even more strongly imprinted.

Cells that fire together wire together – long term memory, is all about new synapses being formed (see figure 19.2) between neurons and new representational circuits

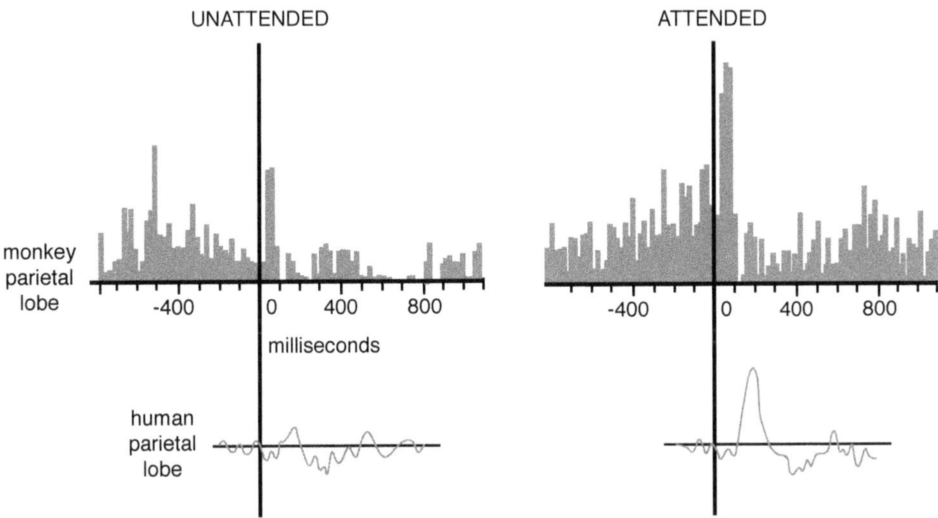

Figure 19.1 The upper traces are the electrical activity shown by a single parietal neuron following a stimulus delivered at a time indicated by the long vertical line. The left side was recorded while the monkey was not attending to the location of the stimulus and the right side was recorded while it was. The lower traces are the average event-related potentials recorded from a scalp electrode over the parietal lobe of a human subject under the same stimulus conditions. Illustration redrawn from: Posner M.I. Raichle ME (1994) Images of Mind. Scientific American Library. A Division of HPHLP, New York, p 21

forming in turn. It's also all about existing synapses being strengthened and those being coupled with others that are weakened. The brain changes, it rewires, it forms fresh connections or loses old ones and this is called neuroplasticity. New 'maps' are formed, new wiring occurs; new memories and new skills accrue. If you've just twisted your ankle for the first time in your life – you will have a new sensory map of that feeling.

Let's have a bit of facetious fun (in a sense it's yellow flags converted into memory biology mechanisms). Or is it a sniff of 'satire'? Maybe that's too intelligent a label here?

So, if you want to make a pain stay and become chronic here are some tips based on memory biology and the formation of new circuits:

- make the pain the main thing in your life...
- give it high value – think about it, concentrate on it, keep coming back to it and concentrate on it again and again

  (Try and get to know every little nuance of its character and behaviour over time and let it worry you about possible nasty things going on. Try and

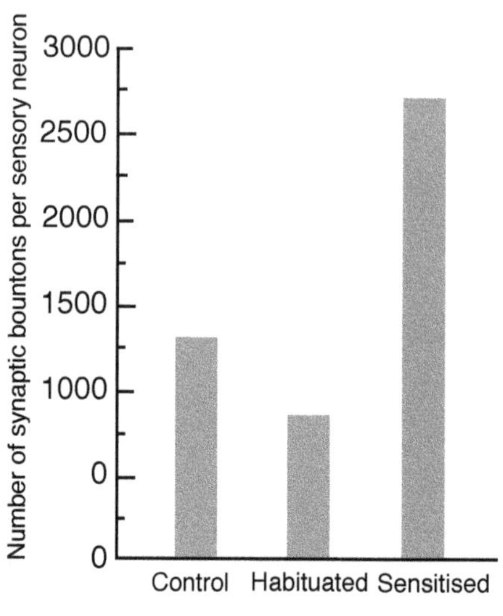

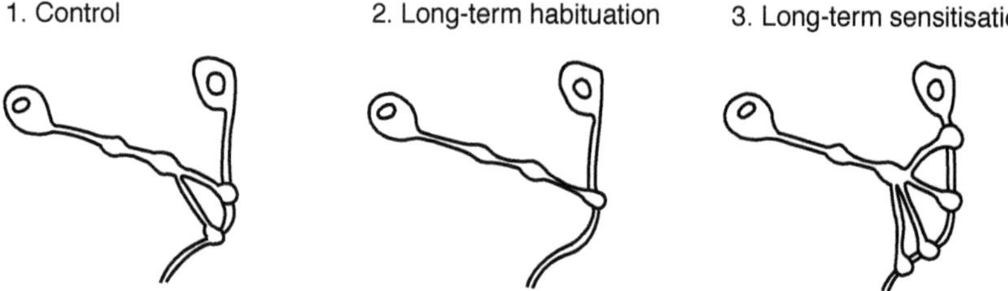

Figure 19.2 Cells that fire together wire together – long term memory is all about new synapses being formed between neurons and new representational circuits forming in turn. Redrawn...

associate it with something that might maim, disable or even end your life. Rate it as 100% torture)

- stop working and functioning and try to lead a life of total boredom – so that you can spend lots of time listening to your body and the pain; don't let distractions like work, hobbies, family and socialising get in the way of time well-spent on concentrating on the pain

- add emotion to it, process it via the 'quick and dirty low road' – try to feel fearful and anxious about it all the time and keep wondering what it is and what it means in terms of threat

- don't listen to professionals who listen to you, who do some testing and who try to reassure you and then give you a simple natural history so you know what normally happens. Much better to listen to the bogey man in your head that's going, 'This is serious, they've missed something. I'm going to suffer for the rest of my life and I'm going to take you down with me if I can'

- listen to your friends and neighbours who tell you stories about someone they knew with symptoms just like yours, who ended up dying of some nasty cancer that wasn't diagnosed in time.

  (Yes, try and seek out information that will worry you about the pain and the cause of it, some alternative practitioners can sometimes be very helpful here. The less they know about real medicine and pathology the more they're likely to help in this. Remember the aphorism: 'A little knowledge is a helpful thing.')

- listen to professionals who tell you it is serious and use words like: 'degeneration', 'stuck', 'trapped', 'out', 'inflamed', 'bad', 'may need an operation', 'could be serious', 'back of a 90 year old'. And who 'Suggest you stop work and look for something 'sedentary'.' 'Stop those active hobbies you enjoy' and 'suggest you think about early retirement to focus on your pain.'
- talk about your pain all the time to others
- seek out information about pain disasters on the internet
- use the internet to self-diagnose rather than listen to the clinician, who's examined you thoroughly and tried to reassure you.
- try and keep as anxious and worried as you can about the pain
- refuse any form of therapy or medication that helps or gets rid of the pain
- feel hopeless and helpless and keep reminding yourself that no therapy's ever going to help
- use supports, sticks, mobility scooters, collars and corsets as much as possible to remind you of your problem and help your body become weak, vulnerable and deconditioned; you know it's best to be sedentary and the dangers of over-doing it
- join a similar minded group of sufferers, so you can all talk about your pain all the time; they'll help you through the week
- twitter about it
- set up a face-book page on your problem
- make sure your spouse/significant other is 'solicitous' – in other words they're nice to you all the time, constantly ask about the pain, don't let you do anything for yourself in case you make it worse and also go out of their way to make you feel hopeless and helpless
- make your pain your new hobby, make it fun and enjoy it, you know it makes sense.

And so on, I hope you get the picture? Of course the opposite is true if you don't want pain to become imprinted (see pink flags chapter later)!

This is all why I often said in my lectures: 'Reassurance is a pain killer' – or for that matter a whole host of top-down inputs that quell, adjust or re-shape our thinking and emotions to become more adaptive and realistic. It's the slow and accurate high road working on the quick and dirty low road again! Top-down manipulating and moulding the bottom-up activity. Reassurance is one thing, but it's got to be followed by re-activation, doing stuff, staying occupied, getting physically going again, good pain coping strategies and pain control and helping yourself etc.

Chapter 19.2
Cortical reorganisation 1

'Somewhere, something incredible is waiting to be known.'

Carl Sagan

Recently a great deal of learning and pain research in relation to what goes on in the brain has been investigating 'cortical reorganisation' – meaning changes in brain maps and it's been fascinating. One of the main areas of focus has been the primary somatosensory cortex the so called 'S1' or 'somatosensory cortex area 1' region. See the top illustration in figure 19.3 where to confuse further, it's labeled simply the 'sensory cortex'!

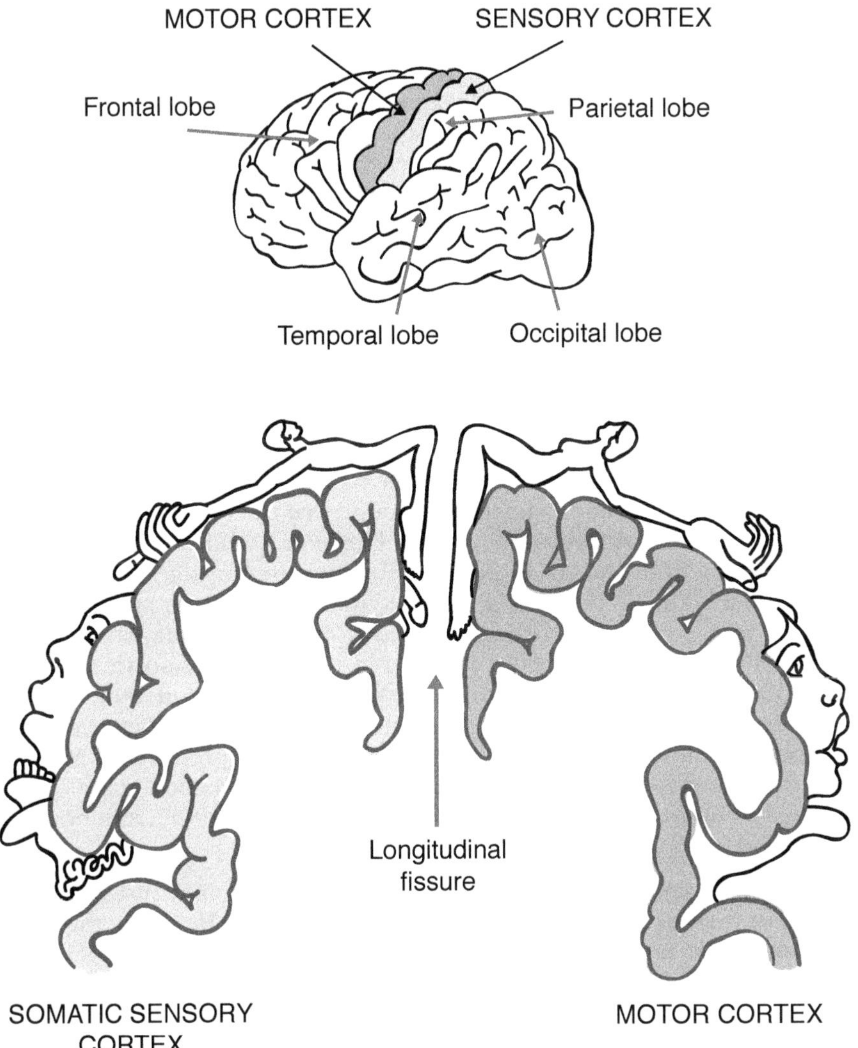

Figure 19.3 'Cortical reorganisation' – meaning changes in brain maps. One of the main areas of focus has been the primary somatosensory cortex the so called 'S1' or 'somatosensory cortex area 1' region. See the top illustration, where to confuse further it's labeled simply the 'sensory cortex'! Redrawn...

Let's get the anatomy straight to start with, because it can get really quite confusing and as far as I'm concerned, nobody seems to explain it clearly. I'm setting up for a failure here for sure!

If you put a flat hand onto one side of your head, with your palm just above your ear and the fingers pointing upwards so the tips touch the head round about the midline – you're roughly over the 'parietal' lobe of the brain and under your hand is the primary somatosensory cortex (S1). The primary motor cortex is just forward of it, in the adjacent 'frontal' lobe. These two areas lie in a long strip of the cortex, that, if viewed in coronal section (figure 19.3, lower illustration) runs medially from deep in the longitudinal 'fissure' (the big gap between the two cerebral hemispheres), then upwards before running laterally and downwards towards the temporal lobe. As you can see from the figure, the 'sensory' map of the body is represented on this surface, starting medially deep in the fissure with the genitals, followed by the foot, lower leg and knee. The rest of the leg, trunk, head, arm then hand follow before the very large face, the teeth, tongue, larynx and a rather small 'intra-abdominal' representation curled underneath at the bottom. The classic motor 'map' of the primary motor cortex has a similar 'topographical' arrangement. Don't forget that things in the brain are predominantly 'crossed over', the left brain has the sensory and motor maps for the right side of the body and vice versa, the right the left.

Several great brain pioneers in the late 1930's determined all this. Wade Marshall was the first to note that touching a cats' skin or moving hairs on it, produced electrical responses in specific groups of neurons in the somatosensory cortex he was investigating. Marshall joined up with John Hopkins Medical School physiologist Philip Bard and together they found that the whole of the body surface was represented in a surprisingly organised fashion. Wilder Penfield went on to extend the study from animals to people. He was a neurosurgeon at the Montreal Neurological Institute in the 1930's. Penfield did operations on patients with brain cancer and epilepsy and kept them conscious during the operation, in order to determine the pathological tissues he needed to excise. To do this, he used an electrical probe stimulator applied to the surface of the brain and found that specific cortical areas produced localised sensations on the patients' skin. After a great many operations, explorations and probing he was able to produce the sensory map that's so well known today and often referred to as the 'Penfield' map[1]. The map is depicted in figure 19.3. His findings were published in 1950, in a book[2] he co-authored with colleague Dr Theodore Rasmussen.

Penfield did the same for the primary motor 'map' next door just anteriorly and organised in a similar medial to lateral strip (figure 19.3). He found that using the stimulating probe in specific areas he could trigger specific movements. One of the great discoveries that Penfield made was that these maps were 'topographical', meaning that areas adjacent to each other on the body surface are generally adjacent to each other on the brain maps. Yes, but take a closer look and you can see that the

1 - For a wonderfully full account of how Wilder Penfield worked with his patients see: Sandra and Matthew Blakeslee's book: The Body has a Mind of its own, Random House, New York. Chapter 2.

2 - Penfield W, Rasmussen, T 1950 The Cerebral Cortex of Man.

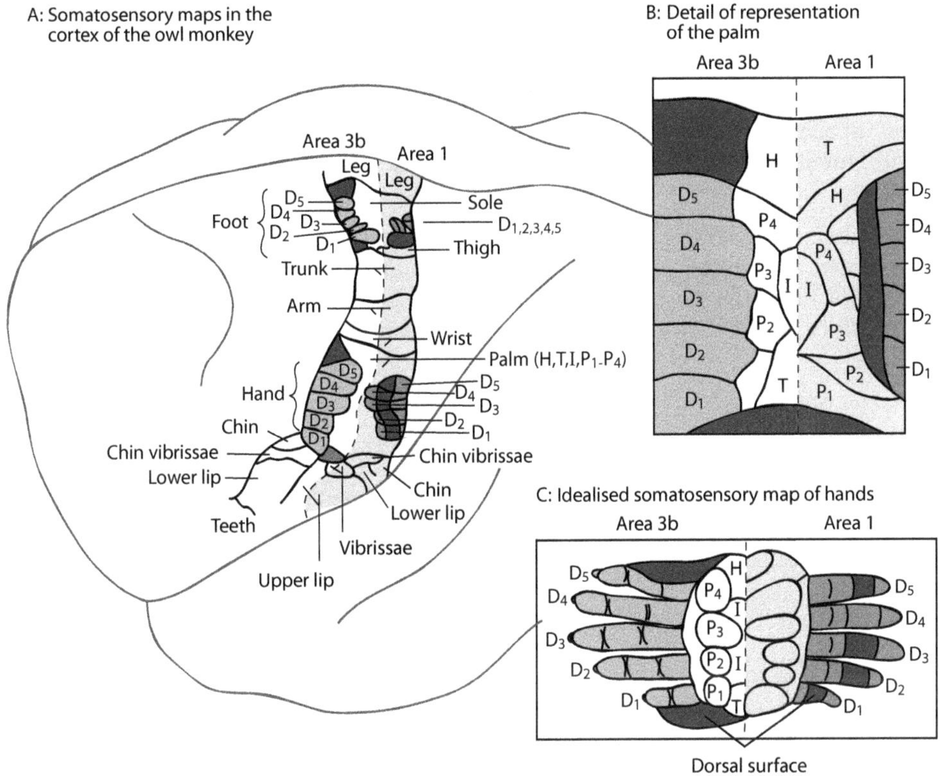

Figure 19.4 Looking down on the somatosensory cortex of one hemisphere of a monkey. Redrawn...

genitals are next to the foot and the hand next to the face! This will be of interest when we look at amputation, moving maps and er, foot fetishes!

Let's just go a little more complicated with the S1 cortex because it's been divided up by brain anatomists. You may not know this but the somatosensory cortex has more than one topographical map, it's actually got four: called 'Brodmann[1] areas' 1, 2, 3a and 3b.

The trendy regions of S1 are areas 3b and 1. (Yes, confusing isn't it: S1 is the whole primary somatosensory cortex which has 4 areas: areas 1, 2, 3a and 3b, and they're in this order: running from front to back it's: 3a, 3b, 1 then 2 – the reason that they're so out of order is that Brodmann wasn't too good at doing accurate vertical sections).

1 - *Dr Korbinian Broadmann (1868-1918) was a German neurologist who divided the brain up into 52 distinct regions based on anatomy and cell type, his numbering system is still in use today! For example areas 17 and 18 in the brain's occipital lobe are the primary visual areas.*

Check out figure 19.4. We're actually looking down on the somatosensory cortex of one hemisphere of a monkey. There are two strips, the one on the left, anteriorly, is area 3b, the one on the right, area 1. Both have topographical maps of the whole body and more or less mirror each other. In the boxes to the right you can see the detail of the palm of the hand in areas 3b and area 1 as well as the whole hand. D stands for digit with the respective finger numbering, P are 'palmar pads' and so forth.

Now, look at the next figure (19.5) which shows the S1 cortex in a little more detail plus a section through it. It also shows the location of the secondary somatosensory cortex (S2) and the posterior parietal lobe. If you look at the section (the bottom illustration), you can see that somatosensory cortex (S1) starts at the bottom of the

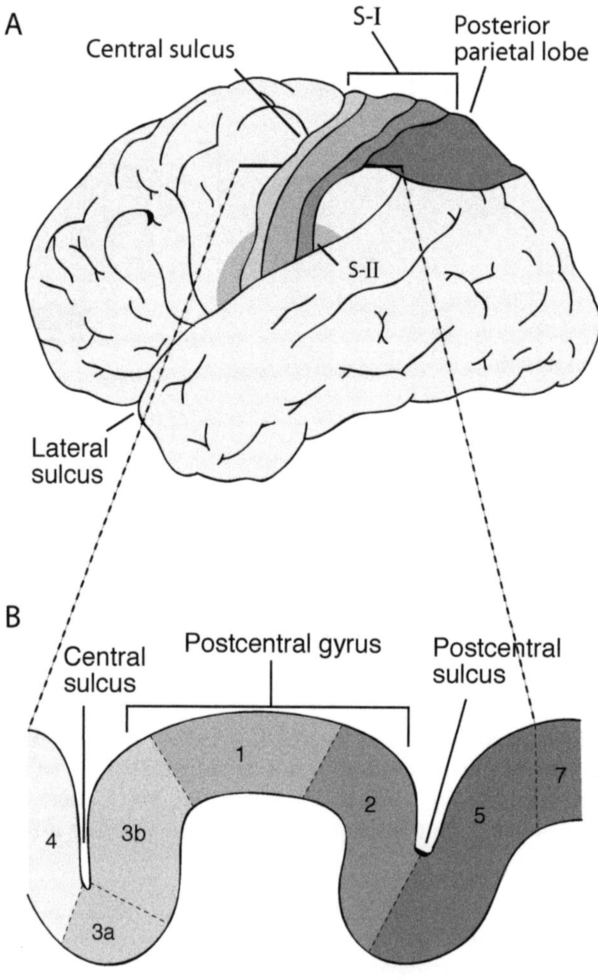

Figure 19.5 The S1 cortex in a little more detail plus a section through it. Redrawn...

long vertical crease called the 'central sulcus' and finishes at the bottom of the next crease called the 'post central sulcus'. Between the two sulci lies the postcentral gyrus. (Gyrus means, any of the prominent, rounded, elevated convolutions on the surfaces of the cerebral hemispheres).

'S1' is divided up into its four out-of-order parts. Starting anteriorly, area 3a lies at the bottom of the central sulcus followed by area 3b, area 1 goes across the gyrus and finally area 2, which lies in the post central sulcus. These four areas equate to four maps, each apparently representing subtly different features of touch and proprioception, but may also include pressure, temperature and pain. For example, sensory information from muscles and joints important for limb proprioception projects to area 3a; area 3b relates to skin information about touch and this information is further processed in area 1.

The point is that if you close your eyes and someone puts an object in your hand, all the various areas work together to form an image of the object in your brain that enables you to recognise it. Think the touch equivalent of the 'Fighting Temeraire'! (See chapter 16.2). For precise touch information, like when 2 point discrimination is being tested, we're largely using areas 3b and 1.

Back to these areas a little later. You might want to re-read it with a gin and tonic or, as Janet Street Porter has recently suggested if you're over 40, a spliff!

When I first found out about these somatosensory maps I wanted to know how they worked them out so accurately. Jump to the 1950's and the invention of microelectrodes – tiny, tiny electrodes that pick up electrical activity in individual nerve cells in the brain. This allowed 'micro-mapping' to happen – which even today is still about a thousand times more precise than any brain scan. Further, microelectrodes can pick up signals that last for thousandths of a second, whereas brain scans can only pick up bursts of activity which last one second in thousands of neurons. Scans miss heaps. The trouble with micromapping is that it's tedious and takes ages. So now we come to a character called Michael 'Merz' Merzenich, who's been described as 'the world's leading researcher on brain plasticity'. Back in the 1960's he would cut away a small piece of a monkey's skull overlying the hand area of S1, exposing about a 1-2mm strip and insert a microelectrode beside a sensory neuron there. Then he'd tap away on the monkey's hand until he found an area of skin that made the neuron fire. He recorded the location of the neuron on the cortex and the location on the skin of the hand and then moved on to another neuron nearby, repeating the process until he'd mapped the whole hand. We're talking maybe 500 electrode inscrtions done over several days and repeated many times on many monkeys. 'Merz' and his co-workers basically produced a refined Penfield map.

Now, the big deal back then was that brain areas and maps were thought to be fixed. The firm belief was that all areas of the brain were formed and connected up during development and growth, but by adulthood they were all considered to be done and dusted for the rest of life. That was it. The function of the brain was 'localised' and hence fixed for ever, no arguments.

Let's flip to some famous research on juvenile plasticity.

Thanks to the work of David Hubel and Torsten Wiesel around that time, it became widely accepted that the juvenile and growing brain was plastic and influenced by the impact of the environment and experience. These two researchers discovered what's come to be known as the 'critical period' of development. For example, they sewed shut one eyelid of a newborn kitten and mapped its visual cortices at different time points. They found that the area that normally processed input from the closed eye failed to develop, leaving the cat blind for life in that eye. What they also found was that the part of the kittens brain that had been deprived of input from the shut eye had begun to process input from the open eye.

So, two things from this: **firstly**, for normal development, environmental stimuli are required – the brain just doesn't end up all ready to work unless it gets appropriate stimuli, at an appropriate time. The environmentally derived stimuli drive the neural network's development and therefore the wiring. **Secondly**, if a part of the brain that would normally develop into a given function doesn't receive adequate stimuli, it fails and a nearby network or map that is developing normally will seize the area and make use of it.

Looking at it this way, there doesn't appear to be such a thing as a redundant area of brain, there's no waste! Like good old Burglar Bill that I used to read to my kids, when he came across something that he fancied and nobody was looking he'd go, 'I'll have that' and he'd stick the object in his 'loot' bag. In the brain, if there's a bit doing nothing the neighbours will go 'I'll have that' and purloin the piece of real estate for their own use. So, your existing maps, if you don't keep them used and healthy are in danger of becoming degenerate and even being taken over. Moral here? Use it or lose it! Or more likely: 'If you don't use it then something else will use it.'

It's important to note, that assigning a single function or 'input' to an area isn't how it is in reality. A single area may have several functions and many different inputs and processing possibilities. Thus, losing one of the functions or inputs may allow one of the others to very quickly step in and take over.

The 'critical period' of development came to be seen as a 'window' of time, during which the area of brain in question was particularly sensitive and plastic to the environment and during which it had rapid, formative growth. Language development for example, has a critical period that begins in infancy and ends between eight years and puberty. That explains why in the UK we're so 'good' at other European Languages! We don't start learning them until the onset of puberty... Doh! Educators need to listen to neuroscientists perhaps?

Now, if you hang around goose eggs so that you're the first thing the hatching goslings see and you're around more or less constantly for about three days – those goslings will '*imprint*' you on their brain as their most important person, their 'Mum' and they'll follow you round from then on. Nice. That's a really interesting critical period 'window' example for you!

So, here's my thought and proposal – that the anti-nociceptive system, the pain-off circuitry has a critical period too, or at least it needs to be 'taught' to wire-up well and work efficiently. The pain-off network needs practice, just like vision or any other sense or skill you care to name. Well, if that's the case, so too the pain-on system? It could well be. I mentioned 'social modeling' in earlier chapters and it seems pretty clear, that when we're young and probably throughout childhood and beyond, we learn from those around us.

Surveys have been done that ask teachers to indentify the children who whine, complain, are absent a great deal, visit the school nurse most frequently and show the most illness behaviours. Unsurprisingly, there's a high correlation linking the children with these illness behaviours to parents who have ongoing pain problems and disability (Christensen and Mortensen 1975). Chambers et al (2002) taught mothers to interact with their children in a pain-promoting or a pain-reducing manner and found significant effects of maternal behaviours on children's perceptions of pain. As an aside, that's why we all need to learn about 'reinforcement' skills from psychologists and get good at using them.

We learn how to behave when we hurt but we also learn 'try-not-to-hurt behaviour' too and my point is, that how 'good' we get at either of them will have an impact at the neurobiological level. Though not proven, it seems pretty obvious to me that the practice we get when we're young may well set us up with an efficient pain-off system (or pain-on system) for the rest of our life.

My maternal grandfather was a dentist. Mum was one of five children, brought up in a pretty no-nonsense but loving environment. The first time I needed a filling at the dentist and because of her experience with her Dad, my Mum goes, 'He doesn't need an injection, just get on with it.' I was probably about six or seven years old. I never thought twice about it, climbed into the chair and suffered the drill for five minutes. It was pretty sharp but as soon as it stopped the pain was instantly gone. On the way out of the dentist I felt fine, in fact I felt pretty good with myself, even though I was a shy skinny little kid with short hair and short trousers. Mum said, 'That wasn't that bad was it?' No, it wasn't and from that day on, all my life, I've never needed an anaesthetic for fillings at the dentist and I reckon my pain tolerance has been pretty high. I give thanks to my Mum's 'cruelty' to a naïve little lad; and a whole pile of other childhood and beyond rough and tumble experiences as well.

The moral is obvious. Send the kids back down the mines and up the chimneys and ban the screens! The 'Elastoplast-free' (Elastoplast is a trade name for sticking plasters in the UK!) world of the modern child, their sterile environment and the wimpy fear of breaking the skin leaves a massive 'pain-off' system experience gap. Maybe we don't even get enough pain-on experience for the pain-off system to practice on!

Just like the one eye blinded cat: no experience equates to no wiring and no wiring leaves no function. So the gap left in your head might just get purloined for some hypersensitivity circuits to make their marks. My suggestion is that you start refusing the injection at the dentist, especially for your kids!

Maybe the cane at school did my pain-off system some good too? After a good caning, in order to try and look 'hard', we used to smile on the way back to our seats! Well some of us who got caned regularly did, but some may well have been traumatised for life and suffered later, who knows?

The trauma-for-life flip-side here is the notable correlations between childhood abuse/negative early life experiences and chronic pain and health problems later on. Correlations are all well and good, but they don't necessarily mean cause and effect. Still, it makes sense that nasty experiences early on and particularly through various critical periods may well disrupt normal development and impact later life.

As we saw in section 6, there's mounting evidence that some chronic pain sufferers have significant degeneration and loss of grey matter, in particular to those areas that may be involved in anti-nociception. Now, this research should come with a big warning on the can, that, at this point in time we do not know what this loss is showing or what it means. That still doesn't stop thoughts like this...

That on-going pain is due to a fault in our wiring-loom and that those who hurt so much are simply not endowed with an adequate anti-nociceptive system...

'Sorry, it's not my fault I hurt. I haven't got a pain-off system like other people.'

But if we do blame the lack of a certain bit of wiring-loom, might that not mean it's genetic? Or could it be due to lack of practice during the critical period for the pain-off system? Or, was it OK before the pain problem started and it was the pain problem that caused the degeneration? Chicken and egg a bit? We don't know. But, it would be great to serially scan a pile of young people in these brain areas and then plot their lives longitudinally to see their pain history and see if any scan changes correlated.

In a recent book sent to me by Mick Thacker, called 'Brainwashed', the authors make a massive case for great care when interpreting what appears on fMRI scans, especially when it comes to blaming so called scan abnormalities on 'complex' presentations. Their concern was with drug addicts and criminals, plus abnormal and antisocial 'behaviours'. One could easily clump chronic pain sufferers into the 'complex presentation' basket and make a whole pile of misguided assumptions from looking at their scans.

I mentioned the trendy gene-blaming tactic for inadequate pain-off systems just now. The love of blaming 'genetics' and absolving ourselves of all blame for our upbringing and past life experiences, has to be put in the context of what genes do, given the environment they're put in. (It's nature **VIA** nurture again, **NOT** nature? **OR** nurture?). Here's a good example of how to understand this.

The genetic **potential** to be super-fat might well be there but not expressed, unless environments change. The 'Pima' Indians of Arizona are great examples of what's called the 'thrifty phenotype'. Remember, a 'phenotype' is the living organism that you observe; it is a result of the 'genotype' starting off in its egg environment following fertilisation, growing and developing and finally maturing into the adult organism. We're all phenotypes then? Yes, we are. So is a receptor protein! Anything that can be classed as a product of gene activity can be classed as a phenotype – from our microstructure to our macrostructure. Thus, a particular receptor is sometimes viewed as the phenotypic expression of the particular gene that was responsible for it. But so too, say, an individual nociceptor, it has a phenotype – with its particular number of synapses, its specific population of receptors and neurotransmitters – *at any given time*. As we've already seen the nociceptor can change its makeup, build new connections and synapses, change the type and quantity of its neurotransmitters and its receptor populations – all depending on the circumstances it finds itself in and the demands put on it. Neuroscientists call it neuroplasticity, but biologists would also call it 'phenotypic switching'. If this process could occur to us as a whole it would be neat. I might be able to change to something or someone of my fantasies? I'm thinking Jimi Hendrix right now but I'm trying not to. It would be cool to be a bird for a day or two, or even a dolphin (there's a new blockbuster movie in there somewhere!).

Now, Pima Indians have the highest rate of type 2 diabetes in the world and are super-fat. Before the white-man and modernisation, this group of people lived in the nutritively challenging environment of Southern Arizona (Desert)! Their phenotype was thin and athletic – they were a race of well adapted hunter-gatherers. They flourished because of their 'thrifty phenotype'. Their metabolism was super-smart at converting any surfeit of calories into fat stores; they thus survived from the meagre food resources that were hunted and gathered. Any little bit extra in the way of food consumption was quickly and efficiently converted into fat 'stores' for use in leaner times, of which there were many in the harsh desert environment. When modern man came across the Pimas they saw them as malnourished. And, as a result of introducing them to the 'normal' western eating style, soon led the Pimas to become fat, with the secondary complications of type 2 diabetes. Today it would be blamed on 'fat genes' but in their naturally challenging environment thrifty fat genes and the resulting phenotype was a massive advantage. Their beautifully evolved food conversion to fat efficiency should be applauded perhaps. It's just that Pimas, like most of the western world, just need to eat very little relative to what they now do.

Don't blame the Pima genes; blame the genes and the environment the genes are in! Nature via nurture! So, some of us may have genes that create the potential for us to be sensitive and more pain producing phenotypes, but those genes may not express in this way unless they're given an environment that triggers them to cause the problem.

I've drifted off a little; we need to get back to the neuroplasticity story. Recap: we've confirmed that neuroplasticity is important and exists in the developing and growing human; for normal development, environmental stimuli are vital for normal brain and nervous system development – particularly in the so called 'critical periods'. I've argued that the growing youngsters of the Western world need more rough-and-tumble and Elastoplast use and less sympathy, so as to provide the right environment for good development of an adequate pain-off system. And you've all agreed to bring your kids up taking on this advice! Start early is the motto. When I was a kid, I was up trees most days, my hands were full of splinters, there were scratches all over my legs (wearing shorts, see, you know it makes sense) and I fell out of the trees into patches of stinging nettles; I got smacked a lot at school (and sometimes at home too!). But don't go ahhhh... my parents were very loving and I was very happy... although school is another story! My parents just kicked my brother and I outside to play in the garden and I was always in trouble for teasing, making a mess or not doing as I was told. In the summer we weren't allowed our pasties unless we'd been for a swim (freezing agony for the first five minutes) and thankfully there were a few trees and places to explore – to get scratched, bleed and hurt a bit.

Chapter 19.3
Cortical reorganisation 2: use it or lose it because someone nearby will Burglar Bill it!

'Tact is the ability to tell someone to go to hell in such a way that they look forward to the trip.'

Winston Churchill

The notion that adults could show brain neuroplasticity was shunned by the great majority of researchers until relatively recently. The localisationists ruled the day and anyone who tried to suggest otherwise just wasn't taken seriously. So, from the early 1960's on researchers like Merznich, who were convinced that the adult brain could neuroplastically change, faced an uphill battle to convince the dogmatic and ruling beliefs of the day. Even Hubel and Wiesel, who'd demonstrated such impressive plasticity during growth and development and who got a Nobel Prize for it, were too rigid in their views to listen to anyone suggesting that the adult brain was changeable.

Merznich did some great work on monkeys, but there was some even more amazing work, which even today has still not received the praise it deserves. And this was done by an American researcher called Paul Bach-y-Rita.

Merznich first; then a bit on pain; then finish with Paul Bach-y-Rita in the last chapter of this section!

As we've seen, Merznich mapped the hand area in S1 of the brain of adult monkeys. He then cut their median nerves, denervating the nerves' distribution to the monkeys forearm and hand. Following this, he set about remapping the hand area of S1. Here, he put his microelectrodes into cells of S1 that prior to denervation were activated when areas of the hand supplied by the median nerve were touched, for example, the middle of the palm. Now, being deprived[1] of any peripheral input from the median nerve, nothing happened when the palm was touched. But, and surprisingly, he found that these cells weren't redundant, they now responded when areas of the skin were touched that were supplied by the adjacent and intact ulnar or radial nerves! It seemed that the input from these nerves had grabbed the median nerves' former map. They'd done a 'Burglar Bill' on it. Merznich actually found that the ulnar and radial nerve maps in the hand area had virtually doubled in size. So, if one area of the brain is not being used, another input or function will grab it and use it – that is the cruel selfish world of 'competitive plasticity'. I like the term that was coined by Gerald Edelman, 'Neural Darwinism', or as the famous DNA scientist Francis Crick said, 'Neural Edelmanism'. That is a massive pat on the back then! Interestingly, Gerald Edelman, who right this moment is still alive I believe, got the Nobel Prize for Physiology in Medicine in 1972. Along with fellow researcher Robert Porter, he discovered the structure of antibody molecules. Later he became famous for his work in neuroscience and philosophy of mind.

Maybe if you stop moving, rest and do nothing because of your pain, your S1 maps that represent the body area that is painful, will take over and expand into the areas involved in processing other aspects of sensation and that aren't doing too much because you're resting – like feeling objects/feeling the environment, as well as into the areas involved in processing the sensation of movement? In my experience, a great many chronic pain sufferers who become physically disabled have poor balance, poor quality of movement and when their muscles are statically tested have this ghastly 'cog-wheel' type contraction (discussed in the 'Kate chapters' section 17). So, when all factors are considered, the presentation amounts to a control

1 - That cutting a peripheral nerve 'deprives' the CNS of input can be strongly challenged – see Nerve root section of this book.

and 'proprioceptive' dysfunction problem? Further, it's now evident that patients with on-going pain show deficits in two-point discrimination. In other words their normal non-pain sensory function becomes impaired.

I've just thought of this: 'use it or lose it, because someone nearby will Burglar Bill it!' Sorry, but it might help you remember it.

Remember, the various areas of S1 (3a, 3b 1 and 2) are involved in processing multiple sensory modalities – we mentioned touch, but also proprioception, pressure, temperature and pain. And, they're all very close together. So, if one input is dominant over the others, like pain might be over proprioception, deep pressure and even temperature (because the sufferer is not moving and putting normal forces and sensations through the area), then the pain processing cells and circuits start to want more cells and circuitry to be involved. And, because those cells that normally monitor movement and pressure in the area aren't doing much, the pain processing cells make a grab for them – a press-ganging Burglar Bill operation if you like.

'Right you 'orrible lot, you're doing nothing, you're all coming with me…'

Remember too, that one of the naughty rules of how to get on-going pain (chapter 19.1) is: 'don't move for a long time, put it in a sling, be careful with it, maybe put in plaster and get mad with it'. Some of you oldies like me, may remember plaster jackets for low back pain? I still see patients who experienced them. They always say it was total torture but, hey, the back pain got better. Passage of time anyone? Or did it really get better?

Now, a slight aside that interests me here and I think, adds to this debate quite nicely. Vernon Mountcastle (see Kandel et al 1995), one of the great neurologists of the 1950's and 60's under whom Merzenich studied, was responsible for a great deal of the early evaluation of the monkey cerebral cortex. He was the one who started doing recordings from individual cortical neurons. He went on to determine that the visual, auditory and sensory cortices consisted of six well organised cellular layers. Further, as far as the somatosensory cortex was concerned, he discovered that the layers were actually divided up into columns containing cells that only responded to a specific sensory 'sub-modality' on a specific area of skin. For example, he found cell columns for say, a small area on the tip of a finger that would only respond to light superficial touch; or another nearby column for exactly the same skin area dedicated to deep pressure. Sadly there's no mention of cells and columns that respond to tissue threat, nociception… and pain! I'm not sure that this has been investigated[1]? Single neuron recording needs to come back into fashion perhaps? So, my thought is that a column for one modality, say pain, may be next to a column for pressure and if the pressure column is underused, or not used because of protective behaviour or immobilisation and the pain one is full-on, then it's likely to overpower and conquer the adjacent pressure column. Neural Darwinism again! No wonder patients who are in nasty on-going hand and arm pain say things like their hand or limb doesn't feel quite like their own and that they fumble with it, or don't write as well. If they've lost subtle sensory sub-modalities due to columns being annexed by pain

1 - Mick Thacker tells me that Giando Lannetti is looking at this using EEG's and calls it the fovea on the finger!

processing, it's hardly surprising. This subtly altered 'representational area' of the sensory cortex can only add to making their neural signature (thinking in Melzack neuromatrix language) representation somewhat different and distorted.

Can you see how important it is to keep the 'other' sub-modalities going therefore? Neural Darwinism a la Louis and any good physiotherapy says keep the proprioceptor columns busy; keep the deep pressure columns busy, keep the light touch columns busy, keep the temperature columns busy. Stop those pain columns coming in and taking over your column dude, square-up. Looks like thumbs up for regular massage and movement, with a bit of hot and cold therapy! Or, even better, combine it with 'keep it moving and part of normal life'. Yes, perhaps, that's all fine early on, but there may just be a little bit more to it than that, especially for more chronic and ongoing pains.

I've used the little column explanation with quite a few patients – now I'm going to add: 'use it or lose it because the column nearby will Burglar Bill it!

Chapter 19.4
Cortical reorganisation 3: sensory discrimination

'I have left orders to be awakened at any time during national emergency, even if I'm in a cabinet meeting.'

Ronald Reagan

There's been a recent trend to using therapeutic sensory discriminatory inputs for the treatment of phantom limb pain, CRPS and even back pain (see Flor and Moseley references).

Here's what Herta Flor (2002) did for phantom limb pain of the upper limb:

'Participants were required to discriminate between electrical stimuli of different frequencies, which were applied to 8 different locations on the stump of the amputated limb. They were trained to discriminate the location and frequency and received feedback on the correct response.'

The patient's sensory cortex arm 'maps' were recorded (fMRI) before and after the treatment task.

So, for me and my patients, this sounds like a highly doctored TENS machine that has 8 wires with 8 small electrodes stuck on the end of each wire. There is a frequency adjustment and maybe even an intensity adjustment for each of the 8 outputs, so that one might be zap… zap… zap… another zappity, zappity, zappity… Another zzzzzzzzzzzzzzzzzzz… and so forth through a variety of 8 reasonably spaced frequencies. The 8 electrodes are stuck all over the stump and the clever TENS machine generates a random current of a given intensity and frequency through one of the electrodes that the operator knows the location of, but the patient has to work out by thinking about where they're feeling it. So, the patient is asked to concentrate and say <u>when</u> they feel the current and then <u>point to the</u> electrode that they feel the current is coming through. Next they have to <u>allocate a particular frequency to</u> the sensation… like 2 Hz; 25hz; 50Hz; 100Hz and so on presumably. It sounds like quite good fun! Probably a bit tricky to start with, but with practice gets easier. Flor's group of patients had practice sessions of 90 minutes on consecutive days for 10 days. So, quite a bit of practice and some intense concentrating and learning seemed to be required. Knowing learning theory I slightly wonder if they had regular breaks (because breaks help).

What they found was pretty cool. That yes, with practice they all got better at it, that their phantom pain reduced by an average of 60% (wow!) and that when they re-examined their cortical maps (more soon), the observed cortical 'reorganization' to be normalised. Significantly, there was a strong correlation between the improvement in cortical reorganization, the reduction in pain and the improvement in sensory discriminative ability.

Further, rather clever studies on patients with upper limb type 1 complex regional pain syndrome by Moseley's group (eg.2008, 2009), looked at more clinically convenient treatment methods. They found that being pretty simple still worked with these normally very difficult to help patients. The study used thirteen patients whose symptoms had been present for an average of fifteen months (+/- eight months). So, most sufferers were pretty chronic, but not terribly so.

Sometimes the way in which research is done is very instructive clinically and also just good for your thinking! So I'm going into it in a little more detail.

Prior to the 'treatment' phase of the study they measured:

1. Pain, using a VAS of 100mm (a line on a piece of paper 100mm long). So worst pain possible equals 100mm and zero equals no pain at all. The average pain rating at the start was 54mm (i.e. 5 out of 10 roughly). The patient had to simply mark along the calibrated 100mm line to indicate the amount of pain they were in.

2. Two point discrimination (TPD): here, they use a caliper accurate to 1mm. The caliper had two points or 'prongs' that could be brought together to touch i.e. zero mm. To do the test they start on zero and press the points gently into the skin of the hand, until the skin just starts to blanch. (I suggest you see what I mean by using the end of a paper clip on the skin of your finger). They prevented the patient from seeing what they were doing with a simple screen. Then in small gradations gradually increased the width of the prongs until the patient consistently said, they felt two points instead of one. This distance was the patients TPD score in mm. The mean score was 43mm when measured in the patients' pain area on the hand.

3. 'Function' using a 'Task Specific Scale'. Here, each patient selected five different tasks that they were finding difficulty with since their problem had started. For example, sleeping, driving the car, dressing, eating. The patients were asked to indicate on a zero to ten scale how well they could currently perform the task where 0 = completely unable to and 10 = able to perform normally. The average score from the five tasks was very poor at 2.2 (+/- 0.8). Note that this is a distinctly 'subjective' assessment of function and that there's plenty of research to indicate that what patients think they can achieve is a lot different from what they actually do achieve. They usually underestimate! (See Waddell 2004; Main and Spanswick 2000).

The treatment consisted of three phases after an initial waiting period phase:

The first phase was called '**Tactile Stimulation**'. Here, patients came in and 5 points were marked on the affected limb. In the research paper 5 points on the hand were illustrated, the hand being where most pain was located. The points were quite close together, each point being kept at approximately that individuals starting TPD score apart. So, one point may be over the MP joint of the hand, the next point roughly 50mm proximal, the next point 50mm medial and so forth. They then took a photograph of the marked hand and printed copies for later use.

They now used two 'probes' made of cork, one very thin one (2mm) and one wide (11mm), to press onto the skin. The upper end of the cork was mounted on a spring loaded cartridge to help standardize the amount of pressure applied to the skin every time. The subjects hand was hidden from view using a screen as before. The researcher then proceeded to use one or other of the corks to press on one of the five areas. After each stimulus there was a rest period of 15 seconds and the whole thing was repeated 24 times which took around 6 minutes. A 3 minute rest followed and the whole thing was repeated 2 more times giving a total of 72 stimuli over a 24 minute session. This was then repeated every weekday and the patients were asked to repeat the session at home once a day. To do this each patient brought in a partner or friend who was trained in what to do. They were given a pen lid and a wine cork to use instead of the fancy cork probes! This phase of the study went on for around two weeks. Every second visit their TPD was reassessed.

Note that this phase was pure stimulation – the patient hadn't got to think or participate, they just had to sit there and take it (i.e. passive therapy!). In fact the researchers didn't want them to focus on it particularly, so they allowed them to listen to music, read a magazine, or do both.

Now, to help with compliance for the 'home' bit, the patients were asked to record what they did in a 'training diary'. Patients were also asked to 'rate' the credibility of the treatment on a 100mm VAS. On the left of the line were the words, 'not at all credible' and on the right 'completely credible'. It's a nice measure of 'salience'. So, the nearer 100, the more the patient viewed what they were doing or having done as being credible and relevant to their problem.

A brief aside:

Think about assessing 'credibility' with your day-to-day patients perhaps?

'Now Dorothy, I've been doing this wiggle waggle treatment to you for around ten treatments now, on a scale of 0-10 how 'credible' does it seem to you?'

'Credible Louis?'

'Yes, do you feel that what I've been doing to you is relevant to your problem and is going to help it?'

'Listen dear, I love coming to see you. It's the highlight of my week, but what you do to me has to be pretty much classed as hocus-pocus, don't you think? But I don't want to be rude or anything...'

'Ah? Oh... Right... Well then... Ahem... er... Well, I was trying to engage the left brain through the medium of elbow pressure on the soft visceral masses that were responding and I felt we were really getting somewhere with the appendix zone.'

'I had my appendix out when I was 19 dear...'

(Sorry for the sarcasm – but I hope you can see what I am getting at?).

Salience, although not really discussed in their paper, is a really important issue. If you're going to learn something, or participate in doing something, like a set of exercises you've been given, or the incredibly boring looking home tasks involved in this research, you're hardly going to make an effort with them if you can't see the point! If you don't make an effort, if you don't 'believe' in it, you're not going to 'learn' it or benefit from it and it's hardly likely going to change anything in your brain for the better! Recall from an earlier chapter 'BO' – 'Belief and Optimism', so important in getting patient compliance and, in changing their processing.

Back to the research...

So, after two weeks of doing all this, the patients now entered the third '**Discrimination Phase**'. Here's where they have to get involved. In this part of the treatment trial the exact same procedure was used, but this time the patient had to concentrate on the stimulus and indicate which point was being stimulated, using the picture of their hand placed on the table in front of them and that had been taken at the very start. They had a choice of the 5 points and these were clearly seen on the hand picture. The patients were also shown the two probes – the 2mm and the 11mm corks and asked to say which one was being used to touch the spot on their limb. As before, they couldn't see their hand because of a screen. So – the patients had to concentrate to say thick or thin probe and also indicate the location of probe from one of the 5 points on their hand picture. All the other conditions were exactly the same as in the 'stimulation' phase. Further, the researchers taught the patients' helper to do the same thing at home but using the pen tip and a wine cork. Again, one clinical session per weekday and one at home for around two weeks. This phase requires the patient to really concentrate and practice – it's now mentally 'active' therapy.

The patients were reassessed immediately after the treatment and again after three months as a follow-up.

The results:

1. Pain at the start was 54mm mean. After the 'stimulation' phase: 51mm mean (no significant change), but after the 'discrimination' phase the mean score was 24mm and this was maintained at the 3 month follow-up. That's roughly 50% drop in pain following some pretty intense daily 'sensory discrimination training'. For these types of normally very difficult to help patients that's pretty impressive.

2. Two point discrimination (TPD): at the start this was 43mm average; after 'stimulation' more or less the same, but post 'discrimination' was 36mm – maintained at 3 month review. The patients had improved their ability to discriminate by an average of 5.7mm (half a cm). It's worth testing the palm and back of your hand to see what you're like. On the back of my hand, my two point discrimination with eyes closed using a paper clip, is roughly 20mm. The key thing here is that, if you practice anything, especially if you feel it's important/salient – you're highly likely to improve at it. The more you do it well, the better you get. It requires effort and lots of repetition though! (I hope you are all thinking, columns competing with each other and here the 'precise-sensory-information' cortical columns are competing with and trying to displace the 'pain-columns' that have dominated. Get out of here you!).

3. Finally '**Function**': at the start the mean score was 2.2 out of 10 (that's really poor), after 'stimulation' there was no change but after 'discrimination' it was 5.5 and again maintained at follow-up. That's a good 50% improvement without any specific functional rehabilitation. Not bad and note that measuring function using specific tasks wouldn't be at all difficult.

The brilliant thing from this is the importance of engaging the brain. 'Top down **during** bottom up', the patient has to be involved in training the reprocessing of their problem. Moseley and Wiech (2009) discuss three possible mechanisms for the improvements:

1. **Distraction**. That attending to the stimulus and what they had to do with it distracted from the pain, or that attending to the area in a 'neutral' and objective way reduced the threat of the various touch inputs – which in turn reduced the pain. Recall the 'threat processing centre' from sections 16 and 17.

2. **Exposure.** In other words, keep doing something that is unpleasant or feared and you can get used to it i.e. desensitizing, or 'wire-apart-depart'? Here, the patients had their painful limbs continuously touched during the treatment and home practice sessions. But, as the authors point out, there was no change in any of the measures following the 'stimulation' period – a time when plenty of 'exposure' to touch was going on.

3. **Cortical reorganisation.** This is the mechanism that the authors favour and seems reasonable in the light of the Flor outcomes with amputees mentioned earlier.

From my clinical/theoretical view point, I'm thinking and seeing the following with regards this treatment approach:

> Long term pain, with long term neglect of the body parts affected by the pain, leads to loss of normal inputs to the brain – like simple touch, pressure, temperature and the sensation of movement. Patients with complex regional pain syndrome (CRPS) are particularly well known for having what is called 'body perception disturbance' (BPD). They have altered perception of the involved limb and altered thoughts and feeling about it. In some to the extent of wanting the limb amputated (more on this soon).
>
> It seems that high levels of activity in nociceptive pathways, combined with long term protective behaviour and therefore a massive loss of touch, pressure, movement, temperature 'input' due to the loss of use and function, may lead to massive changes in the cortical representational maps. For example, cortical cell columns normally devoted to pressure, touch, movement perception or temperature may be taken over by the massive and new processing needs of maladaptive nociception/pain. This may also involve, at a more macroscopic level larger areas, thus 3a, 3b and 1 may shift their function towards being pain processing dominant and expand (or contract), in parallel with the 'new' processing demands and circumstances.
>
> In the 'treatment' patients with upper arm CRPS it seems to me highly likely that the loss of sensory capability is a fair bit more than just two point sensory discrimination. In the clinic, consideration of pressure, proprioception, temperature, vibration, rough/smooth, texture and so forth are important, offering possible treatment/rehabilitation avenues to explore.

Certainly, the Moseley et al treatment method shouldn't be too difficult to set up in the clinic.

There must be a great deal done in 'setting this up' in the patients' mind. This unfortunately is not mentioned in the research. It never is! What on earth did the researchers say to the patient subjects to make this whole thing salient, I'd like to know? For one thing, by not even mentioning any patient explanation of the treatment mechanisms suggests that you don't have to? That means, say nothing, just do the treatment and it and it'll work? Oh, yeah... Come on!

So my suggestion is, that the research is repeated in exactly the same way but that there are two groups. In the first group no pain or treatment explanation is given. In the second it is. The requirement here is for an understandable overview and explanation of the patient's pain mechanisms and how the proposed treatment was going to influence it. My hunch would be that an explanation, a rational 'top-down' narrative for the patient to ingest and digest would be essential, as in all treatments, but especially something seemingly quite so wacky as being prodded by bits of cork on the back of your hand and then trying to tell where you were prodded and how thick or thin the 'prod' was. The patient must have some kind of rationale, understanding or belief about what they're doing if they're going to help to rewire it! I also have a hunch that you could do, or get the patient to do, virtually anything so long as the patient and the clinician thought it was relevant and rational! The word 'placebo' is heavy in the air here and I keep thinking of how impotent treatments can be when they are in the 'hidden' as compared to in the 'open' condition (see chapter 8.1) and the similarity between this and the 'explained' and 'not explained' conditions I'm suggesting here.

As a clinical aside, one of my key clinical things has always been, that whatever I do with the patient or get them to do at home they have to understand and see the point of it. It has to be salient. I want the patient to be involved with plenty of BO! So in the explanation there has to an emphasis on words like concentrate, participate, enjoy, improve and see the point in what you're doing and if you can't then ask...!

Graded re-introduction of function is vitally important and must be introduced as soon as possible. Function may even be the key here, because it provides the very sensory inputs that the body has been deprived of and that need to be reinstated in order to get the pain 'invader' out.

I have fears that there's a real danger of this rather seductive 'pain treatment' overwhelming the bigger and more complex issues that chronic pain presents with. I have similar fears for the 'graded motor imagery' treatment that is also popular at the moment.

Here are a few issues that I have with it. The messages that surround any form of pain 'treatment', focus on lessening or making the pain go away or even fixing the problem, but with little or no emphasis on assessing or managing the physical, functional and psychological issues that may surround the problem. To me, it's back to unidimensional nature of manual therapy and passive therapy in general, where the rationale is that, when the pain is fixed any functional and psychological problems will naturally improve or resolve. The problem with on-going pain is that it rarely if ever fully resolves with 'treatment'. The only way for the patient to reach their full functional potential is to directly address the functional and activity related problems. Evidence from the 'fear-avoidance' literature continues to amass impressive results. Pain isn't directly addressed, but function and feared activities are by using 'behavioural experiments,' graded exposure and 'graded activity' programmes. The key thing is, that pain reductions can be just as impressive with these programmes as it is with 'sensory discriminatory training', but with the addition of functional and physical confidence and much improved health of those who undergo the programmes.

I know which approach and outcome I would prefer if I were a patient. To me, at the present time, it seems impossible for treatments like 'sensory discriminatory training' and 'graded motor imagery' to fit into a multidimensional approach with these sorts of patients. When someone can demonstrate this and also demonstrate that the results of these treatments are as wonderful as we are led to believe, I for one will remain with my kit on by the side-line. I have to say that I have had no success with either method and I am yet to meet anyone who has. I have however had plenty of patients with chronic problems who these treatment methods have been used on and failed, often at great expense too. I am rather saddened because these patients have massive functional loss and physical impairment; they have lost physical confidence; they are low in self esteem and have very low levels of optimism about the future. And, not one of the therapists seen, has taken any kind of rehabilitative treatment or management strategy that the situation is crying out for.

Chapter 19.5
Cortical Reorganisation 4: changing maps

'Anyone who thinks sitting in church can make you a Christian must also think that sitting in a garage can make you a car.'

Garrison Keillor

Let's have a closer look at the 'moving' and 'reorganising' of cortical maps.

I've already discussed how cutting the median nerve to the hand of a monkey halts normal sensory input to the S1 cortex. The now redundant map there gets purloined, or 'Burgler-Bill'd', by the adjacent ulnar and radial nerve sensory input. Thus, the S1 brain maps representing the innervation fields of the ulnar and radial nerve, expand and 'reorganize' to make use of the unused median nerve area. Merzenich also found that if he amputated the middle finger of his monkeys the maps either side of the first and third fingers would do the same, they'd expand and make use of the now 'unused' middle finger map. That was all back in the 1960's, when Merzenich and a few others, were starting to challenge the establishments dogmatic insistence that the adult brain was fixed and had no 'plastic' properties. It took many years and many elegant experiments to convince the general neurology research community that they were wrong.

At the present time cortical 'maps' of the S1 cortex are recorded using electroencephlography (EEG) or magnetoencephalography (MEG). In both of these, electrodes are placed on the skull that pick up very fine electrical signals. It can also be done by using fMRI or PET scanning. So, it's a great deal easier, but far less accurate, than it was back in Merzenich's microelectrode day.

Let's start by over-viewing a little of what's been found with map changes during learning. For example, in violinists, maps of the fingers of the left hand (the fingers used on the violin fret-board), can be compared to those of the right hand (used to merely hold the bow), or compared to normal non-musicians. Concert grade violinists, especially those who practice a lot and from a very young age show markedly enlarged finger maps, in areas 3a and 1 of the primary somatosensory cortex (S1). When a violin or cello players 'fingering' hand maps are compared to normals, they may be as much as five times larger! Likewise, Braille readers. What's also of interest is that when practicing stops these changes disappear (Janke 2009)! I wonder then if we can get patients to stop 'practising' their pain. Yeah, do what most superstar sports folk do – take a winter break, have an 'off season'. We can certainly use learning as an example in our 'explanations' when it's appropriate.

Let's take a closer look. Figure 19.6 shows cortical representation of the five digits of a monkey 'pre-training' – bottom left. This was Merzenich's group again (see Jenkins et al 1990). What he did was train his monkey to deftly and rather skillfully turn a flat disc and if they got it right they'd receive a food reward. The reward only came if the monkey used the very tips of digits 2, 3 and 4 to turn the disc. So 'Merz' then leaves the monkey to keep doing this for days and weeks on end until they become really good at it – they've done it many thousands of times. He then re-maps their brain and as you can see from the figure, the representations of digits 2, 3 and 4 significantly enlarge. Its good old 'use it or lose it – Burglar Bill it'!

Thus, learning, novelty, new anything, including pain can change the brain and its maps. Learning rewires it, it becomes more efficient and if you persist with learning, that part of the brain expands and grabs neighboring brain for its own use. To my knowledge there's no research that's investigated the effect on the function of the area expanded into! Does it have a detrimental effect? For example, if a virtuoso violin player's first finger map enlarges and expands into the chin area – does the

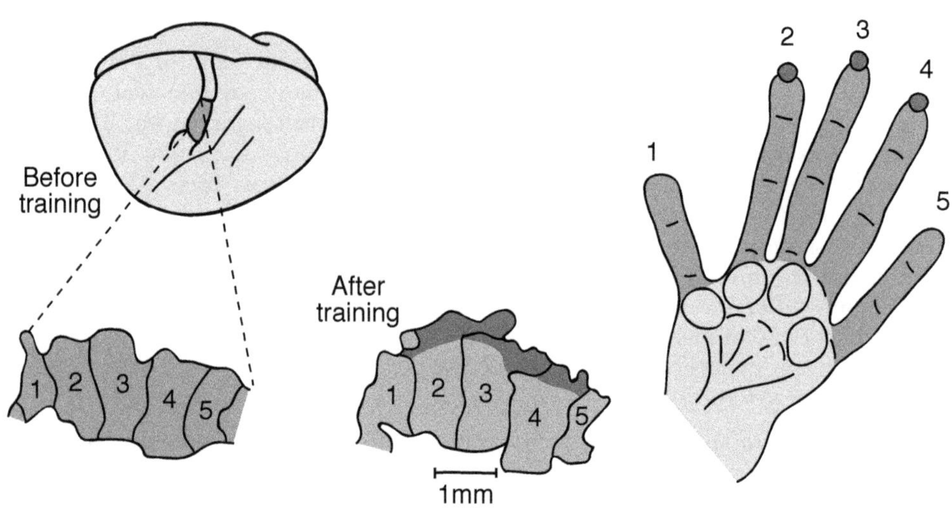

Figure 19.6 Shows cortical representation of the five digits of a monkey. Redrawn from: Jenkins et al., (1990).

chin area lose some sensory functionality as a result? Easy bit of research to do unless someone's already got the answer?

So, as we learn, the 'map' not only enlarges, it becomes denser, more responsive, more refined and more sensitive – as shown by the two point discrimination practice. Some folk who lose both hands learn to use their feet very skillfully, not only do they become incredibly dexterous, but also their sensitivity increases so that they can feel and manipulate with quite extraordinary precision. Surely brain neuroplasticity beyond doubt? This is a good example to use with patients to show them they can change their brain.

I want to have a quick flip to the primary motor maps.

This is the work of Alvaro Pascual-Leone (APL) who used a technique called, 'transcranial magnetic stimulation' (TMS) to delineate changes in the maps of the cortical motor areas. TMS basically 'injects' a little magnetic field very precisely through the cranium, which in turn induces impulses when the field reaches the neurons of the brain. If you do this over the motor cortex you produce an increased tone, or activation, in muscles relevant to the map area stimulated. This tone increase can easily be recorded.

APL took naïve subjects who had never learnt a musical instrument, or to touch type and measured the size of their finger muscle motor maps. He then got them to learn a very simple five finger exercise on the piano keyboard, in time with a metronome. The aim was for them to learn the exercise to quite a fast pace and they were asked to practice for two hours a day for a week. Everyone got better at the exercise of course. In parallel with the practice their motor maps increased in size too. That was phase one. In the second phase, the group of subjects was divided into two; one group continued to practice for another four weeks, the other stopped altogether. The maps were reassessed and as you'd expect, the maps in the group who'd stopped shrank back to the pre-practice size after one week. But in the group who continued to practice, the enlarged finger maps also got smaller, even as the performance continued to improve!

The reasoning goes like this: when you're a novice, the early practice causes 'an exuberance' of neural rewiring but as you continue to practice, you reach a new phase of long term structural change in your maps. Many of the novel neural connections you made early on aren't needed anymore. The skill gets better integrated into your maps basic circuitry and the whole process becomes more efficient and automatic. On the other hand, if you practice every day for many years and you're a virtuoso – you're maps will be enlarged (see Blakeslee and Blakeslee 2007). I reckon that while we see these folk as quite brilliant, like any top musician or sportsman – motor function to die for, it's actually a bit weird, even a bit abnormal perhaps? Let's raise our hats and thanks to neuroplasticity for the mind-blowing achievements that, given a staggering amount of practice, can emerge from the single-minded world of the obsessive compulsive? I know I wouldn't be sitting writing this if I didn't have a fair sized dollop of this 'trait' in me.

Further, if you keep practicing something, you'll have noticed how it gets easier and easier, until it becomes virtually thoughtless – you do it quite naturally, you're in that state called 'flow.' In parallel with this, it seems that the 'motor programme' or 'cell assembly' for the skill you've newly learned and continue to learn, **gets moved in the brain.** In the early 'novel' learning days, the motor-programme resides in the 'higher motor regions' like the 'supplementary motor' area, an area always engaged in any novel and complex or unfamiliar task, where lots of attention and thinking are required (its often a cognitively hard bit too). Later on and with regular practice, it all gets a lot easier and maybe after a couple of months it's a good deal smoother and more **thoughtless and less effort-full** too. At this stage, the 'supplementary motor' area gets used less and less and the whole caboodle is transferred downward in the cortical hierarchy to reside mainly in the 'premotor cortex'. Go on for years with it, like an obsessive compulsive and the programme gets its own room, together with electric plugs, drinks cabinet, music system, light show and double bed! The skill has finally 'arrived' in the 'primary motor cortex'. When interviewed, the most recent arrival, a tune called 'Colonel Bogey,' said, 'Even though I've made it to the place I've dreamt about getting to all these years, I never thought it would be quite like this. Wow, this place must be paradise. What's so cool is that I can look down on all those other tunes struggling to make it in here. They've got no idea how hard it's been!'

I get the very strong feeling that pain representational maps are likely to do the very same thing. To start with, if the practice stops (you heal or you get on with life and ignore it), the map simply diminishes in size and the pain goes. If the pain persists for a few months, it gets 'better integrated' into a nice little package and quietly sent to the sensory equivalent of the premotor cortex, where it still has a chance to get forgotten – albeit a lot harder. But if it goes on and on, it'll end up in the sensory equivalent of the 'primary motor cortex', where it's now such a well ingrained habit and maybe almost impossible to get rid of. Colonel Bogey's resting place perhaps?

This all sounds very logical and neat but there's a difficulty in that some brain representational maps associated with pain show increases in size, but in support, some show reductions in size. It's never likely to be straight forward!

An interesting article by Hashmi et al 2013, sent to me by Steve Robson, my friend and physiotherapy writing colleague, who thinks along very similar lines to me, is supportive of this 'shifting' notion. The article has a bit of a weird title:

Hashmi, JA et al 2013 Shape shifting pain: chronification of back pain shifts brain representation from nociceptive to emotional circuits. Brain, 136:2751-2768

As far as the discussion here is concerned there are a few relevant points from the article that crop up and need stating and expanding....

1. Part of this brain scanning research involved longitudinal observation! Neat!

2. These researchers scanned two groups of patients: chronic low back pain sufferers (CLB) and subacute back pain sufferers (SBP). They recruited 31 CLB's and 39 SBP's. The CLB group had their problem for an average of 13.5 years whereas the SBP's average was just 9 weeks.

3. They scanned the SBP's as soon as they could and then 3 more times over one year – the second scan was at 15 weeks and the third scan was 42 weeks.

4. They divided the SBP's up into 'recovering SBP and 'persisting' SBP and compared their scans to each other and to that of the 'chronic' (CBP) group.

5. As far as I can see, they mashed all the 'brain activity' fMRI results of each group together and using clever statistical analysis of the scans, came out with an overall picture of where all the action occurs for each group at the various stages of observation. If you read the article, you can see that as the numbers of subjects scanned went up, so the number of areas involved increased. If you read the book, 'Brainwashed' you'll know to feel highly sceptical when this sort of thing is done, but I haven't enough knowledge to be able to see any flaws in the methods used. But, I'm wary of conclusions made in the context of, 'these are the areas of the brain that light up when you've got chronic pain and these are the ones for more acute pain'. I needed to say that because I bet my chronic pain scan, if I had chronic pain, would be quite different from yours? The key thing is, that certain areas may be far more likely to flash their lights than others in everyone – but care must be taken not to assume that the list below is all there is to it and that's it!

6. So their amalgamated scan findings showed that in chronic low back pain the areas that 'lit-up' were as follows:
   - the perigenual anterior cingulate cortex extending into the...
   - medial prefrontal cortex, plus...
   - parts of the amygdala, and...
   - the basal ganglia.

In the article these workers labelled all these areas as 'emotion related' circuitry (I'm not at all sure about that. 'Brain-centric'!)

7. The areas that light up in the sub acute (SBP) group were:

    - the anterior to mid insula
    - areas of the thalamus
    - the striatum
    - the orbitofrontal and inferior cortex
    - dorsal parts of the anterior cingulate cortex.

    They labelled these areas as the 'acute pain circuitry' or 'nociceptive' circuitry.

8. Now, I could spend a day criticising this terrible 'pocketing' and 'compartmentalising' but it's pointless. It will go on for as long as man wants to keep trying to find the simple explanation for something very complex. I think these guys are trying to say 'Hey we've found the acute pain circuits and the chronic pain circuits...

9. ...and they're linked up!' So, the interesting thing is, from the longitudinal bit of the research, was what they found was that, as the subacute merged into chronic (i.e. those in the SBP 'persistent' group), their scans shifted from the 'acute pain/nociceptive circuitry' to the 'emotion related' circuitry. Those who were SBP's but were 'recovering' stayed with the 'acute pain' circuitry. The key time was one year!

10. I wish they'd shown some individual series of the scans.

So, even though I've been critical of it, here is perhaps the first evidence of circuits 'shifting' and moving, just like there are for motor learning pathways that end up in the 'primary motor cortex', already discussed. The next thing will be to show that as the individual with pain gets better at it, the amount of circuitry dedicated to it actually gets less and less. The trouble is that a person with on-going chronic pain cannot be in a happy place; to shift out the 'pain' bits from the 'fed-up' bits, seems an incredible task to contemplate. Another problem is that many of the areas on a scan labeled as being 'active' are assumed to be facilitatory – when in fact they could be inhibitory. We still have a long way to go I think, but it is very interesting.

Back to learning...

Researchers have also tackled learning motor skills by using imagination – so called 'mental practice'.

'A violinist who spent seven years in prison and practiced playing in his mind every day, gave a flawless performance the night he got out of jail.'

Did he really, wow!

So, APL (Alvaro Pascual-Leone remember?) repeated the five finger piano exercise with one specific form of practice – 'internally generated motor imagery'. So the subjects, as before spent two hours a day five days a week imagining the five-finger piano key strokes. After one week, this type of motor imagery practice led to nearly the same level of body map re-organisation as physical practice. As the Blakeslee's (2007) point out, 'As far as your motor cortex is concerned, executed and imagined movements are virtually identical.' And this, 'When you imagine movement, your primary motor cortex is inhibited' – all the other motor areas are working full-on, just as if the real movement was taking place! Let's take a quote from Blakeslee's book:

> *'Pascual-Leone determined that the level of performance after 5 days of motor imagery was equivalent to 3 days of physical practice. But, when he added one day of physical practice to the 5 days of motor imagery, his subjects were as good as those who practiced physically for 5 days. Motor imagery can give you a distinct advantage in your training. You can get better with less rather than more physical practice.'*

For the clinic a few tips from all this:

1. It's worth remembering this bit of research so you can tell it to your patients when appropriate!

2. Pain and the awkward stereotypical antalgic postures and movement patterns that accompany pain, if allowed to go on and on will get scribed, etched, or imprinted into the brain just like the skills of those virtuosos. And if you keep mentally rehearsing pain, by constantly dwelling on it, you will further help to keep it there. The patient, who keeps focusing on their pain because they're worried about it and it's become an attention 'habit' are in real danger. Skilled physiotherapy can address this, by getting the patient's physical confidence back and also by helping them with top-down-during-bottom-up tactics, to stop them constantly 'coming back to their pain' all the time.

3. Poor movement quality – often tense movement, needs addressing early on. The aim is to prevent 'tense stereotypical' movement patterns imprinting. As I will discuss later, I like to examine patients and find the biggest easiest most pain free and most relaxed movements possible and – use them. Explicitly get the patient to focus on relaxed easy confident, 'Thoughtless-fearless-movement' and then start using it in day to day life.

4. The use of imaginary movements may be very appropriate in the early stages of graded activity programmes. For example a patient can lift their very painful shoulder to about 40 degrees with very little pain, after that the pain reaches unbearable levels by a maximum range of 90 degrees. As a home exercise the patient found that they could do an active movement to 40 degrees, imagine the arm going all the way up and back down to 40 degrees and then actively down to the side.

Now, amputations, pain and genitals!

The first star here is V S Ramachandran, 'Rama' and his famous patient 'Tom', a 17 year old, who lost his arm after a road traffic accident and then developed a phantom limb four weeks later. Tom's phantom would 'do' things, like reach out to break a fall, or it would annoyingly itch but he was unable to scratch it. Rama knew about earlier monkey experiments, which showed how the redundant arm maps caused by nerve injury/deafferentation had been taken over by the adjacent face maps. Check out the earlier figures (19.3 and 19.4) of the Penfield map and note that the hand/arm representation is just above the map for the face. Because of this Rama did a clever thing with Tom, he blindfolded him and started gently touching him on his stump, over his shoulders and upper torso and asked him what he felt. Amazingly, when he touched his face, Tom said he felt the face being touched but he also felt his phantom hand being touched too. Just under the nose on the upper lip – he felt the index finger, under the mouth – the pinky and the thumb, when his cheek was touched. As a result of finding this out, Tom was then able to scratch the phantom itch by scratching his cheek! When Ramachandran mapped his sensory cortex using MEG he found that Tom's hand and arm map had been 'taken over' by the adjacent face map. Think about it, here's a bit of brain that suddenly has no input (*yes, but... see nerve root chapter*[1] *NR 1*) and nothing to do, so is left craving some form of input. This situation may be very similar to the dorsal horn of the spinal cord, when there's been a peripheral nerve injury and loss of sensory input because of it. Here, the deafferented dorsal horn sensory neurons try to make new connections in their search for the 'input' they crave. Many start to grow new branches that wander about within the dorsal horn. In so doing they may be liable to make new and inappropriate connections. Also, what connections they still have may strengthen, with previously silent inputs activating to make novel ones. The same sort of process may well occur in the 'redundant' maps of the sensory cortex following amputation. Thinking in a very 'specialised way' it may be that neurons, or 'cell columns' previously associated with the processing of light touch, may wire or make novel connections with other modalities like vibration, nociception, proprioception, or even temperature. The result? Light touch may process as pain, or warm, or pressure.

When these early results of Ramachandran's became a bit more public many amputees started coming forward and telling their stories. For example, a lower limb amputee who said that when they had orgasm during sex they felt the orgasm not just in the genitals but also in their phantom foot and leg! Look at the S1 map and it makes sense! No wonder some folk have a bit of a foot fetish then?

---

1 - I have been putting little comments in brackets occasionally saying, 'see nerve root section later' after a comment on 'cutting' peripheral nerves and leaving 'no' input as a result. It is a fallacy that cutting a peripheral nerve means that the stump of the nerve now becomes silent. As I will review in the nerve root section, cutting a peripheral nerve can lead to not only massive maladaptive impulse activity in the stumps of the cut nerves, but also later as the damaged nerve fibres start to try and re-grow. It may well be that cortical areas 'deprived' of their sensory input due to the cutting of peripheral nerves, actually receive a massive and abnormal impulse barrage for a very long time.

From all the research done on phantom limbs with awareness of the limb, but no pain and on phantom limbs with pain, it appears that cortical reorganisation is a key feature. Also, for upper limb amputees, where there is phantom limb **pain,** there is a very strong likelihood of the map of the mouth/face having moved into that of the now lost limb's map area; and the greater the shift of the map the worse the pain problem. To me it's rather odd and hard to reason, especially in terms of cause and effect.

Birbaumer et al's (1997) much quoted study of upper limb amputees is worth noting. His group took upper limb amputees with on-going phantom limb pain and did a brachial plexus block on them. In other words, they blocked the 'sensory' input from the stump. This included the severed nerves that used to supply the lost arm and hand, as well as the nerves still supplying the stump and shoulder area as well.

So, due to the anaesthetic, quite suddenly the brain is prevented from receiving this input. What happens? Apparently, 50% of the amputees with phantom limb pain lost their pain. And when their maps were charted, it was found that the sensory map reorganisation (into the face) had almost immediately reverted back to normal! In the other 50% no change in map was noted and, yes, there was no change in pain! It seems that some phantom limb pains are reliant on peripheral input or peripheral pain mechanisms, whereas others have become truly 'centralised' and 'autonomous' cell assemblies – the pain being generated without the need for any peripheral input. As a little aside, I wish someone would repeat the Birbaumer et al. experiments. I'm an old cynic I guess, but I'm suspicious because of the massive loss of symptoms and the rapid change of the cortical map. Can sensory representations really disappear 'just-like-that[1]?' Still, I'd like them to be replicated really, because my feeling is that these mechanisms are highly likely to apply to on-going pains that haven't suffered limb amputation. I thought this way back when I read the Coderre et al article about central mechanisms (see chapter 5.1). Think chronic RSI, whiplash related pain, even chronic nerve root pain. I remember thinking of these conditions in terms of phantom limb pain, but without the amputation and I occasionally used to explain it to the patients like that! Some found it very useful. The point is, that some chronic pains may be dependent on and triggered by input from the periphery – just like 50% of the amputees who lost their pain with the brachial plexus block... Whereas others, may by truly 'central' and autonomous of the peripheral input. Apparently Steve Gwilym's work on patients who do not get pain relief with joint replacement is suggesting that they have autonomous phantom-pain-like mechanisms.

Now, presentations like chronic RSI, whiplash and nerve root pain may well have peripheral 'generators'. Some may have relatively normal peripheral inputs that are maladaptively processed as pain (due to dorsal horn changes for example) and some may have pure central (autonomous cell assembly) generating causation; the good old 'annoying tune' playing away independently of any peripheral sensory impulse traffic! But all of them are likely to have some kind of 'central' 'reorganisation' map changes to unite them.

I will deal with abnormal impulse generating mechanisms from peripheral nerve in

1 - Mick Thacker tells me they can especially if their basis is not sprouting but masking and masking inputs that were already there!

the 'nerve root' section of the book (see footnote[1] earlier). For now, it's enough to say that damaged axons (i.e. nerves completely severed as occurs in amputation), are very likely to become highly sensitised and capable of self-generating severe and on-going barrages of sensory impulse traffic. Cutting a nerve may render a peripheral nerve to silence, but it may make it scream louder than it ever has.

Central 'map' changes have tended to focus on S1 as we've seen. However, changes in maps throughout the information processing areas of the brain are likely and have been acknowledged; from lower cord levels to thalamus processing; to the secondary somatosensory cortex; the posterior parietal cortex and regions such as the insula and anterior cingulate, in fact all the areas associated with 'threat' and nociceptive processing as already discussed in previous chapters[1].

To back this precept that, 'central nervous system map changes are likely in all chronic pain', is the finding that the S1 maps of chronic low back pain sufferers have been shown to shift towards the leg maps (Flor 2002). Again, the worse the pain and the longer the pain is established the more likely a shift in the map will have occurred. Not only do the maps shift but they also show increased responsivity – meaning lots of neural activity compared to normal, when a given stimulus is applied. This fits with the generally lowered thresholds of chronic pain patients to sensory stimulation. In other words, light touch and firm pressure that would normally be deemed 'non-noxious' and 'slightly uncomfortable' respectably, are both processed and felt as pain i.e. allodynia and hyperalgesia.

Herta Flor's group (see Flor and Turk 2006) did some further work looking at cortical responses of chronic low back pain patients when they received painful 'electric' stimulation, first to a finger (non painful area) and second, to their back at the pain site and in the presence of their spouse – who had already been assessed as being either a 'solicitous' or a 'punishing' spouse! The spouses deemed solicitous are the ones that do everything for the sufferer, respond to their pain behaviour and generally reinforce it. The 'punishers' are the opposite, they tend to ignore their spouses' pain behaviour or castigate them for it, being generally unsympathetic.

You guessed it – solicitous spouse plus painful back stimulation equals greater cortical activation, when compared to, 'punishing' spouse or, stimulation of the hand/finger. The solicitous spouse not only reinforces their partners explicit 'pain behaviour' but also, influences the cortical pain processing too. You can get a similar result if you use verbal responses that encourage higher ratings of pain.

So, tip from the shop floor, if you want to really get chronic pain badly: find yourself a partner who drools over you and your pain, plus have around plenty of friends and therapists who encourage you to report your pain as high all the time. If you want pain to be long lasting and well imprinted, make a meal of it and get others help too…

The investigation of S1 changes in complex regional pain syndrome (CRPS) bucks the trend of phantom limb pain and back pain, in that the S1 representational areas related to the areas of limb pain appear to shrink rather than expand. I guess it

1 - Somatosensory maps that are topographically organised as in 'S1' are common throughout the nervous system, for example in the dorsal horn and the thalamus

could be 'efficient consolidation' as discussed for the motor pattern learning. Meaning, the more practice the circuits get at producing the pain, the fewer neurons and circuits needed. Further, Candy McCabe and colleagues (2003) have found that stimulation of the hand in some upper limb/hand pain affected CRPS patients gives them a simultaneous sensation in their face and for those with lower limb/foot symptoms – stimulation of the foot simultaneously produces sensation in the knee. This seems very similar to the observations of Ramachandran noted earlier and has a very strong scent of adjacent S1 maps coming into the 'processing' picture. When I think about this and my clinical experience over the years, I can come up with many patients who have reported proximal symptoms coming on at the same time as the discomfort being received from my manipulation of their 'distal' tissues. It was like a reversed referral pattern. For example, I can remember several 'Colles' fracture patients reporting building shoulder pain, while I was working away on their hand. Yes, these patients often do have horribly stiff and painful shoulders, but these ones didn't and hadn't reported any pain there, so it was a bit odd. I never had any that reported face sensations or symptoms though, that would have been cool. Maybe they did but they were too flummoxed to mention it. On the other hand, I can think of many patients who've reported symptoms in their back or their feet when I've been working on their shoulders or necks. Is their position on the couch aggravating back/foot? Or me compressing their spinal cord perhaps! Or maybe evidence of 'cortical map wandering syndrome'?

I recently read a small booklet called ***'Do no harm: The people who amputate their perfectly healthy limbs, and the Drs who help them'***, by Anil Ananthaswamy. I found it on the Amazon Kindle website. It tells the story of several people, who have had a lifelong desire to have one of their limbs amputated, because they feel that the limb just does not belong to them. They actually hate the limb in question and find it very hard to feel any sense of normality towards it. The term used for these people is 'Body Integrity Identity Disorder' or BIID. According to the booklet there are three BIID subdivisions: 'Devotees', those who are fascinated by or attracted to amputees, often sexually, but don't want amputations themselves: 'Wannabes', who strongly desire an amputation of their own and lastly: the 'Need-To-Be' group, who have a very real and very fierce desire for amputation.

Some of the sufferers go to great lengths to try and amputate their own limbs. I mention the story of the guy who featured on the front page of the 'Sun' newspaper in the nerve root chapter (NR 1) later. He tied himself to a fence by a railway track, stuck his leg on the line and had a train do the job. Others use tourniquets and then stick their legs in dustbins full of ice/dry ice in an attempt to damage the leg beyond repair, so that Drs have no choice but to amputate the limb. Clearly, elective amputations are not easy to come by, because most surgeons are understandably totally unwilling to even contemplate it. But the booklet reveals the story of 'David' who ends up finding a willing surgeon and goes on to describe the relief and happiness felt once the operation was done! It's a horrid yet spookily fascinating state of affairs.

With our recent greater understanding of 'body schema' and 'body image[1]', it seems that these folk find, from a very early age, that either one of their legs or an arm don't feel as if they belong to them, They come to despise the limb and it becomes an attached yet alien part of them. These people, let's be clear, have no pain, they just find the affected limb to be repulsive and not their own.

As I may have said before, it's a simple exercise to close your eyes and be aware of your body – your head, trunk, arms, legs and even more detail if you so wish; you feel it, you know it's yours, you know where it is and you feel the various pressures of gravity and the touch of your clothes upon it. Imagine for a moment though, that when you close your eyes, even though you know you have four limbs, one of them doesn't come to mind when you do this exercise? Or, if it does, it feels totally alien to you. Incredibly, these BIID sufferers appear to be able to delineate exactly where the amputation should take place on the limb, they can easily draw an exact line where 'they' finish and their alien limb starts.

Body image is an interesting area and one most of us think little about. But, it can become distorted. Think of anorexics who look thin, who are terribly thin, but inside their minds feel fat – their body schema to their mind belies the reality, to the extent that many continue in their terrible quest to try and correct it. It defies logic, but it happens. Think also of paraplegics, quadraplegics and 'brachial plexus injuries', who have limbs and parts of their trunk, that in terms of movement and sensation are cut-off from their central nervous systems by the nerve damage, most people don't think about it, but many of them still have a full body schema when they close their eyes. Melzack and Wall (1997) describe many such cases:

' 'CA', who'd been involved in an accident and avulsed his brachial plexus, described how his completely paralysed arm differed completely from what he felt. While the paralysed lifeless arm dangled by his side, he felt a phantom arm that was placed across his chest. The phantom never moved and the fingers were tightly clenched in a cramped fist with the nails digging into the palm. The entire arm felt 'as though it was on fire'.'

Melzack (1991) described a quadriplegic who felt that when he was lying on his back his legs were sticking up at right angles to his body, even though they were flat on the bed... There was an upper limb amputee whose phantom arm was constantly in a 90 degree abducted position – the patient would often go through doors sideways, so as to allow the phantom arm to go through without catching.

I now come to the clinic and my experience with patients who tell me their arm or leg feels fat, or heavy, or swollen, or somehow shorter than it should be. Yet under close scrutiny it clearly isn't! I can recall many patients who'd be convinced that their fingers were swollen and larger, their rings would no longer come off, or their hands were pink and hot, yet I just couldn't see or feel any difference. It's quite common I think and maybe more common in the more complex and long lasting pain states.

1 - *Body schema is the sense that the body is a whole, and body image is whether the individual 'likes' what they have.*

So, at an extreme end of the spectrum comes our sad friend CRPS (see Gifford 2013, for overviews of CRPS). These are the ghastly pain hypersensitivity problems that often do have swollen arms/legs and trophic changes – their skin is soft and flakey, their finger or toe nails are in poor health, their distal limbs may be bright pink, blue or very pale, they have sweating abnormalities and so forth. All these can occur at various stages in the development of the condition, but also, can often slowly abate too. However, some of the feelings may remain: feelings of swelling, the perception that the limb is swollen or fatter, there may be localised feelings of swelling in the fingers or toes and quite often, patients say that their limb just doesn't feel like it's their own. This isn't uncommon in many pain states.

Those who have worked, listened to and written about these patients in some detail are now revealing that they also have what's called 'Body Perception Disturbance' or BPD. And, like our BIID friends earlier often have a strong desire for their limb to be amputated. It seems that like the examples already given, these patients suffer from some kind of body image disturbance. Jenny Lewis and Candy McCabe (2010), have come up with an excellent BPD questionnaire and in their work they appeal to the general clinical community to give more attention to the presence of this phenomenon.

These CRPS patients report that their limb feels psychologically 'detached' from the remainder of their body, there's a sense of disowning – what they see when they reluctantly look at it is at odds with what it feels like; some parts may be grossly enlarged, others missing, they are often unsure of the posture or location of the limb and may hold it in odd positions which to them feel quite normal. Many not only disown their limb, they are unsurprisingly reluctant to even touch it and avoid thinking about it. Little wonder their cortical maps are so shrunk! None, or very little representational map – no ownership, no knowledge, no part of the body schema neuromatrix or neurosignature!

It would be very interesting to scan the brains of those with Body Integrity identity Disorder (BIID) to see if their somatosensory cortices revealed anything of significance. One would guess that their limb representation would be somewhat diminished.

The sense of our body – our 'body schema', seems to be driven by networks of neural activity in the brain. Melzack's 'neuromatrix', that produces the neurosignature, which in turn, via his sentient neural hub, produces the body self-image we all have. Melzack seems pretty convinced that the body neuromatrix is genetically determined and supporting this is the finding that many of those born without limbs can still have phantoms of full arms and legs, even though they have never experienced them. I must say, I find the notion of a genetically pre-determined arrangement of neurons that represent the body hard to imagine, without some environmental stimulus to direct things. I think the key, as far as Melzack is concerned, is that there is very basic genetic instruction for a 'body image' but that this requires the environment to act and guide its development. I still find it hard to see how this basic genetic instruction can somehow 'contain' a full four limbed body... Maybe I'm missing the point?

I slightly wonder if a few of those born without fully developed limbs actually do have 'full' body neuromatrices. And that their development is directed, not by their own body feedback, but by some kind of mirror neuron effect derived from observing normal limbs in others. This argument is countered by Melzack's observations of phantom limb pain in the very young infant – who've therefore not had the opportunity to observe others.

I have to say that in all these years since I've been interested in all this pain mechanism stuff, I am yet to come across anyone who has an interesting phantom experience. I've had plenty of patients who were keen to have their painful limbs amputated though!

Recently, Philippa had a patient who had no arms, due to her mother taking the drug Thalidomide back in the early 1960's. I got her to ask the lady whether she had 'phantom hands'? Apparently the lady responded, 'Of course I haven't, because I was born like this.' Sample of one – supports my hypothesis!

As I've been discussing, patient's reporting that their painful limb doesn't feel like it's their own, is surprisingly common. In my clinical experience it is very common with nerve root pain going into the arm or leg, for example.

So, to finish here, a note on getting a limb 'back' after or during a pain episode – the absolute key is normal use and to encourage the sufferer to try and avoid thinking about it as abnormal. This involves accepting the weird sensation as the 'new normal' and to try and get on making sure it's used normally. Never tell the patient that it will 100% come back to normal. It might not. Tell them it may or it may not, but give them the positives of other patients, who report the same thing and who just get on with it and accept it, versus the ones who let it screw them up. On a couple of occasions I have told patients about others, who let the problem get to them so much that they ended up wanting to have it amputated. Their problem was that the more upset they got with the feeling, the worse it became and the more upset they got with it again. Yet the opposite occurred for those who accepted it and welcomed the oddness as a part of them. I know it's not good CBT to 'tell' patients like this, but early on, in the acute and sub-acute phases, I think it is, so long as it's not the only thing done and it's done in a very positive way.

While rather blunt, the bottom line is: if it's going to go, it'll go – so best to get on with it… and, if you just get on with it and don't let it bother you… it's far more likely to go!

Chapter 19.6
Cortical Reorganisation: Paul Bach-y-Rita

'The most terrifying words in the English language are: I'm from the government and I'm here to help.'

Ronald Reagan

I'd promised I'd mention Paul Bach-y-Rita (PBR). Why? Because he was way ahead of his time with regards to neuroplasticity and there's a great deal that's of practical relevance to pain treatment and management stemming from his work.

For this story I rely heavily on Norman Doidge's excellent book: The Brain That Changes Itself and a book by Sandra and Matthew Blakeslee called: The Body has a Mind of its Own. If you have a chance, read them both. I would also suggest viewing the YouTube video: http://www.youtube.com/watch?v=7s1VAVcM8s8

PBR made a simple observation: that in nervous systems, all sensory information is made of the same stuff – mere patterns of impulses. To quote him from the video:

> *'We don't see with the eye, we don't hear with the ears, all that goes on within the brain... If I'm looking at you, the image of you doesn't get beyond my retina, from there to the brain it's pulses...pulses along nerves, well those pulses aren't any different from the pulses from the big toe. It's the way the information it carries, and the frequency and pattern of pulses... and so if you can train the brain to extract that kind of information then, you don't need the eye to see, you can have an artificial eye...'*

His first insight occurred in the early 1960's when studying visual processing in the cat's brain. The researchers he was with showed a cat an image and they noted visual processing areas would fire impulses in the brain, but when one of them touched the cat's paw accidentally, the visual area fired again. They then tested sound, the same thing happened – the so called 'visual' area responded and processed other sensory modalities[1]! PBR reasoned that if all sensory inputs were ultimately 'transduced' into impulses, then any part of the cortex should be able to process whatever electrical signals were sent to it. He started looking for 'exceptions' to standard neurology which back then, as I've already said, was dominated by one function, one location and the dogmatic insistence on 'fixed' adult wiring, eschewing any considerations of adult plasticity ever being possible. PBR was certain this was wrong and like Merz, set out to show the establishment that a review of their position was essential. I kind of know what they felt like when I was banging on to physiotherapists about 'central mechanisms' to better explain chronic pain in the mid 1990's. My mate Mick Thacker was on the same planet as me back then too and I'm sure he felt the same way. Pat Wall – same!

PBR believed that given the opportunity, a blind person could 'see' by using another form of sensory stimulus. He proposed and went on to prove that skin and its touch receptors could substitute for the retina – both being two dimensional 'sheets' covered in sensory receptors. It's worth going to YouTube to see the original machine he produced. (Site address above)

He adapted an old dentist chair and on the back rest he put around 400 small mechanical solenoids, to stimulate the subject's back. Each solenoid had a little almost bullet-shaped plunger, that when activated moved forward to press into the

1 - *I hope you can you see why it's so daft to allocate areas of the brain to specific functions like the Hashmi et al. (2013) lot did for acute and chronic pain – discussed and described in the last chapter!*

subject's skin. They were arranged in rows on a sheet that the sitting subject's back came into contact with when they settled in the chair. All the 400 stimulators were routed to a camera, such that when it was focused on a particular object it caused the solenoids to press a pattern relevant to the object into the person's back. In the YouTube film, the blind subject moves the camera around to 'look' at an old fashioned phone that has the receiver taken off and placed to the right of the phone. As he moves the camera around he takes in the various stimuli and very quickly goes, 'It's a phone and the receiver is to the right.' The best way to think of how this works is to imagine someone outlining an object on your back with their finger and then having to guess what it is.

Earlier in the YouTube film it highlights a man called Roger, who had been totally blind for thirty years. This fellow was 'seeing' with the modern equivalent of the dentist chair, solenoid stimulator mat and a camera! The stimulator has been refined to a thin, flat, 3cms square plate that was placed on the tongue. The plate has a great many little stimulatory electrodes and is connected to a bank of three very small digital cameras strapped to the forehead. The digital image from the camera now makes an 'electrical drawing' on the tongue via 625 fine little stimulators. Think of little pulses and think that the tongue has far better sensitivity and tactile discriminatory power than the skin on the back. With lots of practice the results are astonishing. The film shows Roger, blind for thirty years, throwing tennis balls accurately into a dustbin from about 7-8 paces away. It shows how he can see playing cards and know them and also be able to move around a room following parallel lines. Roger of course had to practice a great deal in order to be able to do this.

What's intriguing here is that with practice the brain shifts from two dimensions to three, adding depth and more perceptual complexity. This 'sensory substitution' means that the brain decodes skin/tongue sensation and turns it into pictures – the 'touch' related areas of the brain can now process visually. Or do the 'touch' inputs from the tongue get processed in the visual cortices too, are they passed over there? The answer is yes they do. PBR's research team scanned totally blind subjects who were using the tongue-camera and showed clear activity in their visual cortices. The touch information now processed 'as vision' and, to those researchers when interviewed, they actually feel it should be classed as vision.

As PBR said, 'We see with our brains not with our eyes'. He went on to develop 'electric feeling gloves' with NASA, to be used by astronauts, but they also helped leprosy sufferers. These gloves have sensors on the outside and send impulses, about the object being touched, to areas of the skin on the patients upper arm or torso that are unaffected by the disease and that have normal sensation. Leprosy sufferers, who hadn't had normal hand sensation for twenty years, found that with around two hours of practice they could feel small cracks in the table! One said that he'd been able to touch and 'feel' his wife for the first time in twenty years. PBR makes the extraordinary point of how little input is needed to make something very real and for it to have many dimensions.

PBR's interesting story includes his father, Pedro, who had a massive stroke when he was 65 years old. The Drs and physiotherapists basically gave up on him as his condition 'stabilised' in the early months after being hospitalised. He was unable to speak and had a half body paralysis including one side of his face. The medical establishment had given up. Paul, 'blessed with ignorance' about any form of rehabilitation went to work with him by patiently repeating movements, going through rolling, crawling, all fours, to standing and crawling along walls. It seemed logical to go back to what he could do well and progress from there. Pedro carried on practicing on his own too, crawling on all fours and Paul just kept repeating and making things more difficult as he progressed. **The key was using normal life experiences as exercises[1].** (I've underlined this and put it in bold because, musculoskeletal physiotherapy needs to take this on board far more in my opinion.) PBR and his Dad also worked hard on speech and communication.

Pedro had been a scholar and a poet and after many months of rehab with Paul he started to want to write again, he had to relearn to type again, slowly and in stages. By the time he was 68 his recovery was excellent and he started to teach again, going on until retiring at 70 years old. He was active for seven more years after his stroke and continued to hike and travel until he died at 72. Remember, this was back in the early 1960's, when there were no such things as scans. Amazingly, Paul decided he wanted to find out about his father's brain and he got one of his colleagues to examine it. It showed a massive lesion from a stroke and gained the comment: 'How can anyone recover from such damage?' It seemed that his brain, even with such a massive loss of tissue was still able to re-organise, re-learn and recover. What better evidence for adult neuroplasticity?

Here are some important physiotherapy messages from this:

1. For recovery to occur the patient and the therapist need to be motivated and do a lot of repetition and practice. This is clear from Pedro but also, Moseley's two point discrimination training.

2. No one's going to be motivated unless the things they are doing seem relevant. Remember SALIENCE! Making something salient is down to physiotherapists learning to explain in language and terms the patient can run with.

3. Success breeds success too: a little progress can help and motivates one to do more.

4. Exercises must approximate, at the very least, real life activities. Good physiotherapists should always make sure the patient sees the functional relevance of an exercise. I have to say one of my favourite exercises to criticise here is 'VMO' training and oblique abdominal training. VMO stands for 'Vastus Medialis Obliquus', it also stands for maximum operating speed on an aircraft(V_{mo}) and vegetable marketing organisation! It's the muscle that is massive in many footballers – it's the muscle that works hardest when you lock out the knee under load, in the last few degrees of knee extension, as when you kick a football or climb a stair or a hill. Sorry to be facetious, but please can physiotherapy educators get more of a grip. Why? Because

1 - If you're interested – this is 'enactivism' in action!

exercises designed to work parts of muscles that never work in isolation are non-functional. In my experience those who seem to worship such focused muscle work largely miss the bigger picture.

5. Learning takes a long time and tends to come in quick, slow and, no-improvement phases. You have to keep going through the inevitable plateaus. Learning needs plateaus for what's called 'consolidation.' I draw the plateaus on my recovery graphs sometimes (see section 17), so patients know to expect slow progress or no progress at all from time to time.

6. Learning needs to be rewarding and fun. That means goal setting and goal achievement. It also requires attention and concentration. Find out how long your patients are capable of attending and concentrating for and start there, or even less, to make it easy. I slightly fear that skills of attention are being inexorably degraded given the flicking, changing, screen dominated quick-bite of information world we live in. Sitting reading a book for more than five or ten minutes is becoming a challenge for a great many. Just my opinion, to keep your attention going.

7. The senses can be 'rewired,' or better 'retrained'. You can see with your back, you can see with your tongue, you can relearn to feel through your hands by feeling through your trunk. PBR's father Pedro lost a great deal of his brain to stroke, he couldn't move or speak but with diligent and guided practice he recovered these functions. If these sorts of things can be learnt or recovered, surely habitual pain behaviour and pain processing can too. New more adaptive cell assemblies can be produced that actively and effectively compete with maladaptive ones. There's plenty of evidence for this now, let's embrace it and do it.

In the next chapter we now take a look at stress again, but this time it's chronic stress.

Section 19
Read what I've read

Ananthaswamy A. (2013) Do No Harm: The People Who Amputate Their Perfectly Healthy Limbs, and the Doctors Who Help Them. Amazon UK download.

Birbaumer N., Flor H., et al., (1995) The corticalization of chronic pain. In Bromm B. and Desmedt J.E. (Eds). Pain and the brain: From nociception to cognition. New York, Raven Press.

Birbaumer N.H., Lutzenberger W. et al., (1997) Effects of regional anesthesia on phantom limb pain are mirrored in changes in cortical reorganization. Journal of Neuroscience, 17:5503-5508.

Blakeslee S., Blakeslee M. (2007) The body has a mind of it's own: How the body maps in your brain help you do (almost) everything better. Random House. New York.

Chambers C.T., Craig K.D., Bennett S.M. (2002) The impact of maternal behaviour on children's pain experiences: an experimental analysis. Journal of Pediatric Psychology 27:293-301

Christensen M.F., Mortensen O. (1975) Long term prognosis in children with recurrent abdominal pain. Archives of Disease in Childhood 50:110-114.

Doidge N. (2007) The Brain that Changes itself. Stories of personal triumph from the frontiers of brain science. Viking. New York

Dworkin R. H. (1997). Which individuals with acute pain are most likely to develop a chronic pain syndrome? Pain Forum 6(2): 127-136.

Edelman G. (1994) Bright air, Brilliant fire: On the matter of mind. Penguin. London.

Edelman G. (2004) Wider than the Sky: The Phenomenal Gift of Consciousness Yale Univ. Press. New Haven.

Flor H., Birbaumer N. (2000). Phantom limb pain: cortical plasticity and novel therapeutic approaches. Curr. Opin. Anesth 13: 561-564.

Flor H. (2002) The modification of cortical reorganization and chronic pain by sensory feedback. Applied psychophysiology and Biofeedback:27 (3): 215-227.

Flor H., Turk D.C. (2006) Cognitive and learning aspects. In: McMahon S.B., Koltzenburg M. Wall and Melzack's Textbook of Pain 5th Edn. Churchill Livingstone. Edinburgh.

Gifford L.S. (2013) Topical Issues in Pain 3. CNS Press, Falmouth.

Hashmi J.A, et al., (2013) Shape shifting pain: chronification of back pain shifts brain representation from nociceptive to emotional circuits. Brain, 136:2751-2768.

Jancke L. (2009) The plastic human brain. Restorative Neurology and neuroscience: 27: 521-538.

Jenkins W.M. et al., (1990) Functional reorganization of primary somatosensory cortex in adult owl monkeys after behaviorally controlled tactile stimulation. J Neurophysiol 63:82-104.

Kandel E.R., Hawkins D.H. (1993) The biological basis of learning and individuality. Mind and Brain. W H Freeman and Company. New York.

Kandel E.R. (2006) In Search of Memory. The Emergence of a New Science of Mind. WW Norton and Company. New York.

Lewis J., McCabe C.S. (2010) Body perception Disturbance (BPD) in CRPS. Practical Pain Management: 60-66.

Main C. J., C. C. Spanswick (2000). Pain Management. An interdisciplinary approach. Churchill Livingstone. Edinburgh.

McCabe C.S. et al., (2003) Referred sensations in patients with complex regional pain syndrme type 1. Rheumatology 42:1067-1073.

Melzack R. and P. D. Wall (1996). The Challenge of Pain. Penguin. London.

Melzack R. (1991). The gate control theory 25 years later: new perspectives on phantom limb pain. Proceedings of the VIth World Congress on Pain. M. R. Bond, J. E. Charlton and C. J. Woolf. Amsterdam, Elsevier.

Moseley G.L., Wiech K. (2009) The effect of tactile discrimination training is enhanced when patients watch the reflected image of their unaffected limb during training. Pain 144:314-319.

Moseley G.L., Zalucki N., Weich K. (2008) Tactile discrimination, but not tactile stimulation alone, reduces chronic limb pain. Pain: 137,3 600-608.

Posner MI, Raichle ME 1997 Images of Mind. Scientific American Library, New York.

Ramachandran V.S., Blakeslee S. (1999) Phantoms in the Brain: Human Nature and the Architecture of the Mind. Fourth Estate. London.

Ramachandran V.S. (2012) The Tell-Tale Brain: Unlocking the Mystery of Human Nature. Windmill Press. London.

Satel S., Lilienfeld S.O. (2013) Brainwashed: The seductive appeal of mindless neuroscience. Basic Books. New York.

Waddell, G. (2004). The Back Pain Revolution. (2nd Ed). Churchill Livingstone. Edinburgh.

Section 20

CHRONIC STRESS

Chapter 20.1
On-going pain and maladaptive stress 1. Hyperactivity of the stress response

Back to 'stress' again and back to Hans Selye's General Adaptation Syndrome – the 'GAS' (see section 9).

Recall the three stages he described:

1. The stage of ALARM
2. The stage of RESISTANCE
3. The stage of EXHAUSTION

...and recall that the laboratory rats he observed when suffering ongoing stress, whether the stress was physical (toxicity from the injections, extreme exercise, ongoing high or low temperatures), or mental (him chasing them around every day, caged next to a cat...), ended up becoming sick and that some died.

When he examined them they typically demonstrated: enlarged cortex of the adrenal glands (the part of the gland that produces the stress hormone cortisol); bleeding stomach ulcers and withered lymph nodes and thymus glands – a sign of weakening immune response.

Selye (1982) recognised that animals and humans were often subject to ongoing stress and that for the most part they stayed healthy and coped – the stage of 'adaptation' or 'resistance' as he called it. He described his observations of this stage as *'In many instances the exact opposite of those that characterized the alarm reaction.'* He went on...

'For example, during the alarm reaction, the cells of the adrenal cortex discharge their secretory granules into the bloodstream and thus become depleted of corticoid-containing lipid storage material; in the stage of resistance, on the other hand, the cortex becomes particularly rich in secretory granules. In the alarm reaction, there is hemoconcentration, hypochloremia(decrease in concentration of chloride), and general tissue catabolism, whereas during the stage of resistance there is hemodilution, hyperchlormeia, and anabolism, with a return toward normal body weight.' (see Selye 1982).

'Curiously, after still more exposure to the noxious agent, the acquired adaptation is lost. The animal enters into a third phase, the 'stage of exhaustion', which inexorably follows as long as the demand is severe enough and applied for a sufficient length of time.'

Selye neatly likens the process to our whole lives...

'These three stages are reminiscent of childhood, with its characteristic low resistance and excessive response to any kind of stimulus, adulthood, during which the body has adapted to most commonly encountered agents and resistance is increased, and senility, characterized by loss of adaptability and eventual exhaustion, ending with death.'

The terms hemoconcentration and dilution he uses relate to the concentration of blood cells in the blood. Hyper and hypochloremia relate to the increase or decrease in chloride ions in the blood. Remember that Selye began his research and discoveries in 1936, the quotes above come from one of the last pieces he wrote before he died in 1982. What Selye was observing with hemoconcentration was an increase in white cells in the blood, particularly neurtrophils and macrophages. Accordingly, it seems that the release of cortisol **during acute stress** may help to promote the body's defence reactions, though Sapolsky (1994) is sceptical here and discusses immune system suppression at great length. Certainly the vast current stress biology literature favours immune suppression – that's why stress can make you sick or more vulnerable to being sick (see below). In fact Selye himself showed that the lymph tissue and thyroid glands were hugely diminished in size by on-going stress. That's all correct but it seems that low levels of cortisol may stimulate white cell production. Back in Selyes' day it was well known that therapeutic levels of steroid produced a marked suppression of the immune system and the scientific community used this fact to criticise Selyes' findings and ideas (good science!). But, therapeutic levels of drugs are often given in very high doses and this 'reasoning' may have been overlooked. Selye liked the notion that acute stress should enhance the body's defences but that ongoing stress (the stage of resistance) would gradually deplete that resistance. That the immune response gets depleted by stress is now strongly established.

Since Selye's time a massive amount of research has revealed a great deal more about the detrimental biological, physiological and psychological effects of ongoing stress. Selye was the pioneer, whose serendipitous find all those years ago led to the further unravelling of a psycho-somatic biology, its mechanisms and to the relatively new discipline of 'psycho-neuro-immnolology' (PNI) – which is rational and empirical mind-body stuff. I'd like to emphasise though that while the word 'stress' makes most of us think of mental pressure, it mustn't be forgotten that ongoing physical stress or even better, a combination of mental and physical stress, must always be considered.

The point is – that if you subject any animal to ongoing stress, it may adapt and cope for a while, but if it goes on beyond its coping capacity it will become weaker, less viable and more than likely sicken. The everyday pressures of our hunter-gatherer ancestors were more to do with basic hand-to-mouth survival – dealing with basic needs of shelter, food and water and raising a family. The adage 'stone-age-man-in-the-fast-lane' is often used to describe our current situation. We are living in very different times to our ancestors and those we evolved to cope with. Stressors back then were a whole lot different to those of today, I think you'd agree?

The stressors of the day now... Prolonged emotional and psychological over-load probably sums it up. Witness the 'tiz' that 'we' get into over seemingly minor, almost pathetic issues (if you're like me and 'think like a hunter- gatherer' and compare our current situation to theirs occasionally).

'I hate my shape… my buttocks sag too much, (the mirror's doing my head in).'

'What are the neighbours going to think?'

'I've waited twenty minutes now for the Dr.'

'Mel said I smelled, he said I had 'BO,' I'm devastated. I'll ask the Dr, urgently.'

'I've got impossible work targets.'

'I don't earn enough to pay for me TV license, me fags, me bottle of gin and me cat and dog food or the petrol for me BMW.'

'My youngest isn't doing very well at athletics, he keeps getting beaten by that Carl kid and they didn't pick him for the soccer team again, he's devastated and I'm going to need to see my therapist.'

'Mummy, do I need to see a therapist too?'

'It's time I got married and settled down.'

'I should never have got married I know now.'

'There's been another robbery and I'm not going down the town again, those thugs are everywhere.'

'Arghhh – traffic-jams, mortgages, deadlines and relationship problems, life's not worth living. Don't even mention politics...'

History will look back at this short age we live in and wonder what the hell went wrong I reckon. Say a little thank you for the amazingly clean and fresh water that comes out of the tap from time to time and try and reflect on how lucky we all are in the 'Western world'. Sounds a little partronising!

Good old Robert Salposky tunes it all in for us throughout his brilliant book:

'Junk Food Monkeys and Other Essays on the Biology of the Human Predicament'

Which is now called *'The Trouble with Testosterone and Other Essays on the Biology of the Human Predicament.'* The essays are fascinating, read them after you've read his *'Why Zebras don't get ulcers'* book if you're interested.

Back to the task...

On-going stress can cause disruption, or what's called 'dysregulation' of the stress system. Think about the classic stress response and we tend to think of 'fight-or-flight' – high alert, instant ready for action to save our skin. Imagine being in this state of heightened arousal nearly all the time and often for no obvious reason? A state of constant anxiety for no obvious reason is neatly termed 'floating anxiety'. Anyone with it is likely to have a 'dysregulated' stress response and their stress response is said to be 'hyperactive'.

That is pretty straight forward, we can all think of those twitchy edgy people who can't sit still, can't sleep, are constantly restless, have one track minds and so on and so forth. But, as we should all come to expect from biology, there's a response that is the exact opposite, down at the other end of the 'stress dysregulation' spectrum and here the stress response is said to be 'hypoactive'.

What's clear is that ongoing stress can lead to poor health, Selye's stage of 'exhaustion' and for many it can lead to disease or at least increased vulnerability to it. On-going stress reduces the efficiency of normal recovery processes, it weakens our normal 'coping' mechanisms and any vulnerability or susceptibility that we might have may express itself. Here I always think of a patient of mine who had an identical twin sister (I mentioned her before). She used to come to see me occasionally with various aches and pains, she wasn't arthritic but she was 'jointy' and she was prone to things like tennis elbow, plantar fasciitis, stiff shoulder, neck, back... but she got along pretty well. She talked about her sister who had full blown rheumatoid arthritis and was now in a pretty bad way with it (mid 50's). The point I'm making is that here are two people with the same genes but whose lives took different paths, one very stressful at the wrong time, the other though stressful at times, was altogether more comfortable and well balanced. The stressed sister's coping capacity was compromised and allowed the disease that they were probably both susceptible to – to express itself and go on to disable her.

So, not only does on-going stress weaken our capacity to cope, it also has the capacity to upset our normal stress response and 'dysregulate' it – which then may go in one of two directions, that is towards hyperactivity, where the normal stress response gets greatly amplified, or towards hypoactivity, where it is dulled.

An important consideration here is that on-going pain is an on-going stressor with plenty of potential for producing stress system dysregulation. The direction in which the stress system dysregulates for any given individual may well be down to long-established, early, or even genetic, predisposition.

Let's take a look in more detail:

Features of hyperactivity of the stress response

When I first started reading about stress, in the early to mid 1990's, 'hyperactivity' of the stress response was strongly linked to 'fight or flight' and the biology of adrenaline and cortisol – all the stuff that Selye was famous for bringing to the world's attention. The psychiatric literature called the type of mood disorder associated with high levels of cortisol and adrenaline and the 'fight or flight' response, 'melancholic depression' with the following clinical features:

(Think about your patients or yourself when you're under stress as you read through, it makes it more fun!).

- hyper-arousal and redirection of energy – can't sit still
- anxiety – queasy stomach, dry mouth, pounding heart
- ill at ease
- vigilance, becomes hyper-vigilance – always focused on the thing that's of concern.
- increased startle response, 'Oh you made me jump!' is our everyday experience here – but imagine it all the time
- insomnia
- cognition/thinking, attention and memory all obsessively focused on one thing, often with depressive ideas; poor concentration on other things; poor ability to memorise anything; and difficulty solving everyday problems

- excessive cautiousness and anxiety
- loss of interest in food, sex, hobbies, socialising, life... 'Look at him, used to be the life and soul of the party, he's become a chronic misery guts.'

Now note in addition the 'Features of stress' listed by Hans Selye. As you go down, again, think about how you react when you are stressed, as well as thinking about your patients!

- general irritability, hyper-excitation or depression
- pounding of the heart
- dryness of the mouth and throat
- impulsive behaviour, emotional instability
- overpowering urge to cry or run and hide
- inability to concentrate
- feelings of unreality, weakness or dizziness
- tendency to fatigue, loss of the joy in life
- floating anxiety – afraid but do not know exactly what we are afraid of
- emotional tension and alertness – 'wound-up'
- trembling, nervous ticks
- easily startled by small sounds
- high pitched nervous laugh
- stuttering and other speech difficulties
- bruxism – (grinding of the teeth, often at night)
- insomnia
- hypermobility – up and down all the time
- sweating a great deal
- frequent need to urinate
- diarrhoea, indigestion, queasiness, occasional vomiting
- migraine headaches
- premenstrual tension or missed menstrual cycles
- pain in the neck and lower back
- low or excessive appetite
- increase smoking, drugs
- nightmares
- neurotic behaviour
- psychoses
- accident proneness.

When I used to teach this stuff I'd ask the group what they felt when they were stressed, 'Think about how you feel before an exam, or something that makes you nervous?' I'd always tell them about how I felt before giving a lecture at a conference, 'Dry mouth, shits, fidgety, memory loss, fear of failure, desire to run away, tearful, increased smoking, loss of appetite, why the fuck am I doing this?... etc...'

Then I'd go, 'Hands up those of you who feel 'X' when you're wound-up?'

Where 'X' would be any of the features in the above lists.

What I really wanted to point out was that their stress 'reaction' and their symptoms of being stressed were not the same as those of the person next to them, or to that of their patients. One person might get a dry mouth, the next a headache or stiffness across their shoulders, others might get pounding of the heart and go all sweaty, others go for back pain and maybe the desire to eat a box of chocolates. The whole thing was quite revealing, but the key issue was that for some patients, whatever complaint they were presenting with, stress could amplify it or even add symptoms to their clinical picture. This will be discussed further in the 'Vulnerable Organism' section later.

Another thing I liked to emphasise was that, 'Just because you experience stress like you do, in your specific way, doesn't mean to say that others will be the same as you.' I'd also then say, 'And, just because you can bend forward and touch your toes and then put your forehead on your knees doesn't mean that everyone should be able too!'

It was also a good point in time to admit, that in the past, I had probably given many of the symptoms of stress a 'musculoskeletal' categorisation, when in fact they may well have been a part of that person's stress response.

Melancholic depression has been associated with chronically activated (hyperactivated) hypothalamic-pituitary-adrenal (HPA) and sympathetic axes. That means increased cortisol and adrenaline.

An increase in CRH (corticotrophin releasing hormone) levels (see section 15) and hence an increase in cortisol in the blood has been implicated in the following conditions:

(Again, think about your patients – many may have bits or 'hints' of these, and so do you and I!)

- anorexia nervosa
  (At a basic you and me level, when some of us are stressed we go off food and stop eating. I know that's not quite the same as the distorted body image that these individuals suffer, but it's a point about how stress can lead to loss of weight. It's called cachexia when associated with chronic illness states)
- panic anxiety
- obsessive compulsive disorder
- chronic alcoholism
- excessive exercising – associated with infertility and hypogonadism

  ('Don't blame me love, it's all the exercise…')
- premenstrual tension syndrome
- hyperthyroidism
  (Note symptoms here: increased metabolic rate, increased cardiac output,

hypertension, rapid pulse, increased sweating, intolerance of heat, insomnia, excitability, nervousness, irritability, weight-loss, sweaty palms and menstrual irregularities. A great many patients report that they're on some sort of thyroid drugs. It's a pity that medicine doesn't register a bit of a wider perspective and go beyond the isolated organ abnormality perspective. The bigger picture may well present a dysregulated stress system and stress response – with the potential for a multi-dimensional approach. That may mean offering help with coping and managing stress)

The wise stance is, that it's all far more than one or two chemicals and one or two pathways, but the underlying thing of importance is on-going stress and stress system dysregulation.

Let's now look at the diametrically opposite state.

Chapter 20.2
On-going pain and maladaptive stress 2. Hypoactivity of the stress response and a bit more

Features of Hypoactivity of the stress response

This is where on-going stress leads to a massive dulling of the stress response – not enough cortisol, not enough adrenaline. It's as if the stress response can't cope anymore, packs up and goes into hibernation, it becomes 'desensitised'. In the psychiatric literature a hypoactive stress response is associated with 'atypical depression'. When you review its features it doesn't seem particularly 'atypical' however. It turns out that there were two reasons for it being labelled 'atypical':

1. Historically it was first identified with its 'unique' symptoms after melancholic depression had been described, and...

2. Its response to the different classes of antidepressants that were available at the time was different from melancholic depression. Mono-amine oxidase inhibitors (MAOI's) worked, but tricyclic antidepressants didn't. Just so you know: MAOI's are obviously drugs that inhibit the activity monoamine oxidase, in so doing they prevent the breakdown of monoamine neurotransmitters, keeping levels of them high in the nervous system and therefore increasing their 'availability'. Put simply, MAOI's keep levels of the neurotransmitters adrenaline, noradrenaline, melatonin, dopamine and serotonin high in the nervous system! The chemicals of excitement! Let's boogie!

Take a look at the features of 'atypical depression':

(Again, amuse yourself and do a bit of self analysis and maybe think about your patients too?)

- hypoarousal – apathy, lethargy, passivity, can't be bothered, no energy, you've all been there and you probably combine it with...
- polyphagia – an abnormal desire to consume excessive amounts of food, yup, whole boxes of chocolates, digestives, éclairs, might as well finish the cake, one more drink, so that you...
- increase in weight and then you feel...
- fatigued and therefore...
- sleep all the time!

That's Sunday afternoon for most people.

A hypoactive stress response has been associated with the following disorders:

- seasonal depression
- chronic fatigue syndrome or TATT – tired all the time
- fibromyalgia
- hypothyroid conditions

(Here we are medicalising it nicely down to one chemical i.e. not enough thyroxine! Hence, patients on thyroid tablets! Thyroxine is a hormone that stimulates metabolism of course. So, the features of not enough thyroxine are: decreased metabolic rate, loss of hair, facial oedema, coarse dry skin and hair, complaints of cold due to increased body temperature, decreased perspiration, slow pulse, tiredness, slow thinking processes, lethargy, sleepiness, weight gain and menstrual irregularities and of course 'atypical depression' and importantly musculoskeletal pain!)

- some forms of obesity
- post traumatic stress disorder (PSD)
- vulnerability to autoimmune disease.

Hence, hypoactivity of the stress response – the HPA axis, means a decrease in measurable corticotrophin releasing hormone (CRH) and a subsequent decrease in circulating cortisol. Not enough cortisol equates to not enough control of inflammation or the immune system. Thus, 'hypoactivity' of the stress response is associated with development of 'auto-immune' related conditions like rheumatoid arthritis, multiple sclerosis, fibromyalgia and chronic fatigue. Atypical depression is common in human rheumatoid arthritis (RA).

Esther Sternberg's research

If you have time, it's worth reading...

'Putting the mind and body back together again', Chapter 4 in Esther Sternbergs' book: 'The Balance Within: The science connecting health and emotions'

Esther is one of the post-Selye pioneers of mind-body-body-mind biology, with a particular interest in understanding the brain and mind in relation to rheumatoid arthritis. Her book is a wonderful narrative of the history of mind-body-body-mind science and the state of the art here too. I'll summarise a little that's of interest from this chapter.

Researchers use various genetically pure 'strains' of rats to study disease. Two famous strains are 'Lewis' and 'Fischer' rats, 'Lewis' being susceptible to auto-immune diseases like RA and MS (multiple sclerosis). In RA, the immune system 'attacks' the joints and in MS, the myelin in the nervous system suffers and inflammation is generally poorly controlled in both. 'Fischer' strain rats are the exact opposite – they're resistant to auto-immune disease and they're highly resistant to inflammation. Through some wonderfully diligent research, Esther and her team discovered that the susceptibility and resistance were down to the relative reactivity of each strains stress response.

Lewis rats, being the 'susceptibles' had **dulled** HPA responses to streptococcus bacterial stressor material (protein from bacterial cell wall) they used to test this. In fact, the reaction to 'strep' cell wall would go on to produce RA in these rats! So, a dulled or 'hypoactive' HPA axis means less cortisol, or rather corticosterone for rats and therefore less control of inflammation and their immune responsivity.

In contrast, the resistant Fischer rats were found to have marked **reactivity** of their HPA axis and therefore plenty of corticosterone to dampen any immune/ inflammatory response.

Research into the **behaviour** of these rats, when stressed, went as predicted from observing their stress responses. Fischer rats showed high stress-behaviours and Lewis low, remaining relaxed and unperturbed. I hope you can see I'm making a link between, the Fischer strain of rat and the hyperarousal/melancholic depression 'attributes' in humans and between, the Lewis strain of rat and the hypoarousal/ atypical depression human attributes.

So, here's some interesting but slightly tenuous links, Lewis rat = high susceptibility to RA and they tend to be laid back, lethargic, apathetic can't be bothered kinds of rat. In human RA sufferers some workers have noted a link to atypical depression, in other words, to the lethargic, apathetic and 'the can't be bothered' kind of human. RA however isn't as simple as this, so great care required with this over-simplistic view!

A key thing that came from the research was that interleukins, like IL-1, were found to be major stimulants to the HPA axis. The pathway runs like this:

Expose the organism to a stressor – for Esther's team it was strep bacteria cell wall protein, but it could just have easily been a real infection or a tissue injury – an inflammatory/immune response kicks off. This then causes the release of interleukins into the circulation, which enter the brain via the blood-brain barrier and soon reach interleukin receptors on CRH neurones in the hypothalamus. These CRH neurones in turn fire and get the HPA axis ball rolling, with subsequent release of corticosterone/cortisol from the adrenal cortex into the circulation.

In Lewis rats there's a genetically determined sluggish HPA response and this is found to be due to the lack of responsive CRH neurons. In the Fischer rats the CRH neurones make too much. So, if you don't want RA or any auto-immune disease – pray that you've inherited a tendency to poor CRH responsiveness and a dull HPA axis? Must be a good thing surely?

Well, think about nature: a dulled out, lethargic, can't be bothered, chilling in the sun type rat soon gets scooped up by a hungry Buzzard and that's the end of that. Much better to be the flighty, cautious always on the look-out type? Well, not really, go too far that way and you just can't settle to get anything productive done! Somewhere in between may be best?

There's another thing with regards the low cortisol, chilled, lethargic and dulled out characteristic. Cortisol/cortisone is vital in that it controls excessive immune activity. Too much immune and inflammatory activity can kill you very quickly; inflammatory chemicals damage epithelial cell walls causing them to leak; with a massive loss of fluid from the circulation; rapid loss of blood pressure and death! The condition is called 'septic shock' and it requires early and quick recognition and a massive dose of steroid to counter.

Let's have a pause for clinical reasoning's sake...

> We are all on a stress responsivity continuum – stressy, jumpy, tense and wound up, on the toilet all the time at one end, lethargic, sleepy, dozy, overweight and can't be bothered down the other. With the evidence from the Lewis and Fischer rat experiments, there's probably a significant genetic component to it, or more accurately, a genetically determined pre-disposition to being pushed one way or the other on the stress continuum by what life throws at us. My own tendency is towards the stressy, anxious end but I've also a bit of the can't be 'arsed 'give-up- and-die' bit from time to time too. Put me under pressure for a long period and I lose a little weight and look for an occasional roll-up rather than eat. You might go the other way.
>
> A patient with ongoing pain who has a tendency to 'hypoactivity' is going to take one hell of a lot of motivation to get going, whereas the hyper may overdo it! That's the theory, but it's not my clinical experience, I'm getting flashes of 'hyper' type patients and think that they've been the most difficult of all! They try what you suggest, if it doesn't work straight away, that's it, or, they do it, it makes them ten times worse and, that's it!
>
> For the 'hypo' getting some motivation, excitement and novelty going may be hard, but it's got to be a good thing. Don't start them off on the frightening fairground rides or bungee jumping followed by the boot-camp! Start easy build slowly, graded exposure!
>
> For the 'hyper', they can't keep their mind in one place for a moment. So, it's chill/relax/yoga/meditation, leave the job, the wife/husband and ride off into the sunset to find an adrenaline-free paradise. Again, while 'relaxation-exposure' might be the best thing to do in theory, it is in fact the last thing they want to do and when they are persuaded to try, they're hopeless and soon give up. 'I went to the yoga class like you said Louis, Oh the bloody time dragged, all I could think about was all the things I had to do. Five minutes of that and my head was done in and the bloody class went on for an hour and a half. I was a gibbering idiot by the end.' 'Oh, well, maybe we could do some Tai-chi together?' These are the patients that it's a major achievement to get them to do diaphragmatic breathing for more than 3 or 4 breaths. I'm being facetious, but you should know what I mean. Just think of the 'far end of the spectrum' type patients.

In summary, it's worth thinking about some of the physiological effects of stress system dysregulation:

For ongoing **hyperactivity:** think suppression of the immune system and also of inflammation and the healing processes. As already discussed, the clinical utility of this is that stress slows or puts healing 'on-slow down' or 'on-hold'. The earlier stress chapters provide plenty of evidence here. And this can be shown to the patient, as a start to get them to see the importance of winding-down. A suppressed immune system may also result in an increased risk of infection. Also, and again as already discussed, think ongoing stress means high ongoing circulating cortisol and if it drifts on for long,- this means 'catabolic' or 'breakdown' of body tissues. For example, muscle wasting and weakness, bone thinning as in osteoporosis and poor skin, hair and nail health. Many ongoing 'pain' sufferers report feelings of 'weakness' and describe 'heavy leaden legs' when they do even modest exercise. This catabolic aspect may well be a factor in the back of our minds, although the best view to take is one of disuse and deconditioning for the patient.

For ongoing **hypoactivity:** think about autoimmune disease like RA, less cortisol means less control of the immune system and the healing system perhaps too. These processes may run amok and therefore be less efficient as a result?

It wouldn't surprise me if there wasn't a link here to osteoarthritic inflammatory flare-ups as well. Stress researchers tend to think of OA as purely mechanical, or wear and tear. To me, many patients presenting with 'degenerate' backs, necks (for example, spondylosis), knees, hips etc. have periods of relative stiffness but are comfortable; they can also have periods of flare-up, which are very likely to relate to localised inflammatory flares in the joints, in many ways similar to RA. My observation of a great many of my patients over many years, is that they go through long lasting and repeating flares of pain-on and awful for a while; followed by pain-off for a while and later, the whole pattern repeating. Eventually however, their joint settles down and becomes quite manageable, perhaps a bit noisy, of limited range, stiff to get moving after resting and obviously enlarged and often deformed (think knees, feet and hands!). To me, this is almost a milder version of the pattern of RA, where flares go on and on for many years, eventually leading to the classic inflammatory 'burn-out', leaving the joints horribly deformed and 'arthritic' but far less painful. I'm thinking of the classic 'swan neck' hand deformities in RA and of a patient with the disease, who continued to play the piano throughout her disease process. She could still play very well, even with marked swan neck deformity in her hands, which was quite incredible. She was lucky to have large hands, which may have helped a bit.

Again, I plead for long term observational research here so that we have a much better knowledge of 'natural history'. I've been lucky in a sense that I live in a relatively small community and 'following-up' patients happens all the time – in the town, pubs, on the water, beaches, golf-club etc.

The influence of stress and emotional state on joint pain 'flares' in OA and RA seems to be quite strong. Certainly emerging links of increased pain and on-going pain and disability to psychosocial factors, would support this. Biologically increased and on-going stress (psychosocial) may well equate to loss of control of inflammation through the 'hypo' dysregulation effect. It may not be, but hey, why not, it's worth thinking about and it gives us a possible 'explanatory' route in with the patient, if that is deemed helpful or necessary. It gives us a good reason for a possible management strategy that would help i.e. to deal better with the obvious psychosocial factors you've picked up from your ABCDEFW (psychosocial evaluation).

If OA, then why not other related conditions like the 'enthesopathies' – the ligament/ tendon bony attachment site problems, whose underlying 'cause' could well be uncontrolled low grade inflammation? An 'enthesis' is a tendon or ligament to bone attachment site. Think of conditions like plantar fasciitis, epicondylitis, bursitis and tendinitis – like the focal tenderness of the tendo-achilles insertion on the calcaneum. I'm also thinking of the vast number of localised pains in the region of the knee medial or lateral collateral ligaments, that are often associated with early degenerative changes. The warning though is to not latch on to thinking that just reducing an individuals' stress is all that's necessary! Make it a possible part of overall management when appropriate. Let's not be like the pressured GP's who after a five minute consultation go, 'Mrs Jones, you're stressed, you need to relax more, I'm going to prescribe you these tablets that will help you become so spaced out you won't know what day it is, or that you ever had a problem...'

As I've highlighted, a major thing here is that we should note the great individual variation in response to on-going stressors in our lives. What's your tendency towards – hypo? Hyper? Or have you got a touch of both? Doesn't it depend on the way you've been stressed, how long it's been going on, the type of stress; maybe the way those around you react to your situation is a factor and so forth.

What does pain and the accompanying stress do to a person?

This isn't going to be a huge literature review or expert summary, just some comments in the context of on-going stress to maybe make us think.

Pain clearly limits life in some way and is bound to have some kind of psychological impact, more especially if it goes on and on and doesn't get better when they said it should! We are all different of course. For example, in the early acute phase of a pain problem, if a patient finds the experience particularly stressful, they may well be starting the process of stress system dysregulation. Past experiences of stress or an on-going 'stressy' life may be factors too. Think Selye's stage of 'resistance'. We can cope with on-going pressures for a while, but eventually the systems 'batteries' run down and we enter the 'exhaustion' stage. Remember too, the parallel with Robert Post's work on manic depression and the concept of 'kindling'? (See section 6). Here, early psychological stressors were found to lead to a mild depressive episode that soon cleared, but as time went on so the episodes became more and more frequent, lasted longer and often began for no reason at all. It seems that past stressors had left their mark, influencing how future stressors would be dealt with. The strengthening, but maladaptive mental-pathology circuit had 'kindled' from small, seemingly modest beginnings, into something that was much more problematic – a thing that had a mind of its own. The stages of alarm – to resistance – to exhaustion can be applied here too. Earlier, when I discussed kindling, I noted the similarities to the way chronic back pain can sometimes develop. For some of us, it may be that we grow better at coping, almost hardened to the stress of life, but for others it's the reverse – we become more and more vulnerable.

The yellow flag/psychosocial literature states that a significant predictor of poor outcome is psychological distress associated with the pain. For example, in my clinical work over the years I have found anger and blame, in relation to accidents, a very common and particularly difficult issue. Whiplash related pain patients, often years down the line are still angry with the 'idiot' who went into the back of them.

'They got out of their car and shouted at me, they didn't even apologise.' Is a frequent comment that sums it up. Many RSI sufferers are tormented with anger and even hate directed towards their managers; for forcing them to work at high levels for long hours, for very little pay and little appreciation. The atmosphere coming from inside these patients' heads can be very caustic. Imagine what their stress systems have been doing for so long!

I vowed long ago, that if I ever run into the back of someone I will get out of my car (if I can!), speak nicely to the driver whose car I hit and apologise, sincerely. Sod the insurance companies and lawyers who tell us to 'never admit liability'. I want to do the decent human thing and say sorry. I know that the simple gesture of apology can be so very important. I'd even go as far as to use the word 'healing'.

Anger associated with injury and long lasting pain is very destructive. I got my first insight of the research into this by reading:

Fernandez and Turk's 1995 paper: The scope and significance of anger in the experience of chronic pain.

But the best chapter of all on how to deal with distress and anger (and all yellow flag issues too) is:

Main and Watson's 2002 chapter in Topical Issues in Pain 3, 'The distressed and angry low back pain patient'.

On-going pain becomes more and more puzzling and more and more a case for concern for a great many. Time itself can act as a positive feedback for pain, the longer it goes on, the more distress, the more pain.

Here's yet another list! This time it's of sources of patient stress/distress, related to you, the clinician and your treatment. It's for patients with on-going pain; but it rounds on us to think of these things early on in acute problem management, to prevent them being a part of the problem later.

The patient may have frustration, anxiety, distress, and be demoralised because of:

1. Ineffective treatments.

2. Expectations and hopes of treatment success being dashed, by lack of response, or being made worse.

3. Cocky practitioners offering confident cures – but failing...

4. Confusion from multiple Drs/practitioners giving a whole host of different reasons or different diagnoses for the pain. 'The Dr said it was arthritic and I had disc problems, the chiropractor said my pelvis was badly out and the physiotherapist said I had core instability.'

5. Complex and potentially frightening medical language that hasn't been explained properly.

Like 'spondylosis', 'degeneration', 'chondromalacia patellae' which is one of my favourites; but best of all is 'Osgood Schlatter's disease' when given to a budding your soccer player, who's up for a trial at Plymouth Argyle football academy in two months time, 'Dad, how did I catch that?'

6. Lack of diagnoses and poor explanations.

7. Being told nothing is wrong, with the implication that you're making a fuss or making it up – that it's all in the head.

8. Inappropriate advice to rest, or to stop weight-bearing – especially the therapist or Dr who says 'stop', 'don't' and 'prescribes with authority' all the time.

   The only way you'll realise you're doing it is if you start listening, hearing and analysing yourself! Clinical reasoning talks about 'metacognition' – the ability to think about your own thinking and reasoning. When I first got into understanding pain all those years ago, I realised that my constant 'pain' talk and my constant requests for the patient to tell me about their pain, had to be stopped. It was difficult and I had to keep reflecting on the words I was using, as well as the words I was about to use. In more patient orientated styles of management, that include 'behavioural' and 'reinforcement' techniques of communication, a big change is often required. I am still learning, but to begin with I had massive thoughts about how I needed to phrase things with the patient. Thinking about your own style of communication, what you say, how you say it and how you respond to the patients thoughts and words is a big step in the right direction and, probably the most significant step to improvement a clinician will ever make – once they have mastered good basic skills!

9. So, a great deal of the time we may inadvertently be saying things that can be quite detrimental. Making the patient worse through what you say and through your treatments, what you're doing, is called 'iatrogenesis.' In medicine, the word is generally used to mean an 'inadvertent adverse effect' of the treatment given. It's very much linked to physical (surgery)/ physiological (drugs) issues. For example, the patient who had a hip replacement and ended up with a drop-foot because the surgeon nicked or over-stretched their sciatic nerve. 'Whoops, sorry, that was inadvertent of me.' For us, it may well be too much force too quickly, but mostly it's the subtle communication related 'iatrogenics' that slip in. Take some time out to read the following, and note that if you want the Topical Issues in Pain series cheap, they're now available as e-books for around £2-3.00 each.

Suggested reading on this from Topical Issues in Pain series:

- *Topical Issues in Pain 1: Chapters 8 and 9 by Suzanne Shorland; and chapter 13 by Vicki Harding.*
- *Topical Issues in Pain 2: Chapter 7 by Toby Newton-John.*
- *Topical Issues in Pain 4: Chapter 5 by Caroline Hafner*
- *Topical Issues in Pain 5: Chapters 3 and 4 by Steve Goldingay; Chapter 6 by Jennifer Klaber Moffett, and Chapter 7 by Penny Mortimer.*

On the topic of more classic medical 'iatrogenesis' or, inadvertent detrimental effects caused by drugs, which biologically should be viewed as potential chemical toxins and therefore 'stressors' to the system I've just Googled: 'Death rate from NSAID's' and got this:

The July 1998 issue of The American Journal of Medicine stated the following:

"Conservative calculations estimate that approximately 107,000 patients are hospitalized annually for nonsteroidal anti-inflammatory drug (NSAID)-related gastrointestinal (GI) complications and at least 16,500 NSAID-related deaths occur each year among arthritis patients alone. The figures of all NSAID users would be overwhelming, yet the scope of this problem is generally under-appreciated."

And again a year later (June 1999) in the prestigious New England Journal of Medicine there is a similar statement:

"It has been estimated conservatively that 16,500 NSAID-related deaths occur among patients with rheumatoid arthritis or osteoarthritis every year in the United States. This figure is similar to the number of deaths from the acquired immunodeficiency syndrome and considerably greater than the number of deaths from multiple myeloma, asthma, cervical cancer, or Hodgkin's disease. If deaths from gastrointestinal toxic effects from NSAIDs were tabulated separately in the National Vital Statistics reports, these effects would constitute the 15th most common cause of death in the United States. Yet these toxic effects remain mainly a "silent epidemic," with many physicians and most patients unaware of the magnitude of the problem. Furthermore the mortality statistics do not include deaths ascribed to the use of over-the-counter NSAIDS."

Now, how many deaths per year from 'recreational' drugs that so get the headlines? Let's consider ecstasy because of all the powerfully emotional parent campaigns to 'stop its use' and make young people 'more aware'. I couldn't agree more, but from a brief internet search, comparisons of ecstasy deaths with those that Dr's and the pharmaceutical industry produce 'inadvertently' are worth noting.

- for ecstasy, government statistics for the UK between 1993 and 2006 show an average of between 17 to 33 deaths per year depending on the type of ecstasy used

- for NSAIDs, it's 1,200 deaths per year, so that's a cool 36 fold worse than ecstasy

- NSAIDs apparently cause approximately 3500 hospitalisations and 400 deaths from ulcer bleeding per annum in the UK in those aged 60 years and above.

We don't allow euthanasia in this country yet, do we? Hmmm!

My point is, that on-going stress/distress can come from many other quarters. Think in all dimensions and go back in time too. Don't forget, as noted here with NSAID's and ecstasy, toxicity is a stressor to the system. Not just the drugs we're prescribed but those we like to use recreationally too!

Figure 20.1 neatly sums the pain-stress relationship. Follow round the flow chart.

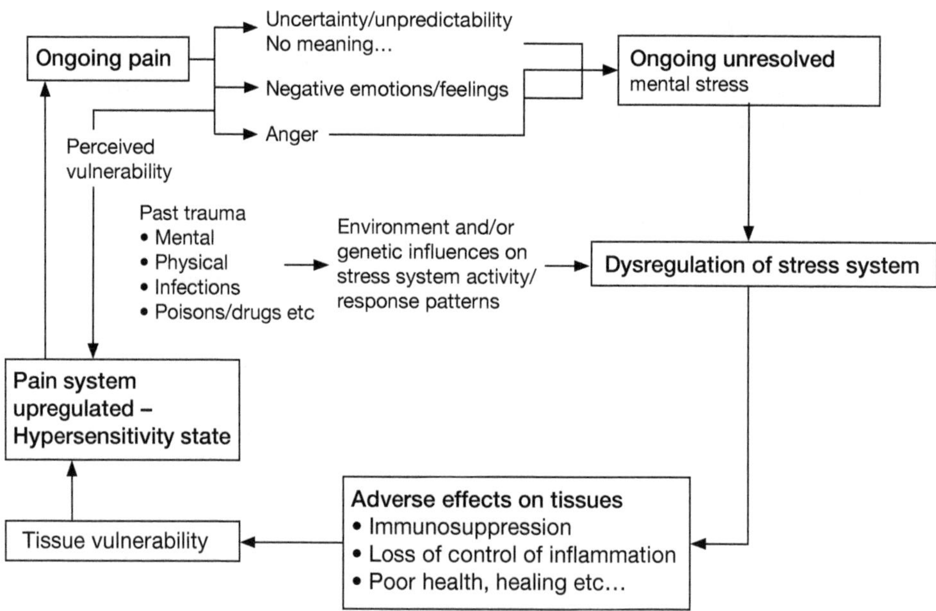

Figure 20.1 The pain-stress relationship

'On-going pain' in the top left corner can be associated with uncertainty and unpredictability, with negative emotions and feelings and not uncommonly with anger too as discussed. There are many more issues too – use the useful 'yellow-flag' mnemonic ABCDEFW to review other possibilities here (see later chapters). The pain sufferer may well have on-going and unresolved mental stress related to their life and to the stress of the on-going pain as well. As time goes on, the patient's capacity to cope dwindles and they slide from coping (physically and mentally) to the stage of resistance, to the stage of 'exhaustion' where their coping capacity is at its limits – mentally and physically. Eventually, the stress system dysregulates as a result of the downwardly spiralling process. Thinking in terms of what's been discussed above, this can result in; immunesuppresion, loss of control or poor control of healing and inflammation, weakened tissues, and poor health and so forth. The 'body-sampling' areas of the brain soon get to know that the body is deconditioned and vulnerable. The result: the pain-on system gets up-regulated, the pain-off system down-regulated. The patient becomes 'hypersensitive' and prone to new pains, spreading pains and pains that are a fantastic puzzle to those who want to find straight-forward answers in the tissues that hurt.

Note, in the smaller print in the middle of the chart are 'other' factors that may be further factors in priming the dysregulation of the stress response. Past traumas – think mental and physical factors every time. Think significant illnesses in the past – like infections and toxicity too. Underlying all this are genetic factors that may play some part in determining our relative stress response direction and our relative reactivity.

Section 20
Read what I've read

Fernandez E., Turk D.C. (1995) The scope and significance of anger in the experience of chronic pain. Pain 61: 165-175.

Goldberger L. and Breznitz S. (1993) Handbook of stress: Theoretical and clinical aspects 2nd Ed. The Free Press. New York.

Gifford L.S. (2013) Topical Issues in Pain volumes 1, 2, 4 and 5. CNS Press, Falmouth.

Main C.J., Watson P.J. (2013) The distressed and angry low back pain patient. In Gifford L.S. (Ed) Topical Issues in Pain 3. Sympathetic nervous system and pain. Pain management. Clinical effectiveness. CNS Press, Falmouth.

Martin P. (1997). The Sickening Mind. Brain, behaviour, immunity and disease. Harper Collins. London. Simply brilliant.

Sapolsky R. (1997) Junk Food Monkeys and Other Essays on the Biology of the Human Predicament. Headline Book Publishing. London. Now called 'The trouble with Testosterone and other essays on the biology of the human predicament.' Into stress and understanding life? These essays are a must read!

Sapolsky R. (1994) Why Zebras don't get Ulcers. A guide to sress, stress related diseases and coping. Freeman and Company. New York. The best book ever on stress and humans.

Selye H. (1978) The Stress of Life. McGraw Hill. New York.

Selye H. (1993) History of the stress concept. In Goldberger L. and Breznitz S.(Eds.) Handbook of stress: Theoretical and clinical aspects 2nd Ed. The Free Press. New York. (Note that Selye actually died in 1982, which was when the first edition of this book came out. Selye's chapter was clearly added for this 1993 edition and he tells his own story beautifully).

Sternberg E.M. (2001) The Balance Within: The Science Connecting Health and Emotions. Palgrave. New York. (Esther's father worked with Selye in the University of Montreal – in the 1950's and she knew him well as a youngster).

Thayer R. E. (1996) The origin of everyday moods: Managing energy, tension and stress. Oxford University Press. New York. A great perspective on mood and stress and one of the better self-help books which don't help type books!

Watkins A. (1997) Mind-body medicine. A clinicians guide to psychoneuroimmunology. Edinburgh, Churchill Livingstone. Good for nerds!

Whybrow P. C. (1997) A mood apart. A thinker's quide to emotion and its disorders. Picador. London.

Nerve Root

Sections 1-5

Section NR 1

PERIPHERAL NERVE MECHANISMS

Chapter NR1.1
Adaptive and maladaptive pain and the nerve root

Clinically the notion of maladaptive pain has become of central importance to how I tackle pain problems. When assessing and observing patients I also 'background' reason, meaning it's ticking away in my head, about maladaptive or adaptive in relation to things like inflammation, the patients reaction and 'behaviour' in relation to their problem, their attitude and understanding of it and so forth. It's a simple helpful/unhelpful dichotomy that some may question but that I think is of vital importance.

For example, thinking about a patient's pain: if it is maladaptive, it is unhelpful and hence my clinical role might be to do my best to help the patient get rid of the pain as quickly as possible. Or, and just as importantly, if the tissues are safe to start loading – my role is to begin showing the patient how to return to functioning and moving normally again. It's easy, usually very helpful and important to teach the patient about adaptive and maladaptive pain – simply because most patients (and often most clinicians, therapists and health workers) response to pain is that it means stop what you are doing, be careful and avoid it. It also can, understandably, mean something is wrong and needs diagnosing and fixing and that the worse the pain, the worse the problem must be.

A common patient response is:

'I've been given pain killers by the Dr, that doesn't fix anything, pain killers just mask the pain and are not going to make anything better. In fact, if I lose the pain without it being fixed, I'll damage it further and make it even worse.'

The result is that a great many patients don't like, or see the point of taking painkillers. As we've already seen in the placebo chapter – such a 'they won't help me' attitude is likely to significantly diminish or even reverse the effectiveness of any painkiller via the nocebo mechanism. A big clinical point is, that the brain of the patient has to be set up to accept and welcome a pain killer and, for that matter, any input or therapy that is attempting to control pain!

The public notion that something needs 'fixing', while understandable, is also problematic. Figure NR1.1 shows a slide that I used for a great many years when trying to explain the biomedical model in my lecture programmes. I often still use it with patients.

Graph A, shows the biomedical model in all its glory – where there is a direct relationship between the amount of symptoms and the amount of pathology. It's how any engineer would design a fault finding system – the bigger the problem the bigger the alarm. Graph B, is medicine at its best and how the public like to think about it – like a car mechanic! Fix the cause of the problem and the symptoms get better. It works reasonably well if you've got Syphillis or a broken leg! But even here, the common observation of any clinician working in acute services is that severe trauma or disease often passes with surprisingly little pain for the amount of tissue abnormality. Our 'detection' and reporting system is pretty smart, but it's definitely fallible. Graph C, shows how symptoms can get worse and worse, even though the pathology may be getting better and better! That seems crazy, but, (and a big but), it's the situation which a great deal of the work us 'aches and pains' clinicians, see every day. From my observations it seems that clinicians readily accept

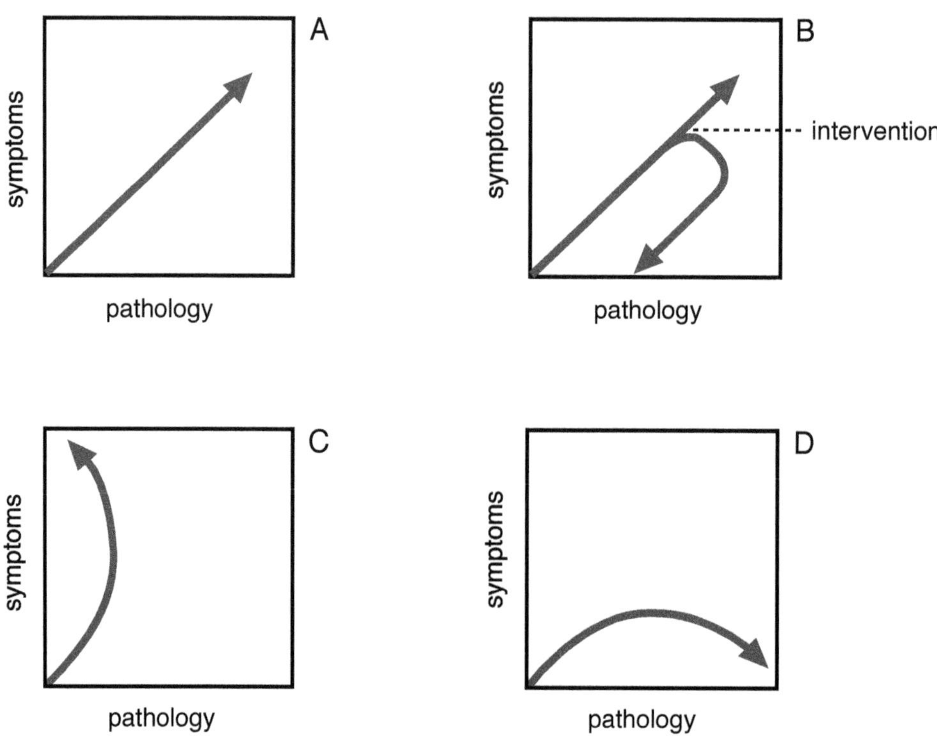

Figure NR 1.1 Failure of the pathology model to predict back pain. Redrawn from Haldeman S. 1990 Spine 15 (7) 718-724

this in theory, yet in practice they don't! Clinicians remain fearful of pain, they can't convince themselves that it may be out of proportion to any injury or pathology, or just remaining stubbornly high, after healing and repair has concluded. A high level of pain creates therapist fear, that results in reticence to get the patient to start to load or use the tissues and that fear is easily passed onto the patient. The manual therapy legacy of 'Severity' and 'Irritability' equating to 'go cautiously' – powerfully remains! Even though the biology of these 'terms and conditions' are so much better understood, clinicians tend to remain stuck in the safety of Graph A.

Like Graph C, D spectacularly exposes the frailty of the 'pain equates to harm' relationship, by showing how symptoms may improve even though pathology may be getting worse and worse. A more realistic 'gig' for symptoms and worsening pathology, is the good old 'Toblerone' effect that's already been discussed. If you spend many years observing degenerative joint problems, which invariably and inexorably do get 'pathologically' worse, variations in pain, or 'Tobleroning,' is what you'll observe. Degenerative pathology plods on, yet symptoms wander about, following the whims of weather, mood, stress, toxins in your food and drink, your activity and inactivity or whatever else you may care to associate it with. My metastatic bone disease does exactly the same. Pain tells fibs, is invariably inaccurate and has a mind of its own – pathology or no pathology, injury or no injury.

I'd like to clarify a few issues around the notions of adaptive and maladaptive pain for a moment, then later review why I'm highlighting them in a chapter on peripheral nerve pain mechanisms and nerve root related pain.

Clinically there is a great danger in using this sort of adaptive/maladaptive logic too simplistically. Here is a list of 'be-carefuls':

- be careful not to oversimplify adaptive or maladaptive – that it's either one or the other (what I'm after, is thinking in degrees of maladaptiveness, or adaptiveness, so you might review a patient and think that their pain is 80% maladaptive and 20% adaptive, meaning the tissues aren't perfect, but the patient should have far less pain than they're reporting)

- viewing all recent or acute pain as adaptive pain and all on-going chronic pain as maladaptive

- assuming that adaptive pain is real pain and maladaptive pain is not real pain – the patient is malingering, amplifying and onto a tidy compensation claim

- classifying maladaptive pain/chronic pain as having a 'central' pain mechanism to the exclusion of all other mechanisms and similarly, classifying all acute pains as a 'nociceptive' mechanism.

All pain problems vary from moment to moment. This means that your acutely twisted ankle can be modest and adaptive one minute, but a moment later, you may be moaning and going on and on about how bad the pain is. Is your pain problem flipping from adaptive to maladaptive? Or is it doing what might just be to your advantage at that moment? 'Louis, your pain always goes when you want to play golf!' Pain, it seems, has cleverly evolved how to fib, especially if it gets in the way of something deemed important by the brain that owns it! Washing up to be done after supper? 'I think I need to lie down for a minute, my back's playing up again.'

Pain learns to know when it needs to shut up. Think things like danger/fear, pleasure activities like say fishing, fleeing, fighting and important opportunities to try and pass genes on to the next generation that also begins with an 'f'!

Pain also learns to know when it needs to make its presence felt. Some folks have a good balance of their 'on' and 'off' systems, whereas others it may be skewed to 'on' (footballers) or 'off' (rugby players). We all have a bit of a footballer and a bit of a rugby player in us; we all have our 'average' place along the spectrum. My observation is that most patients, especially as their problem enters the chronic category of things, tend to err towards the soccer player end, but with skilled listening, examining, explaining and rehabilitation a good many can be shifted towards the rugby player end!

Acute pain can easily be 'out of proportion to the damage done'. Two people, with the same injury, report vastly different amounts of pain, inflame quite differently, react behaviourally and emotionally quite differently and heal quite differently. I would suggest that a great many patients we see have adaptive – pain, inflammation, reactivity, distress, anger, anxiety, pain behaviour etc. Plus a variable dollop of maladaptive – pain, inflammation, reactivity, distress, anger, anxiety, pain behaviour placed on top and in between! The variable processing and biology that I've discussed in previous sections is testament to this. The 'Toblerone' fluctuation can be applied to any issue you wish to observe; its life, inconsistent, constantly trying to adapt and up and down.

A major issue here is being able to accept the variability of these issues, but at the same time have a masterful, somewhat emotionally detached, unidimensional view of the strength and capabilities of the tissues. The idea is to quietly disregard the pain and behavioural 'noise' that surrounds the presentation and skilfully assess the relevant tissue strength, robustness and its capabilities. This is mostly done by a consideration of the whole individual and their history in the context of tissue healing and strength, because adequate physical testing is usually prevented by the pain.

'The pain you've got is mad – your tissues are quite capable of running from here (Cornwall) to John-O-Groats (northern most tip of Scotland) if they had to.' In the right context, you can say this sort of stuff and the patients appreciate it! In the wrong context, they'll think you're a nut and you'll never see them again. I sometimes add this 'You'll probably hurt like hell but you won't do any long- term damage as a result, I promise!' I'll then maybe tell them a story that involves a patient who had long term pain, who had taken a great deal of care and been wary and avoidant; who, on hearing that it's all 'OK', goes out and does something ridiculous like run a marathon and afterwards, never felt better. And, contrary to what the Drs said, there was no long-term damage as a result. Their new and reinvigorated life moves them into a much healthier and better place – the need for on-going 'treatment' soon disappears.

It seems to me that clinicians often don't get to know exactly what patients want from them. Ask them! Often, a major thing is not only understanding and knowing what's wrong, but also whether or not they should be worried about it, or whether they should ignore it and get going.

The other thing is that if you're going to tell a patient that it is safe to start loading and get going – you have to be confident and they have to be confident in you. If you haven't a clue as to what is going on then you are stuck with a 'where's your pain, lets treat the pain' approach.

Try to see a maladaptive to adaptive continuum or spectrum. For example, at one extreme there's a tissue situation that appears perfectly normal but there's a vast amount of pain, disability and related pain behaviour. Somewhere in the middle, are presentations where there is observable and assessable tissue damage (healing/weaknesses/impairments), but the pain and the functional/disability 'presentation' is rather out of proportion to that required and may even be preventing adequate use and loading. For example, think about a knee that has early degenerative changes, little evidence of significant inflammation and a modest loss of range, but a disturbing and disabling amount of pain with marked loss of normal function. These are the patients who have stopped doing their regular walks, can't get comfortable, find it constantly annoying, are avoiding more and more and may well be taking lots of pain killers and anti-inflammatories. They have come to the conclusion that the more they do the more wear and tear they'll create and therefore it's best to do less. Doing less feels more comfortable and this confirms their hypothesis.

Compare these types of patients to those that have as bad or sometimes significantly worse, degenerative changes, who are still running, walking and being active – with little pain or perhaps a bit of post exercise/post rest stiffness.

Back to the spectrum I was discussing.

So, at the other extreme of the maladaptive/adaptive pain spectrum, we could consider a situation of massive pathology or injury and little or no pain. Look at the pictures of the feet (fig NR 1.2)! The one on the left I called 'The lady who walks the cliffs'. The one on the right is 'The lady who walks in the woods'. Both have obvious and severe degenerative changes. These are fantastic pictures to show patients who are starting to let their 'degenerative joint' diagnosis reduce their activities, because of fear of the consequences. Pictures of degenerative feet are brilliant for educating patients about OA and wear and tear. Active but ghastly, degenerate feet like these two pairs, clearly illustrate how function can be maintained and life needn't be so painful. You just need to get the patient to link this up to their 'back' or 'neck' or whatever area you're dealing with. I have countless patients in my head, they have seen these pictures and then done really well with a graded functional programme. Right now I'm thinking of a lady who was virtually housebound but with guidance took about a year to get up to walking five miles. It took time, but she did it and she's maintained it too.

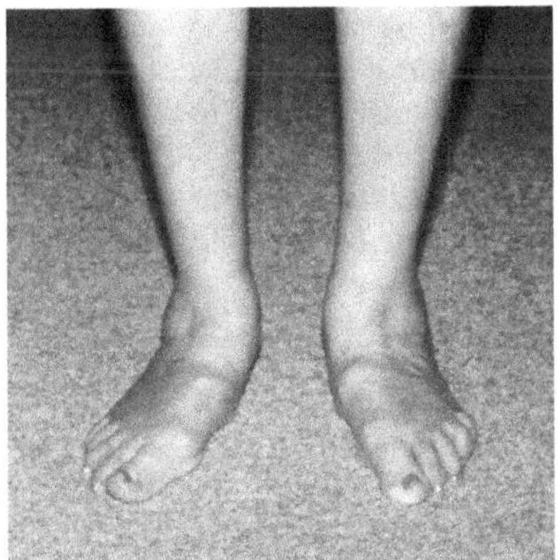

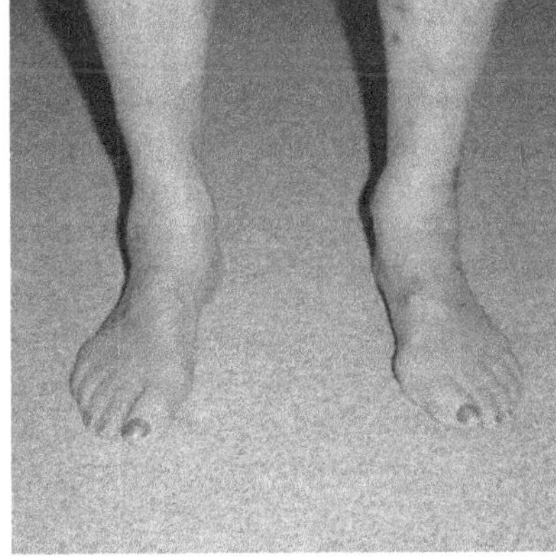

Figure NR 1.2 - The lady who walks the cliffs (left), The lady who walks in the woods (right).

We now have better explanations for the reality of maladaptive pain. For example, where it is viewed in terms of aberrant neural activity and processing, from all levels (peripheral, nerve fibre, central etc) or, at the 'biomedical' or tissue level, where it may relate to maladaptive levels of inflammation and therefore of levels of nociception. But even here there can be huge discrepancies!

We mustn't dismiss the notion of amplifying the amount of pain for some kind of gain. After all, pain behaviour, for the most part is meant to do just that. It gets us looked-after with help and support, safety and comfort, rest and decreased stress and allows us time to selfishly focus on ourselves, take a bit of care and get better. The intention is to create the best conditions for healing to be at its most efficient. Amplifying pain from time to time may well be an adaptive strategy!

'Yeah, keep your pain, you get a big pay out!'

You know, I do think it's OK to have these 'naughty' rather politically incorrect thoughts, but there must be balance! Don't be a pain fascist and disbelieve everyone with on-going pain. Chill, because if you don't believe them and don't like them, you won't be able to help and you're likely to burn-out. The trick, if you don't believe them, is to not mind them, accept them as you find! I've had many patients who I could easily have accused of totally exaggerating their pain, but have got on and accepted their presentation, the way they were behaving and reacting and then helped them a great deal. **The patient in front of you is what you have to deal with and try and help.** This includes managing and dealing with what you perceive as their exaggerated pain behaviour.

Next: **central mechanisms are present in all pain presentations**.

That's from the first instance, to milliseconds, seconds and minutes after an injury, through healing to recovery and probably for ever after too. Modulation – meaning changing the impact of nociceptive activity, changing what we feel and changing how we react is, as I've already discussed, massively down to changing central mechanisms. As I've also discussed though, central mechanisms can become maladaptive: for example, loss of central inhibitory controls and spontaneous firing of central neurones; the formation of memory like pain representations, or cell assemblies that continually access consciousness via their continued activity. This helps us understand the behavioural and topographical madness of some pains. But is not the only mechanism operating – **all mechanisms are playing a part**, that's why pain is such a difficult prospect for a purely biomedical tissue and tissue 'impairment' focused 'fix-it' approach.

I'm afraid I'm rather maddened by those who purport to be pain experts; telling us that precise pains, mechanically patterned pains, with clear-cut responses in relation to forces applied should be classified as 'nociceptive' in nature. Sorry, rubbish in my opinion, here's why. Recall the amputees mentioned in section 5. Central mechanisms/or processing mechanisms can account for incredibly precise phantom pains: in-growing toe nails, corns, blisters, ulcers, phantom joint morning stiffness and even 'inflammatory joint aches' that fluctuate with the weather. The pain of an arthritic joint is so often classed as mechanical, but here is stunning evidence that there's a central representation in place. There has to be in all pains.

Let me be clear: vague or precise, acute or chronic, mechanically patterned or not, all can be accounted for in terms of all pain mechanisms and all need to be considered. A mechanically patterned 'tissue' problem can be well endowed with maladaptive central processing pain mechanisms. I've had a great many patients with precise mechanically patterned pain, which soon goes when they agree that there's little wrong, except that it's over-sensitised. They then take less notice of it or have less concern over it when it comes.

What's this got to do with peripheral nerve related pain? It's this: that I think peripheral 'neurogenic pain' – meaning pain that derives from injury, disease or abnormality to peripheral nerves, is in large part maladaptive/out of proportion to the damage done –***from the very start***. Hence, nasty acute sciatica, for example, is a pain that is way out of all proportion to the tiny area of 'damage' done.

I believe this is quite a controversial statement. I know that it has shocked and puzzled many therapists who I have discussed it with, in my time as a lecturer. It stems from the incorrect notion that all 'acute' pains are natural, normal, believable and have to be representative of what's going wrong; and that, all 'chronic' pains must be abnormal and hard to believe.

The logic of applying this 'maladaptive' label to acute nerve pain is that for us and the patient, getting rid of the pain as quickly and as efficiently as possible, is a very valid thing to do. I quite firmly believe it may even be helping to 'cure' the problem, or at the very least, prevent the potential for maladaptive and on-going peripheral and central mechanisms from being set-up.

Taffy's brachialgia

Taffy was 60 years old when he came to me with pain that ran from his left scapular down the whole left arm to his hand. The pain, a deep horrid aching, was also in his armpit and radiated into his chest to the lower border of his left pectoral muscle. He had a numb tip of his middle finger, loss of triceps power, no triceps reflex and was in constant agony. The problem was of ten days duration and all the painkillers the doctor had given him hadn't done a thing. Most distressing was that he couldn't sleep at all, lying down was a disaster. He had been sitting up all night and was quietly going crazy with the pain. He'd do anything to be helped.

Patients with this sort of desperate pain can often receive desperate treatments, from practitioners desperate to help them quickly. The result: strong traction, forceful manipulation and so forth. None of which make sense and none of which are likely to help and all of which are potentially quite dangerous, or they're 'latently' very provocative; meaning they walk out of your clinic not bad, but later that day or the next, the whole thing gets ten times worse again. These patients are very easy to make quickly worse, but very hard to quickly make better.

The underlying problem, as I'll review, is electrochemical. So at best, strong physical treatments or exercises may provide enough of an endorphin release to quell things for a few hours. Ultimately force is likely to aggravate the situation and shouldn't be done; clinical reasoning dictates that this is not wise action. Don't believe those who say they walked in doubled up and walked out cured – it just does not happen, it's a myth. In the thirty plus years of practice I've never seen a patient walk in doubled up with 'true' sciatica and walk out 'cured'. Although seeing them again years later, they tell me how they remember this very thing happening! Patients either don't remember or like to 'fib' a bit because they like you and were impressed.

Normally 'Taffy' type pain and problems are ghastly for several weeks before starting to wind down and take anything from 8-12 weeks or sometimes up to a year to improve and get better. Again, I have never seen one suddenly get better, like the disc went back or the nerve became un-trapped!

Usually what I do with the Taffy type patient is enough of an examination to confirm a nerve root, 'try' some gentle mechanical inputs – because in some you can find relieving postures, movements and techniques that start the process of 'helping'. I also use TENS or any form of electro-placebo input that isn't going to make matters worse as far as is possible. As far as the 'Shopping Basket' approach (see later) is concerned attending to the 'Pain Compartment' is the issue with the highest priority. Quite often physiotherapy just doesn't have potent enough treatments to help. This is when you need the help of a friendly Doctor.

With Taffy it all hurt and it all made it worse, so I wrote a letter to his Dr giving the findings and the diagnosis and asking for better medication (I usually emphasise codeine/or stronger opiates). Off Taffy went with my letter and he phoned the next day, 'I've got 'Dihydrocodeine' and I'm still in agony'... 'Give the tablets a couple of days' was my response and ring me again tomorrow. I didn't hear from him so I phoned. His wife answered.

'He's asleep. The Doctor saw him this morning and gave him an intravenous 'pethidine' injection. It knocked out the pain and it's knocked him out!'

Taffy rang me two days later to say he had slept for the most part of two days and that his pain was at least 60% better. He was coping fine. Note that most Drs will tell you that opioids, like pethidine, are only likely to be helpful for eight maybe twelve hours and therefore there's not much point in using them for severe acute pain. Well, not necessarily, my observation with a great many patients like Taffy and also via my own personal experience with spinal and pelvic metastatic disease causing neuralgia – constant very high levels of nerve pain, if it's hit good and hard with effective opioid analgesia, the relief can last a lot longer than predicted and to great effect. It's as if it somehow permanently tunes-down the central 'hyper-excitability' state, or even dampens the actual 'ectopic' pacemaker site (more later) on the aggravated lumbar or cervical nerve root, leaving the patient with a lot less pain, never to return to such high levels as the current episode.

Taffy and I kept in touch and he came back for a couple of visits over a three month period and I did all the usual physio things that were required! He worked hard on his muscle strength – which was weak triceps... but I got him to exercise the whole arm and scapular to cover all the C7 innervated muscles and it recovered well. The reflex remained absent and the numb finger tip gradually came back over about six months. The point is, that the aggressive early analgesia worked well and I hope you can see that getting rid of the pain, is a very valid way of speeding-up natural recovery with this sort of extreme pain. Our problem as physiotherapists (or other clinicians) is that our pain relieving treatments are just not potent enough or long enough lasting in these situations. **Powerful medication is worthwhile – hugely. Get your Doctor onside!**

Quelling the pain helps to cure the problem and this is what I tell my patients. There's good research to support this and there are plenty of examples in chapter 15.4 to explain to the patient. When you know and understand pain mechanisms it all makes sense! When you know and understand stress biology it all makes sense to...

The big point though, is that I'd like all clinicians to consider that nerve pain, like nerve root pain that we all see day in day out, is, from the very moment of onset, maladaptive pain. It is pain that is out of all proportion to the tiny little nerve bruising and injury that probably starts it off. That means, aggressive analgesia, backed up by anything that feels good to the patient. For example, I've seen many patients (mostly not quite as bad as Taffy) who've found my manual testing with cervical traction very relieving. So, I often do it using the machine and I set it up in the position that the patient feels most comfortable. This usually means a lot of fiddling with pillows, angle of pull of the rope, body position etc. It's the same for lumbar nerve roots too. If it feels good and helps do it... but don't keep doing it week in and week out and ripping the patient off! For a start, make sure it's alongside a physical recovery programme that's commensurate with the usually slow recovery pace of nerve root problems, plus lend them a traction kit if traction's useful!

Many patients are more than willing to use a home traction kit. Big warning: many of the commercial ones that I have seen pull the neck into extension. However, the over-the-door ones aren't bad because you can get the patient to slump in the chair to increase the amount of flexion. My preference is biased to lying, because it is a far more relaxing position for the neck and whole body, than sitting or slumping in a chair!

Most of my patients find the best position for lying traction to give relief in is somewhere from neutral to almost full flexion. A big note, please don't listen to McKenzie therapists who are obsessed by 'centralisation', that usually means a) end of range and b) movements that favour intervertebral foramen and spinal canal narrowing. I'm all about comfort, relaxation and pain relief – it's calm and easy and like I said, that's more towards flexion. I frequently give patients neck traction in about 20 degrees off full flexion and even advise them to try sleeping with three even four pillows when they're on their back.

No harm done and a great many tell me that was the best advice I gave them. As soon as the pain settled they got back to using fewer pillows when they were ready to.

The traction I give is 'comfortably to the point of pain relief'. Occasionally there are one or two patients who want it stronger and stronger, because they want the bloody thing 'pulled out.' I'm quite happy to pull hard on some grizzly farmer's neck (for reasons you should be able to work out by now), but when I feel things are getting silly, I stop. For those of you who are wondering how much traction the neck will take it is worth looking at Cyriax's old books, where you can see the little plump man putting his whole body weight behind his traction. The patient doesn't slip off the couch because he has two physios holding onto their ankles for dear life! When I first started in private practice in 1988 I had quite a few patients who'd been seen by Cyriax. It was interesting to hear their stories, those who'd had his strong traction and manipulation regretted letting him do it. One or two who'd been injected said it was beneficial for a few months. None were really enthusiastic!

To get back to the home traction story... the end result was that a patient of mine began making me some simple halters and spreaders, plus pulley system. The pulley had a simple door jamb attachment like you get with the commercial home shoulder pulleys. The patient simply closed the door on the bit of rubber at a few feet off the floor, lay on the floor with a couple of pillows, put the harness and halter on, grabbed the end of the pulley cord and started pulling until they felt relief. They could adjust the angle by moving away from or nearer to the door and I encouraged them to experiment with this, with the goal of looking for a similar angle to the one that worked when they were with me.

I had a great many patients volunteer that being in traction was the only way they could sleep. These sufferers rigged up the traction kit in a spare room, threw a mattress on the floor and found the set-up incredibly helpful – spending a fortnight or more there!

If you're wondering, the traction kit had a simple lock out system that engaged when the cord was taken out to the side, a sharp tug released it. I had about five kits and used to lend them to patients all the time. Some of the more 'handy' patients rigged up a spring balance between the pulley and the door attachment to give a reading of the amount of pull. You'll find plenty in your local fishing shop.

I have a great many amusing stories about patients and their home traction experiences, as you might imagine. Pleasingly, none have been negative in the sense of halting or worsening recovery, but a few have involved a household member forgetting what was happening on the other side of the door! The moral of these stories is: always set your traction kit up using a cupboard door.

Apparently, if you lie on the floor your dog won't leave you alone and starts licking you all over... continuously... and gets concerned and goes weird... If you add a traction kit to this scenario the dog will pee on you and call an ambulance! (or so I've been told!)

For some patients, the home traction area of the house became a temporary saviour. It was here they could get relief from the unrelenting restless agony and it was here that they could fall asleep comfortably, for long enough to feel a great deal better.

Long live the home made recumbent traction kit, plus pillows and mattress, for cervical nerve root pain!

Chapter NR 1.2
'Normal' peripheral nerve sensitivity and why such a focus on 'nerve root' pain?

(I wrote this chapter when my health wasn't so good and that coming back to it now, when my health is even worse, I realise that it's rather all over the place in places! So, I'm sort of warning the reader that they may occasionally go... 'What's he going there for; this chapter's supposed to be on normal nerve sensitivity...' But thanks for hanging in with me!)

Most of the literature on pain that is related to peripheral nerves states that a normal nerve is not sensitive. But, when it is injured it becomes mechanically sensitised and sensitive to being tapped, as in Tinel's sign; sensitive to being pulled or stretched, as in the SLR; which, when applied to a patient with 'classic' sciatica will often reproduce the sciatic pain or a component of it.

I kind of agree that a normal nerve is pretty insensitive but also disagree and here's why:

In places, normal nerves do produce a nasty sensation when tapped with a finger tip, think of the 'funny-bone' sensation we all get from time to time. I'm sitting here now and getting showers of pins and needles over the dorsum of my thumb by rapping my finger on the superficial radial nerve about one third of the way down the lateral aspect of the radius. Anyone who has played volleyball will know what I mean. I can also do the same for the peroneal nerve, where it wraps around the head of the fibula and the tibial nerve, in its groove just posterior to the medial malleolus, is particularly noxious. So, if you can tap in the right place, a normal nerve is mechanically sensitive. It's just not as sensitive as it can become, if injured or abnormal in some way. My suggestion is that in order to be able to make sense of Tinel's test in the injured, pathological or 'abnormal' state we all need to know what happens in the normal state. Find those nerves and get tapping!

Functionally, the point is that it wouldn't be helpful for normal nerves to be too mechanically sensitive. They're being stretched, bumped and squashed all the time with normal movements, activities and postures, especially so in places where they're vulnerable to stretching and squashing. Nerves are fantastically adapted to carry on functioning in quite adverse conditions without complaining, but, because they're so important, it stands to reason that they do have a degree of sensitivity to un-physiological and hence threatening forces and movements[1].

Now, my complaint is that there's a big hole in describing and explaining nerve root pain and its behaviour satisfactorily. Although I am full of admiration for books like 'The Biomechanics of Low Back Pain' by Adams et al. (most recent edition is 2012) and the neurodynamic books I've read[2], they all leave me pretty nonplussed and disappointed as a clinician interested in the commonest nerve related pain problems seen in the clinic. Hence this 'Nerve Root' section of the book.

This Nerve Root section is my 'spin' on the cause, generation and behaviour of nerve root related pain. It will include some important biomechanics of the nerve root, in relation to normal posture and movement. What fascinates me is that the spinal biomechanics actually meshes quite well with some aspects of clinical presentations.

1 - There are plenty of excellent 'neurodynamic' books that give all the nerve palpation and nerve testing techniques and should be studied.

2 - I have never opened or read 'The Sensitive Nervous System'.

Having said that, I have to acknowledge the dangers of presenting my own bias and favoured hypotheses. All I can say is that after years of observing predictable clinical presentations, in parallel with scouring the literature surrounding nerve root related problems for better explanations I have come to a point in time feeling quite satisfied! I would be thrilled for someone to follow up with challenging or supporting clinical research trails based around the material presented in the next few sections and chapters. My first problem is to convince the reader and researcher! I hope I'm able to help you see what I mean and I'd also prefer to avoid leaving you thinking I'm a bit too cocky and arrogant for your liking!

Let me now continue looking at 'normal' nerve mechanical sensitivity, the scene needs to be set.

Stretching a normal nerve, as in the upper limb tension tests or the SLR and slump tests, for a great many 'normals' are not at all nice when taken to end of range. Anyone who has done a neurodynamic course and practised the various tests and been practised on, will know that normal nerves, when stretched during these manoeuvres, always produce quite unpleasant mixes of sensations[1]. It's good that they do, because to over-stretch a nerve and to then injure nerve fibres is a serious matter. In-times-gone-by, nerve injury was probably life threatening, especially if a significant neuropathy resulted that caused significant loss of function. Luckily though, the 'threatening' nerve stretching combinations of movements we learn in these tests, while quite easy to achieve on someone else, are rather sensibly not a part of normal day to day movement. On the nerve root courses I used to teach, we used to have practical break-out sessions and learn a few of the tests. Sometimes, during the sessions I'd quietly step back and take a look around at what everyone was doing, particularly noting the positions of the models and thought... What the hell are we all doing to each other? If you step back and look at someone doing say, an upper limb tension test 2a median nerve bias... or someone in full slump with one leg up, foot dorsiflexed and their head right down... and then think about normal movement and normal life... what you're seeing is almost movement madness! Why on earth would a human, in their normal day to day life want to go there? Luckily, we don't go there and our nerves are preserved from injury!

Look, I do appreciate that you might not have quite my sense of humour about some of the things we physios do to each other! So let's think for a moment about how nerves are most commonly injured in day to day life. First up, nerve injury to the point of neuropathy is pretty rare it mostly occurs or accompanies quite severe injury, for example, when a hand goes through a pane of glass. I'm now thinking of a brachial plexus injury and which usually involves incredible traction forces during an accident. When I first qualified, the patients I saw with brachial plexus neuropathies were often the result of a motorbike accident. The motorcyclist was knocked off their machine, they then hit the ground hard on their shoulder and at the same time the side of their head, so that the neck was forced into extreme side flexion away from the shoulder. The point I'm trying to make is that nerve injury from stretching

1 - And if you get several different therapists to do it to you you'll notice a vast difference... the spectrum goes from, the clumsy, ham-fisted and sweaty-betty's at one end, to the light and dainty but, possibly ineffectual at the other!

is relatively uncommon because nerves are well protected. But before we take that as gospel, let's have a look at my hamstrings...

This I think is an illustration of how well nerves are protected.

If I keep my knees locked straight while standing and then bend forward, I reach to just below my knee caps. I always have. The result is that if I want to pick up anything from the floor I bend my knees, or I bend and squat, or drop down on one knee, always have and always will!

'Tightness' in the back of my legs stops me. Simple, tight hamstrings! Hang on, analyse what I feel. Bend forward with knees locked straight. It's a deep dragging sensation going from my buttock/ischial tuberosity area down the back of my thigh into the calf and a bit in the foot too. Now, you folk with flexibility won't understand this, but if I try to bend to the floor keeping my knees straight I can't, but If I let the knees flex about 20 degrees I can reach. What do I feel now? It's pure 'nice' muscly pulling in the hamstrings, quite unlike the horrid 'nervy' dragging sensation right down the leg. It's easy to differentiate the two in normals and in many patients by the **type of sensation** produced.

It seems that bending the knees takes the stretching pressure off the sciatic nerve and it shifts it onto the hamstrings. The result? When I bend I never keep my knees straight, they naturally, unconsciously bend and the sciatic nerve remains happy. Any good observations in the clinic reveal this movement pattern time and again with patients. And time and again it gets the 'You've got tight hamstrings' comment from therapists, as if it was abnormal in some way, even bad!

I strongly believe that my tight hamstrings protect my sciatic nerve and also, that the natural sensitivity of my tight sciatic nerve causes it to protect itself by altering my movement patterns.

Try doing an SLR to as many normals as you can. Do it the standard way with a straight knee and get the subject to report precisely what they feel and remember it and then repeat the test but with a bent knee, keeping it maintained at about 20-30 degrees of flexion. Take it into normal resistance and ask what the subject feels again, in comparison to the test with the knee straight. In many, especially those with tight hamstrings like me, the sensation with the bent knee is clearly in the hamstring and that with the straight leg is far more nervy, being diffuse, vaguely nasty achy and spreading from the back of the thigh well down the leg into the calf. To me and to neurodynamic testing logic, that has to be a nerve stretching sensation and one that can often be easily changed with foot movements. The exception to all this are those normals who are very flexible and of course patients with very nasty sciatica and a very limited SLR. Yet even here, SLR, with flexed knee taken into abduction and lateral rotation shifts the sensation away from the nerve pain towards pure hamstring muscle stretch sensation. If you want to investigate this, you have to be clear about focusing on the symptoms and comparing the symptoms the subject is getting. Another way of doing the 'hamstring' stretch test is to flex the hip first (usually well past 90 degrees and get the patient to then hold their own hip in comfortable flexion), then extend the knee until you can see and feel the hamstring tightening. In the clinic I find this test to be excellent for clarifying a hamstring problem vs a sciatic nerve mechanosensitivity. It's also a good position to perform static contractions of the hamstring in.

Investigating the normal responses to this two test 'stretch' differentiation and its validity would be a simple and great research project for someone?

So, a clinical tip is to be aware that those patients/normals with naturally tight hamstrings could well have naturally tight sciatic nerves; it also means – be careful with strong stretches with straight knees, well that is my advice and yes, it's un-physiological! If you want to stretch, then do it with a bent knee and with the addition of hip abduction/lateral rotation too, if necessary. Oh, and make sure the patient feels a hamstring stretch localised to the muscle, rather than a right down the leg nerve pulling feeling. And, yes, I have given patients minor neuropathies by over-stretching nerves! That was in the days when 'mechanical' thinking dominated manual therapy approaches. Thankfully the integration of pain mechanisms has changed things for the better.

I hope I've convinced you and maybe even the research community, that normal nerves are sensitive. If you have anyone that doubts this just do an upper-limb 1 tension test on them, make sure you get the scapular in full depression before adding the other arm components. Try not to be 'rough' with your handling! You can criticise me but I have seen some very well known manual therapists being horribly rough. If I was the patient I know I'd be saying 'Sorry sunshine, I think we better stop there before you do something you or I might regret, I don't think this is for me.' I'd quietly dress and walk out, pleased that my peripheral nervous system was still intact. The next thing from this is beware of those who teach you – that's at under and post-graduate levels. And lastly, when practising with each other, steer clear of your colleagues who are rough and forceful if you can. Last rule here, never volunteer to go on stage as a model for some guru to demonstrate a technique, especially if it's a strong one!

Squashing or compressing a nerve is generally much less thought about clinically, but is highly likely to be a far more common way of injuring a nerve than by elongation. If you ***gently*** squash a nerve (or ***elongate it***) you also compress its blood supply and in so doing prevent adequate circulation from reaching it. Over time, the nerve becomes ischaemic/hypoxic and one of the first things noticed are pins and needles, later followed by loss of sensation, numbing of the area supplied by the nerve and transient paralysis. You've all fallen asleep with your arms above your head and later woken wondering where your arms have 'gone', eventually you locate them but dramatically find you're unable to move them back down, dang! Once you do get them down again, circulation flows back, great waves of pins and needles follow and soon they come back to life! The other example I like is when you fall asleep on your stomach with both arms under your torso flexed at the elbows and even at the wrists too. For some, this is a habitual sleeping posture, which again can wake you with the same feeling of numbing limb-loss, inability to move or a variable amount of pins and needles. In this posture, nerve compression and hence circulatory compromise is likely to be occurring at the intervertebral foramen in the neck – on the side you turn your head to; also at the elbow, think compression of the median and radial nerves anteriorly at the elbow but also elongation/stretch (which if you think about it also compresses, or increases the pressure in and around the nerve) of the ulnar nerve on the other side of the joint axis; at the wrist, where flexion compresses the median nerve in the carpal tunnel and stretches the radial nerve on the back of the wrist.

Relate this to, for example 'Phalen's test', a pretty standard 'carpal-tunnel' test where wrist flexion is held for up to 30 seconds and if pins and needles, pain or numbness are produced in median nerve distribution it indicates the likelihood of carpal tunnel syndrome. Wrist flexion makes the carpal tunnel smaller and so compresses the median nerve along with all the flexor tendons there too. But so does wrist extension, a test that has been called 'reversed Phalen's'. I'd like to note that this test is quite often 'positive' in quite normal people (another research project!). (See carpal tunnel refs)

Any sustained position will produce a state of hypoxia, in all the tissues that are compressed and all the tissues that are stretched on either side of the joint axis! I think I'll write a new testing manual called 'neural hypoxia tests' or 'neural compression tests' in order to redress the balance that has favoured neural 'tension' tests for so long!

Here's one, sit on a hard chair for up to twenty minutes, sustain and don't move. This is a combined test for compression and elongation of the nerves that cross the buttock (posterior to hip joint axis) and compression of the nerves that cross the hip anteriorly. To emphasise the anterior compression fully flex at the hips while sitting. I hope you can see that I'm being a bit of a facetious knob and that many other tissues don't like sustained postures either. Mind you, as I mentioned in the nociception chapter, they're remarkably tolerant in some people.

If anyone wants a research project – I'd love it if someone would look at sustained testing on a large number of normals and record and report on what they found. Preferably, could you look at sustained neck rotation and side flexion plus combinations of the two, it doesn't need to be firm pressure or nasty to the neck, the same for the low back, also, sustained wrist flexion and sustained sitting with crossed legs... and more! A great many folk find their foot going numb when they sit on their legs or sit cross legged for any length of time. It's not 'bad' circulation, it's simply that person's blood supply being compressed and cut off to the nerves and other tissues supplied.

So, contrary to what the pain biologists and researchers say, life and clinical observation and a not too profound logic, tell me that normal peripheral nerves are wisely sensitive – to stretching, as well as tapping, or other forms of direct force that threaten them. One important 'direct force' is prolonged pressure on nerves – hence their sensitivity to hypoxia. If nerves don't like the situation they are in, they have the ways and means of letting you know so you can do something about it! In turn, and lowering our reasoning to a 'reductionist' level, this means that normal peripheral nerves have the means for transducing mechanical (stretch, compression) forces, as well as hypoxic conditions (chemicals), into electrical impulses. As I'll show, this also means that the injured nerve has the potential to increase this basic and normal response, just like any other tissue does – hence becoming more sensitive **to mechanical forces and hypoxia.**

In my early 1990's 'aches-and-pains' days I thought that a useful way of thinking about 'peripheral' pain mechanisms was to think in terms of two aspects:

The **first** I used to call '**nerve-end generated pain'** – meaning pain that derived from the stimulation of the end terminals of nociceptive fibres, like Aδ and C nociceptive fibres as I've already discussed in the nociception chapters. For the most part 'nerve-end pain' requires any one of three basic stimuli to the tissues that the nerves innervate. These three stimuli are:

1. Nasty physical forces.
2. Extreme temperatures.
3. Inflammatory/metabolic/hypoxic chemicals.

The **second** type of peripherally generated pain, has its origins somewhere along the length of the nerve fibre itself, you could quite correctly call it **'axon' generated pain**, a term that many continue to use.

I still think it's quite a good distinction because 'nerve end' or what's now called 'nociceptive' pain, gives rise to more 'normal' or 'familiar' pains. Think skin and then think, burn, pinch, cut, splinter, graze, maybe you've even experienced some nasty chemical burn or wounding too. In all these injuries the pains are pretty straight forward, being 'familiar' and for the most part, relate well to the type of wounding that has occurred. This logic also follows for most 'sprains and strains' of muscles and joints – there's inflammatory aching and the nasty sharp pains with movement, that all reflect the nature of the injury and the tissues involved. In a broad sense, what I'm getting at is that 'nerve end pain' is familiar to us and seems to be straightforward, whereas 'axon' or peripheral neurogenic' pain is far more complex and puzzling in its presentation.

Together, the **quality**, **behaviour** and **type** of pain that arises from peripheral nerve injury, as I will argue in later chapters, are a major diagnostic feature of peripheral neurogenic pain.

So, if the pain is a bit weird, unusual, out of the normal 'box' then it might be worth thinking 'nervy' thoughts!

The notion that normal nerves are insensitive is daft, they need to be sensitive and they have the means. This is maybe via two mechanisms, one surprisingly is a 'nerve end' mechanism, the other must be axon related, but I know of no research here.

We know that the connective tissue of peripheral nerves has its own nerve supply, just like a ligament does. These nerves are called 'nervi nervorum'. They're little branches that come off some of the sensory axons and branch, to reach out and supply, with their 'nerve ends', the surrounding connective tissue of the nerve. Thus, the collagenous epi, peri and endoneurium has a sensory nerve supply, just like any other tendon or ligament does.

I don't know of any experiment that has tried to specifically stimulate these nerves in an 'awake' individual, so that we can know what type of feeling is produced. It may well be that it's these little fellows that are largely responsible for some of the 'normal' nerve sensations that I've been describing.

If you are confused, it's best to go back to your peripheral nerve anatomy and look at a section through a nerve. What you see is connective tissue in vast quantities and a surprisingly small amount of conducting tissue. The bundles of conducting tissues contain many hundreds of thousands of individual nerve fibres. With all this in mind, think about any forces going through this structure and you will start to appreciate the importance of the connective tissue on the one hand, but the vulnerability of the nerve fibres on the other. As you will see in the chapters that follow, we know a great deal about the injured axon; how it has the potential to create massive impulse barrages, therefore the means to cause quite awful, yet remarkable pains; but we know nothing about a normal axons ability to create impulse barrages when mechanical forces come to bear on them. I think it can react, but it may not be able to. One thing is certain though – normal nerves are sensitive!

Chapter NR 1.3
Nerve pain mechanisms 1

There are ascending levels of explanation for pain deriving from peripheral nerve

As you may have gathered, way back in chapter 1.1, my early experiences with 'pain' patients and particularly those with sciatica like Karen made me extremely frustrated with what I was taught and what I read in standard textbooks. What I saw in the clinic was certainly nothing like what I heard from lecturers, speakers and writers over the years and to be honest it still isn't.

Here are some examples of what I struggled with. The 'vagaries' and madness of nerve and nerve root pain – like sciatica and brachialgia!

- pain all over the place and 'out-of-the-dermatome it's supposed to be in' – just like 'Karen'
- pain clearly sciatic, but all movements virtually normal
  (No 'mechanical' pain-on, pain-off patterns when moving during my examination, yet patient reports clear postural and movement related provocation)
- during physical examination, all movements normal, then five minutes of sitting chatting with me suddenly the pain goes mad – arghhhh!
- very little to find with examination of neural tension tests – yet problem clearly nerve root
- the very common observation of leg or arm pain being hugely provoked by extension and these patients finding lumbar/neck flexion the most relieving
- guru therapists constantly saying or implying, that flexion is dangerous and should be avoided and that extension was safe
  (It was the 'old cut the knuckle and if you keep bending the finger, you keep the wound open explanation'!)
- but the great major of patients, came in moving and standing flexed; they preferred to lie on their side curled up in flexion and often used the curled up kneeling position to get relief
- hence, being upright and good posture making it all a great deal worse
- verve root problems that feel a lot better after a bit of pushing about, but it all flares later and they're in agony for days after
- patients with simple back pain, who've been manipulated or who have been made to do forceful end range exercises (think McKenzie style extension), who sooner/later develop radiating pain and sciatica
- patients with sciatica or nerve root related pain radiating down the arm, who cannot think of a particular physical cause
- symptoms moving about and changing a great deal
- radiation of pain into places the sciatic or brachialgia textbook descriptions never mention (eg. like the testicles, anterior thigh and stomach for sciatica or, for low cervical nerve root pain, radiating into the axilla, the anterior chest,

pectoral area and the whole of the upper quadrant)

- one patient with a nerve root problem tells me they don't like to move, the next is on the move all the time, they can't sit still or sleep – restless in extremis
  (Yet, both have the same looking scans, both have loss of sensation, power and reflex and diagnosis of nerve root impingement – but they could come from two different planets!)
- sciatica or brachialgia – with no referral into the leg
  (for example, pain just in the medial border of scapular, but on close neurological examination there's loss of power and reflex, at C6 or C7 levels; or, pain in the SI area or buttock often coming with a 'piriformis' syndrome diagnosis, who have obvious neural tension signs and often modest or obvious neurological deficit; for example, one or two repetitions of calf-raising appear normal, but repeat testing reveals a significant loss of endurance compared to the non-painful side – scanning reveals clear root impingement.)

This list could go on and I hope the reader is nodding their head in recognition of some of these clinical presentations and conundrums?

I am now going to look at what I see as ascending 'levels' of explanation for the symptoms, signs and presentations that I'm familiar with in the clinic; which I think, give good answers to many of these questions and puzzles I used to have.

The 'levels' start down at the level of the gene... and work up through receptors and ion channels, ectopic impulse generators on axons and their sensitivity; repetitive firing capability; heightened sensitivity; chemicals; abnormal synapses and impulses; hypoxia, inflammation; stress chemicals, disc extrusions and so forth – all the way up to looking at the biomechanics of the nerve root in normal, injured and degenerate spinal states.

If you can take on board, what I've managed to in the last thirty plus years, especially what I managed to make sense of in the early 1990's from the pain literature, for sciatica and brachialgia or nerve root related pain conditions – I hope you'll find the puzzling presentations described above a lot easier to make sense of?

Nerve root pain... the lower levels!

Recall from the chapter on nociception (section 11) that changes in sensitivity relate to changes in receptor function, whereby sleeping or refractory receptors become active, but also to the production and insertion of new receptors and ion channels in the cell membranes of the terminal fibres. In damaged peripheral nerves the process is similar but can be far more devastating. Here, because this process occurs along the damaged nerves and on the axon, it can result in massive spontaneous activity and very weird patterns of impulse activity too.

As always, there are usually one or two researchers whose good sense and writing serve us well. Our man here is Professor Marshall Devor and I would recommend the 2005 chapter from the 5th edition of The Textbook of Pain:

Devor M (2005). Response of nerves to injury in relation to neuropathic pain. In: McMahon SB, Koltzenberg M (eds) The Textbook of Pain 5th edn. Churchill Livingstone, Edinburgh 905-927

And also:

Devor, M. (1990). Sources of variability in the sensation of pain. Recent Advances in Restorative Neurology: 3 Altered Sensation and Pain. M. R. Dimitrijevic, P. D. Wall and V. Lindblom. Basel, Karger: 189-196.

Devor, M. (1994). The pathophysiology of damaged peripheral nerves. In: Wall PD, and Melzack R(eds) The Textbook of Pain. Churchill Livingstone, Edinburgh 79-100.

Devor M, Seltzer, Z (1999). Pathophysiology of damaged nerves in relation to chronic pain. In: Wall PD, Melzack R (eds) The Textbook of Pain 4th edn. Churchill Livingstone, Edinburgh 129-164

It was the 1990 article and 1994 chapter that kindled my clinical understanding of 'peripheral neurogenic' pain. Thank you Professor Devor! You helped make a confused, budding pain therapist more understanding and less fearful of neurogenic pain.

Ask this simple question to the non-medical public 'What happens if you cut through a nerve?' The answer is invariably 'You'll be paralysed.' Not only that, the bit the nerve goes to will feel 'dead' and lifeless. Marshall Devor calls these obvious symptoms of nerve injury **'negative symptoms'** meaning there has been a loss of some kind, though **Positive symptoms** can occur too. When a nerve is cut, we may get odd sensations and pins and needles ('paraesthesias' and 'dysaesthesias'), as well as pain for no reason at all (spontaneous pain) or relatively massive and long lasting responses whenever we gently move or are touched in some way (allodynia and wind-up). Clearly when you cut a nerve it doesn't necessarily silence it completely, in some people it can go mad.

The end result may mean on-going symptoms, ghastly sensitivity and for some, devastated lives. I sometimes ponder the advances made in treating and managing this sort of pain since those 'ah-ha' days in the 1990's and realise that really, nothing much has changed. That's gloomy! But, the good news is that just like frozen shoulders, nerve and nerve root pain has a natural history and for most, the mad nerve or nerve root gradually adapts and eventually settles down. Good management is essential, but I would just love it if a low side effect, low toxicity cheap and simple intervention could be found that stopped the pain in its tracks. I guess if evolution couldn't manage it, we're hardly going to find an easy answer! I do like the intravenous pethidine route remember it worked well for Taffy!

Investigators into peripheral nerve generated pain, like Marshall Devor, usually use rats or mice. They expose nerve trunks near the spine or in the legs and do one of several things:

1. **Ligation and transaction.** Here, a peripheral nerve, usually either the sciatic or saphenous nerves, is exposed in the leg, ligatured (tied with a fine cord) and then cut through just distal to the ligature. This effectively destroys many axons and leaves the proximal surviving

component of the nerve cells. The surviving neurones are said to be 'axotomised'.

2. **Partial lesion of the sciatic nerve.** In this experimental model, a ligature is passed through between one third and one half of the nerve, this is usually done to the sciatic nerve in the upper one third of the thigh. The ligature is pulled tight, which in effect transects the proportion of the nerve ligated. This model thus produces a 'partial' nerve injury (here, some nerve fibres will be axotomised, but some are saved).

3. **'Spinal' nerve transaction model.** The nerve lesion is produced near the spine and is essentially the same as the previous model. The location of the lesion is illustrated in the figure NR 1.3. This is not a nerve root lesion as it's little too far distal, but it's the nearest thing! Note the ligature proximal to the cut. Also, note the cut is specific to the L5 nerve trunk, because it is situated before it joins the lumbo-sacral plexus where it mixes with nerves from other roots, here the L4 is featured.

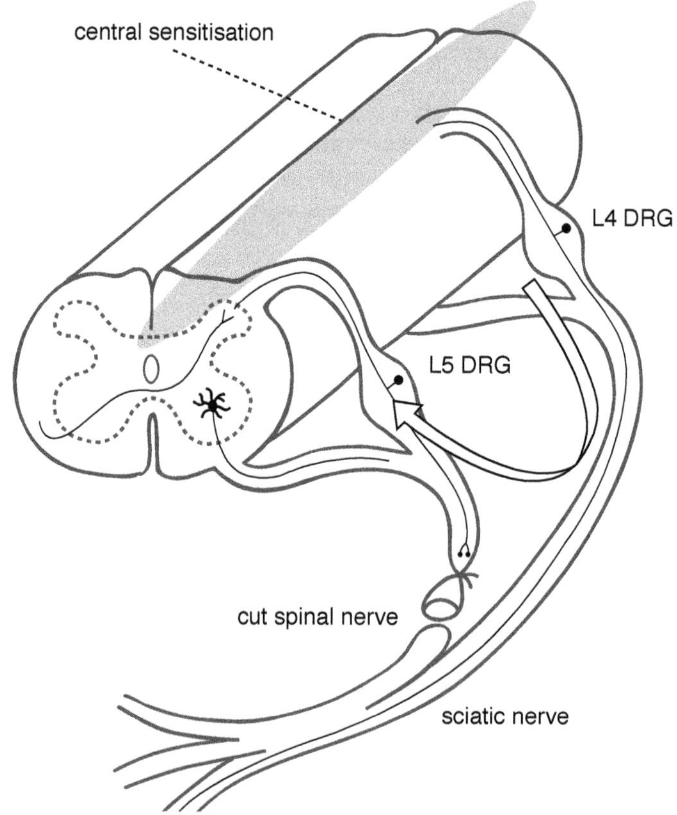

Figure NR 1.3 'Spinal' nerve transaction model.

4. **Chronic constriction injury of the sciatic nerve.** Here, the sciatic nerve, usually at mid thigh level, is ligatured loosely to produce only a modest constriction effect. This light ligature causes the development over time of intraneural oedema, whose swelling is prevented by the ligature and results in a 'self-strangulation' effect. This type of insult produces a degeneration, or interruption, in nearly all large myelinated and a great many of the smaller thinly myelinated Aδ fibres. A large percentage of C fibres afferents survive.

All four of these models lead to the animal exhibiting behavioural signs of pain – hence, they demonstrate 'autotomy' or self mutilation behaviour (they gnaw away at the part that hurts); as well as signs of increased mechanical and thermal sensitivity in the territory of the injured nerve. In other words they're demonstrating allodynia, or heightened sensitivity to normal non noxious inputs. The animals also show signs of on-going pain, such as limping and guarding of the affected paw and limb and, non-pain symptoms such as abnormal nail growth and abnormal skin temperature regulation (similar to symptoms of complex regional pain syndrome).

It's interesting that in humans we rarely witness the equivalent of 'autotomy' behaviour. But most of us will have experienced and probably observed the often constant fiddling, moving and testing that occurs when there's pain or altered sensation of some kind. Think how you fiddle with your face when it's been numbed from the dentist. Think also how we all 'fiddle' with our pain, we rub it, hold it, we play with it, in an attempt to change it. We don't exactly 'gnaw' it though, or do we?

You may remember the meeting I had with Pat Wall to discuss the memory biology. What I didn't mention was that soon after we'd started talking he said to me, 'Did you see the front page of The Sun today?' For those of you who don't know, 'The Sun' is a right wing 'Tit and Bum' UK newspaper, – the last thing you'd expect a Professor Emeritus to be reading! He went on to describe what he'd seen and read. The front page headline was 'How I used a train to cut off my leg' – see the picture in figure NR 1.4. The story is fascinating, but the long and short of it was that the pleased looking fellow had smashed his leg up in a motorbike accident and was patched up over many months by various orthopaedic surgeons... and against the odds they'd managed to save his leg. Sadly though, he went on to suffer with chronic unremitting pain and all attempts at treating the pain or rehabilitation failed. So, one night, after an argument with his girlfriend, he went and lay down next to the nearest railway line and placed his troublesome leg across one of the tracks and waited. In due course a train came along and obliged him with its massive force. And here we see him on the front page of The Sun – with a rather pleased-as-punch look, but also a sad victim of chronic pain and this rather dramatic self-inflicted remedy for it. It would be interesting to follow him up, because one would expect some kind of phantom related problem to arise. But, and it's a big but, this guys brain is pleased with what he did and what he achieved – could that make a difference? I think it could well do. On the other hand, the fact that he had so much pain prior to the amputation means that there must have been a substantial and strong central imprint. Also, the trauma to a great many nerve trunks of the leg could well have added further to his pain problems via extensive 'ectopic' foci forming. A few months ago I wrote to The

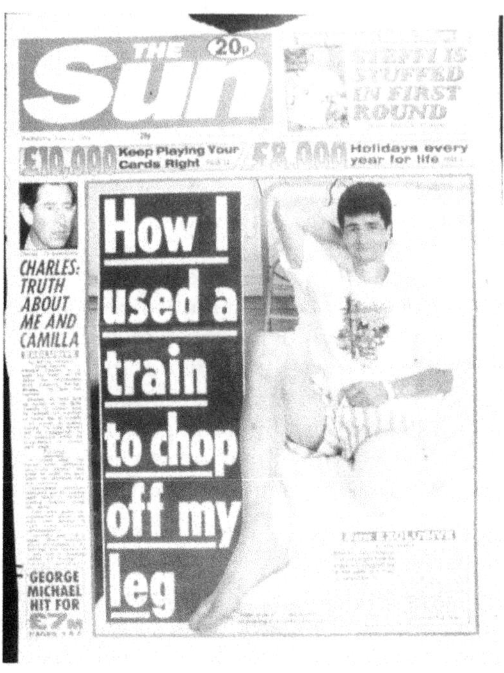

THE Sun 20p

STEFFI IS STUFFED IN FIRST ROUND

£10,000 Keep Playing Your Cards Right

Holidays every year for life

How I used a train to chop off my leg

CHARLES: TRUTH ABOUT ME AND CAMILLA

GEORGE MICHAEL HIT FOR £7m

Figure NR 1.4 'How I used a train to cut off my leg' The Sun Newspaper headline.

Sun, then, nearly twenty years on from that edition of the paper and asked them if they would follow the story up. Sadly, I haven't even received an acknowledgement!

It wasn't exactly 'gnawing' but what he did seems very similar to what those mice and rats tend to do.

I have witnessed one person who wished to remove his painful limb – this was a 'demonstration' chronic pain patient on one of David Butler and my five day 'Dynamic Nervous System courses' in the mid 1990's. This guy wanted to saw his arm off and wished he had the guts to do it. What was brilliant with him was that the pain explanation I spent time doing with him, appeared somewhat, to change his thoughts about the pain and the problem. Sceptical me goes – yeah, but when the euphoria dies down... the pain nags on. I wonder what happened to him too?

Let's return to business...

Recall that when an axon is cut through, the distal part of the nerve is cut away from its connection with the spinal cord, individual nerve fibres are irrevocably separated from their vital cell body's and the distal portion degenerates and dies. That's the 'Wallerian' degeneration we all learn about as students of neurology. Most neurology texts state that the proximal axon, its cell body and central terminals survive, but sometimes the reality is that injured cells can still die away. This may go on for many months. When 'lower' order sensory nerve fibres die, neuroscientists use the term 'deafferentation'. 'Lower-order' means below the level you're focusing on. Here we're focusing on the dorsal horn, so lower-order sensory fibres means, C, Aβ and Aδ neurons.

Loss of sensory input to the dorsal horn leaves the second order neurones missing their normal sensory inputs. Naturally, they want to know where their normal input has gone and some start on a quest to find them and re-connect! It's usually to no avail and the result is often the formation of new and inappropriate connections that adds to the already dire processing nightmare. Deafferentation and the subsequent effects are thought to factor in increased central sensitivity and on-going neuralgic pain.

To me, it's rather sweet that central neurones will go and try and find their lost peripheral siblings. 'I've lost my tissue input and I don't know what I shall do.' It's the nice side of Claudia (our second order central nerve cell), trying to re-establish the presence of all her fawning contacts from out of town. The dark side is the new and inappropriate connections and reactivity it's called 'deafferentation-supersensitivity'.

You know I often wonder about the influence of top-down here? It would be great if you could have two rats and were able to compare what happened in this schemed-up deafferentation situation. Tell the first rat that the sensory input post injury has now gone, accept it, chill with it and don't let it bother you, it may never come back, learn to live with it. If it does come back that'll be cool, just don't get uptight because it feels a bit weird, get used to it and get on with your life. Try not to bite or saw it off or go to the nearest railway... brave up, you'll be fine. Now, the second rat's really pissed that it can't feel it's paw very well and you encourage it to keep getting wound-up about the loss of feeling and the weird sensations, 'Hey, young ratty, how's the pain today, still numb, where's it numb, where's the pain? No better? ... hmmm that's bad..?' (Whoops, sounds like normal physio talk!)

So, I'm wondering if the way we react to a situation might just have an effect on the central 'deafferentation' re-wiring that can go on. Let it bother you and the descending messages are continuously, 're-wire me, fix me, come-on do something down there' – turn the sensitivity up high, see if you can hear anything that might find them... The thoughts then translate to some kind of a trophic stimulus – even down at this first synapse at the cord level. My betting is that it's bound to!

Interesting speculation perhaps! Well it is to me!

Once the lab researchers have cut through the nerve or ligatured it, they then put recording electrodes into the surviving proximal stumps and monitor the electrical 'talking' that goes on. Also, and quite amazingly, using things called 'gene-chip' devices, they can record the activity of individual genes in the cell bodies of the injured nerve fibres and they find that several hundred genes alter their activity following nerve injury! This means that some genes and therefore their protein production are turned on, resulting in an increase in protein products. Of course, some are turned off, leading to protein product decrease and this must be included in the tally.

Sever an axon and here are some of the things that happen:

1. ***Wallerian degeneration, as already stated. Degeneration means*** that there are lots of breakdown chemicals wandering around. They issue, for example from; the dying distal fibre; from the axon; from the now liberated cell contents and from the smashed up, degenerating myelin. Schwann cells and macrophages (remember the 'big-eaters'!) go to work and do the refuse collecting and clearing up operation. The result is that the area is awash with breakdown products and chemical messengers. Think: the cytokines (interlukins), but prostaglandins, ATP, and histamine and many more too. Think also, that these chemicals, given the presence of appropriate receptors – have the potential to produce impulses and pain. Note that after Wallerian degeneration the neurolemma is left behind (that's the outer wall of the tube that the axon and its myelin sheath ran in). It patiently waits, in anticipation of the arrival of the newly sprouting and regenerating fibre to grow into it and, to eventually re-connect with its original target tissue. Like Salmon returning to their river of origin, nerve fibres seem able to 'home' to their correct neurolemma and endoneurial tubes! Sample, scrutinise... respond! Brilliant! Sniff out your destination little bud, look for its special chemical signature and off you go. Reconnection, via regeneration, is an amazing attribute of peripheral nerve fibres. Let's look at the 'bud'!

2. After the 'cut' the proximal surviving nerve fibre seals off where it's been severed and swells slightly becoming an 'end-bulb'. Within a few days this end-bulb starts to form a variable number of little sprouts, whose role is to go in search of the old tube. If this is found the remaining sprouts die back, or as Devor puts it, 'get culled', so that all the focus can turn to supporting the growth in the correct direction and to the appropriate destination. If these sprouts are unable to find their target, as often happens when there's scar tissue in the way, or the separation of the surviving distal nerve sheath is significantly large – a 'tangled-mass' forms called an 'endbulb neuroma'. Think amputation and you've got it! There's nowhere to go! 'Yeah, but, I'm still responsible for the big toe yeah?' Inject a local anaesthetic into a neuroma of an amputee and you can stop their phantom foot pain. Dribble some noxious chemical onto it and you bring it all back. I sometimes use this sort of example to help patients understand referred pain.

3. Observations of disrupted nerve trunks and in particular of nerve fibres, that haven't undergone Wallerian degeneration and are still 'in-continuity' (the light ligation model (4) above), reveal the formation of 'microneuromas'. These may form not just where the axon is injured, but also anywhere along the length of the axon. Thus a 'sick' nerve fibre, which is highly likely to still be in contact with its target tissue, can develop them. Similarly, observations of cell bodies of sensory fibres in the dorsal root ganglion (DRG, in figure NR1.3) show, that if there is any evidence of the environment there being below par, the formation of distal microneuromas on the related axons is highly likely. Examples of situations that can cause the DRG environment to become below par are: inflammatory metabolites – think diffusing through

from any nearby injured or degenerate spine structures; or as the result of hypoxia, which may easily occur when there is loss of space around a nerve root via disc bulges and extrusions, degenerative outgrowths/osteophytes, enlarged facet joints, narrowed foramina, inflammation with local swelling, direct compression of nerve root or indirect via compressing of vascular plexii that supply the DRG). The DRG is of course a major component of the 'nerve-root' area.

Now, back to 1974 our famous pain scientist Pat Wall with colleague Gutnick, recorded massive impulse activity from electrodes placed in the dorsal root ganglion of nerves that had been severed distally. Mechanical stimulation of the distal nerve increased the firing and anaesthetic block using lignocaine stopped the firing.

Later studies, according to Devor showed that increased firing could be produced by stimulating:

- where there was nerve entrapment
- any neuromas and microneuromas at the site of injury or along the dysfunctional nerve
- regenerating sprouts
- areas of demyelination
- inflamed nerves (neuritis)
- nerves of subjects with diabetic neuropathy and with viral nerve infections.

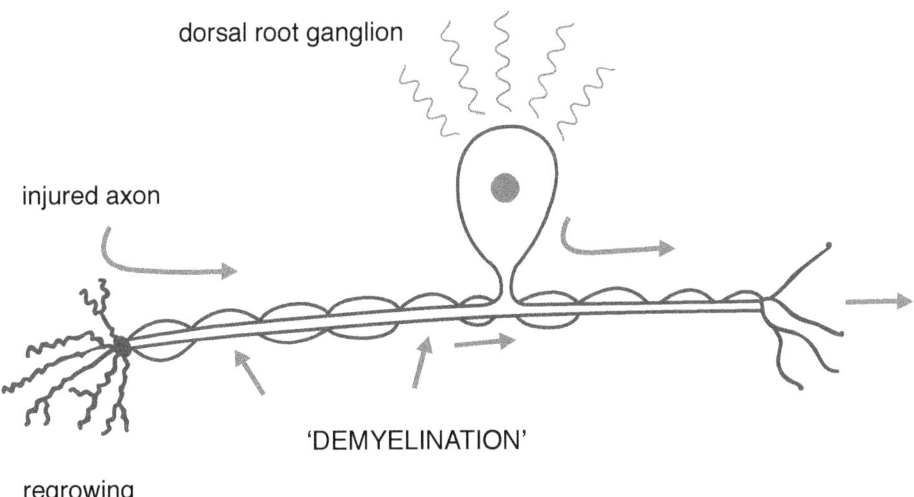

Figure NR 1.5 The dorsal root ganglion of a nerve that has been severed distally illustrating the areas of demyelination, the regenerating and re-growing sprouts and all the arrows indicating increased impulse activity.

Take a look at the slide I did of this from my early pain teaching days (figure NR1.5). Note the 'steam' coming of the cell body in the DRG, the areas of demyelination, the regenerating and re-growing sprouts and all the arrows to indicate, increased impulse activity.

Wall and Gutnick were the first to show that damaged nerve fibres didn't just stop firing and go to sleep. They showed that there was a greatly increased likelihood of increased impulse activity, the so-called 'positive' symptoms that Devor describes. This was of huge significance, in an era where many chronic pains were being treated by cutting out the nerve supply to the areas of pain! Wall knew that the results of these types of surgery for on-going pain states were often ghastly for the patient and he now had ammunition to pelt at those doing the ghastly operations. Did he pelt? Pat Wall was the master of acerbic criticism, often aimed directly at his dogmatic medical colleagues!

The observation was also, that the trains of nerve impulses recorded were of a wide variety and often on-going after a single very modest physical, electrical or chemical stimulus. There could be sudden bursts of activity and then silence and unresponsiveness, or continuing bursts, or simply long on-going trains of impulses – all of which can easily be related to the pain behaviour of any nerve injury related pain-sufferer.

All the above sites are said to be, 'ectopic' sources of impulses and hence of pain. So, the warning label on the can is, beware the positive symptoms of nerve injury! They can be nasty, stubborn and terribly long lasting. These microscopically small structures are responsible for symptoms way out of proportion to their size and status – MALADAPTIVE PAIN! Even POINTLESS pain! A tiny damaged and re-growing or 'poorly' axon, giving more pain than any ghastly musculoskeletal or bodily injury can! Wow!

In my lectures, I found that it often helped the participants to view chronic arm or leg pain as a form of phantom limb pain, but without the amputation! The same peripheral and central mechanisms occur – hence, axotomized and damaged peripheral nerves, plus massive central processing and representational changes occurring, as a result of the massive impulse trains that arrive there. It is Shane gone completely mad with Claudia ardour!

Chapter NR 1.4
Nerve root pain mechanisms 2: a clinical breather

As I noted above it's not uncommon for a patient with a 'nerve root' problem to be at a total loss to give a physical cause for it. After all most of our day to day pains relate to some kind of activity (or lack of), or some kind of stress, strain or injury. A pain that appears out of nowhere can be of some concern, good clinicians should be background pondering possible serious pathology/red flag issues. However, in the world of common-or-garden aches and pains, nerve root symptoms often do appear for no apparent physical reason. For me, rather simplistically but practically OK there are two major thoughts here:

Firstly, could the symptoms relate to some kind of degenerative joint problem? Degenerate joints often do become spontaneously irritable, or inflamed and hence painful. This is reasonably easy to spot or assess with peripheral joints but with spinal joints it's a little less so.

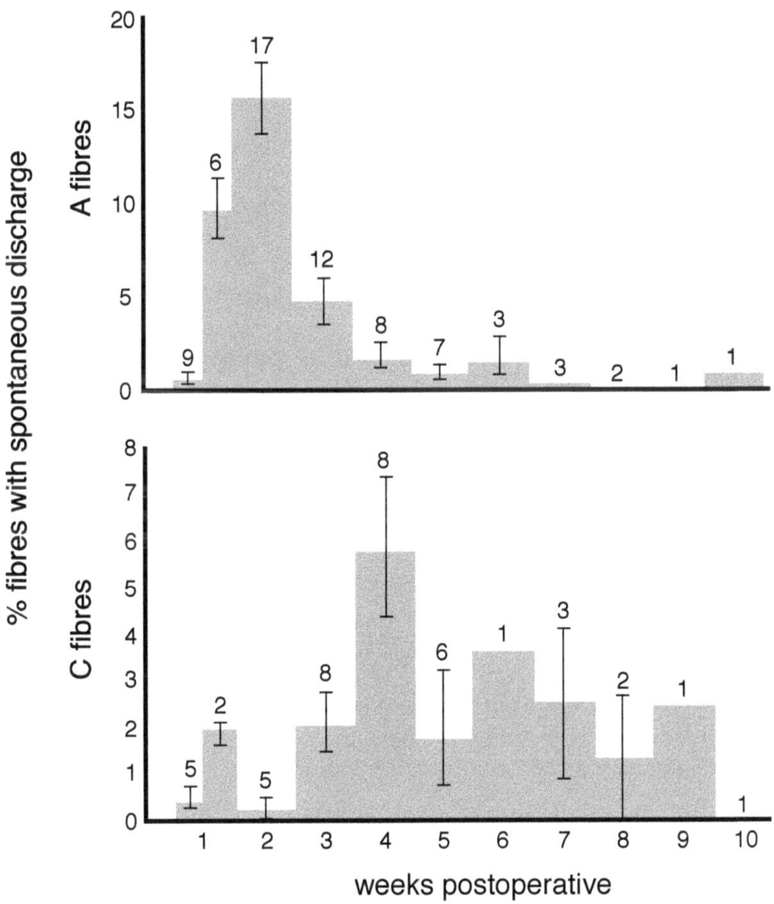

Figure NR 1.6 The activity of Aδ fibres and C fibres ten weeks following fibre injury. Redrawn from Devor's chapter in the 5th edition of The Textbook of Pain 2005.

Or secondly, could there be peripheral nerve involvement? Eh? Yes! Figure NR 1.6 is from Devor's chapter in the Textbook of Pain. Early research focused on the ectopic activity of Aδ and C fibres because they were the 'pain' fibres and largely ignored the Aβ fibres, because they were 'low threshold' and hence not considered to be concerned with damage and disease reporting. (I'll discuss Aβ fibres and ectopia in a little while!).

The top graph shows the activity of Aδ fibres over ten weeks following fibre injury. (I love this observation over such a long time period – it's so clinically useful for us!). Note, very little activity for the first week, then it's massive for the following two weeks after which it starts to settle and really peters out from around five to six weeks on.

The bottom graph is for C fibres and shows a rather modest level of activity for the first two weeks – but thereafter, virtually for the next couple of months, the activity is quite intense. Around the one month mark seems particularly nasty.

But, look at the delay in onset of activity! Aδ and C fibres may take a great many days or even over a week to get going and have the potential to cause pain. Get the patient to think back a bit further, ask too if they've been manipulated hard at some point, or whether they've been asked to do repeated extension exercises over and over again? Or, whether they've done some unusual or awkward physical activity? It's certainly my experience **that the two forms of management for acute and sub acute pain are quite strongly associated with back pain becoming nerve root pain!** But, it's often after a delay of anything from a day or two to a week sometimes more. Yes, it could have happened anyway and that's important to understand too. **My clinical observations over the years, has led me to having the view that every 'simple' back pain has the potential to be a nerve root problem!** That's why for the most part I've adopted a 'graded exposure' approach to all pain problems – acute and chronic. Going at something with force or to full end of range while provoking pain, even if it 'centralises' was what I did a long time ago, but not anymore. It's not worth it and, the results aren't impressive. Lose faith and it stops working anyway!

The good thing about this observational research reported by Devor is that by week ten activity has virtually stopped and this fits with most nerve root patients that I see. Well, roughly... and, sort of! What we often forget with these experiments is that they're done on small rodents whose lifespan is at best two to three years. Thus, if a mouse lives for two years – ten weeks is about one tenth of its life! So the ten week equivalent in humans would be six to seven years! Imagine being pissed-off with nerve pain for a tenth of your life! Rats are, but we humans shouldn't be, ten to twelve weeks or a little more, isn't that big a deal.

Still, whatever the ageing physiology and inter-species differences – the timescale feels about right for clinical observations! It's likely that the metabolism of a nerve in humans and rats goes on at much the same pace. Ten days for them is ten weeks for us then? It seems to fit.

When I discuss nerve root problems and their natural history with my patients, I often include some or all of the following (in palatable patient form):

1. Nerves in, around and emerging from the spine are pretty hardy – they get squashed, stretched and pinched during normal movements, but for the most part never complain and never let you know. They're largely insensitive to normal and often quite intense physical forces. They're surprisingly strong![1]

2. Sometimes nerves can become sensitised by injury, they can be squashed or stretched to such an extent that they do get injured and then react – just like a joint, ligament, tendon or muscle does. But unlike these structures, which begin hurting more or less immediately or at least within a few hours of injury – nerves can take time to become sensitised and cause pain. Experiments done on rat nerves show that increased sensitivity from physical injury may take up to a week or more. (Use this where the patient's pain came on for no apparent reason and as I said, it also gets them to think back a bit further for some possible activity related reason).

3. It may not always be like this – sometimes nerve pain can develop over several hours or a day or two and be clearly linked to an injury or overstrain. (Your explanation obviously has to fit with the story of onset that the patient gives you!). Sometimes the nerve root pain starts very suddenly, though this in my experience is less common, unless there's a past history of similar pain – meaning the nerve and it's pathways are 'pre-sensitised' in some way. (Memories may fade, but it takes a lot for them to disappear completely).

4. Once a nerve is sensitised it can start producing masses of electrical impulses, out-of-the-blue, for no reason at all. This means that pain can come on for no reason and just carry on for no reason and be very hard to stop. It also means that pain can come and go suddenly for no apparent reason – patients' may get sudden bursts of pain and then it's gone without having done anything! Acknowledging and normalising the nature and behaviour of nerve pain can be very helpful to worried patients.

5. The nerve may become very sensitive to movement and physical forces – hence many movements, even small movements causing a great deal of pain.

6. Nerve pain once started often runs on and on for far longer than normal strains and sprains type pain.

7. Nerve related pain can also cause referred tenderness, this means that tender skin, muscle, bones – while in actual fact are quite normal, can hurt horribly when touched or pressed on. (I may then use the shingles example or the angina one (see earlier chapters)).

8. Nerve pain can be easier to understand if you think of an old electrical wire where the insulation has perished and there's short circuiting happening.

1 - *I think Dave Butler reported that the old nerve anatomists and physicians used to treat sciatica by surgically exposing the sciatic nerve in the back of the thigh and hanging weights on it. They reported that the nerve could often withstand as much as the patient's own body weight before it snapped!*

A small movement of the wire and there's a crackle and flash! Care here though, because you don't want to leave the patient thinking their wiring has had it and it needs replacing! As discussed, talk of 'bad' can do harm!

9. Nerve pain is often a bit strange, patients use terms like sharp, shooting, burning, knife-like... jabbing, crawling, deep bony toothache... I've known patients who've had such weird pains that they've been embarrassed to describe them to their Doctor.

Here's my most famous one! The guy's a fisherman in his late 30's and we're getting along fine. I'm asking about his pain and he's giving me the area – over his right scapular and then I ask him what it feels like?

'Louis, I've not had the guts to tell anyone yet what it feels like – because I find it hard to believe myself and I certainly wouldn't believe it if someone else told me. I know if I told my Dr this, he wouldn't believe it.'

'Go on.'

'Take a big needle, like the ones we use to mend our fishing nets, thread it up with some steel wire, like the wire traces we use to catch sharks. Now, start sewing – in here, out here, all the way down here.'

What he was showing me was an in and out stitch; starting by piercing his skin in the upper medial corner or the scapular, going deep into the skin and the underlying muscle, following the medial border of the scapula down to its tip and then back up the lateral border. He went on.

'So the wire's got an end sticking out here... (the upper medial scapular corner) and here (laterally round about the back of the shoulder joint), now, grab the ends and start pulling them to and fro, like you were working a saw.'

He took a deep breath and said 'Believe it or not, that's what my pain feels like 90% of the time.'

It's hard to even contemplate the biology of a pain like this. You might dream of it happening, but not the faintest way would you dream of actually feeling it!

Let's continue...

10. The pain is often hard to give a precise location – it's vague, dull, diffuse and often deep. It can move around from one place to another.

11. If nerves that go to muscles are injured – those muscles may get weakened. (This can be seen as a rather negative message, but the patient may well have weakness and this needs explaining and also reassuring – more on this later). A clinical and personal aside here that maybe of interest. Recently I've had a great deal of 'sciatic' type pain from spinal and pelvic bone metastases. Accompanying the pain has been enough of a neuropathy to weaken my right calf to the extent I could only just go up on tip-toe and I virtually lost a decent functional push-off. The weakened calf became incredibly sore to touch and sore to use. It felt like I'd been overworking

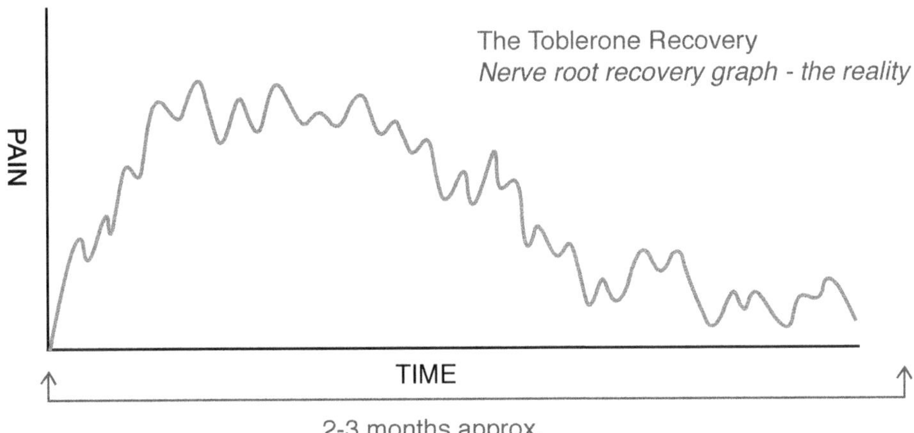

Figure NR 1.7 Nerve root recovery graph showing the normal progression and variation of nerve root pain build up and recovery.

the little bit of strong muscle that was still functional and had overstrained it. Was it referred pain or was it a true injury to that little bit of 'over-working' calf muscle? An interesting thought?

12. If nerves that give you skin sensation are injured – you may get pins and needles or even numbness in the area supplied by that nerve. (Again, no need to say this to the patient if this isn't part of the symptom picture but if it is, or it's picked up during the examination it needs explaining and reassuring, 'normalising' – again, more later)

13. The normal progression and variation of pain is shown in my graph (figure NR 1.7, review section 13 and the Toblerone recovery). The key elements are: the early phase where the pain builds up and up, it may start in the back and spread down buttock into the leg, or just be in the buttock/leg or any combination. It may come on out of the blue, or be related to an obvious incident – the steepness of the graph indicates the rapidity of pain building, so this angle can be adjusted to fit with the patient's story. Or, you can tell them about the huge variety of presentations. Patients do talk to their friends and may hear completely different stories from them. The key is to 'normalise' the crazy presentation and behaviour of it all. Crazy is normal here and to me, crazy presentations steer towards strong maladaptive 'neurogenic' mechanisms – be they peripherally or centrally generated, or more likely, both.

14. The next phase is what I call 'the really nasty phase' and it's often when the patient seeks help. This phase is usually in the realms of two to four weeks, but not uncommonly even longer (see figure NR 1.7). The better the pain and the 'yellow-flags' are dealt with in this phase the shorter the period

and the better the overall outcome. It's very much a 'Toblerone' ride as is shown.

15. After this three to four week nasty phase, the horizontal nasty 'tobleroning' starts to slant downwards and the patient becomes aware of improvements. This downward line/wave goes on for many weeks and may even last for up to a year at low levels. I do tell most patients this – yes it's negative, but it's the reality. But what I do is back it up with something like this:

    Just as you might with a frozen shoulder, you say...

    'The good news is that it gets better, the bad news is that it can take quite a long time. Most Drs will tell you that it takes 6-8 weeks for a sciatica to get better – that's not really the case. In my experience it's usually anything from 8-12 weeks or longer and it may even linger on for a year or more! The good news, as you've seen from the graph, is that it does get better, especially if it's well managed and I can help you here. Now, you may think I'm being a bit grim with all that but the worst thing I can say to you is that I'll fix it in a few days or a week, or, that it should be better in about ten days. What happens here, when you're not better, you get very concerned that something is seriously wrong and you get even more worried; you may go back to the Dr; or go to lots of different practitioners, who give different spins on the problem; you may get forceful treatment and risk making it far worse.. . It's far better to EXPECT it to go on for quite a long time and adjust to things, but then, if it does get better quicker than we said – you'll be pleased. Now I mentioned a 'year or more' just now, most folk get over the worst of sciatica in this round about three month period and they're pretty much better, only getting the odd flashes of symptoms, or a day or so bother from time to time. But they cope with that well and eventually these last few bits and pieces fade away.

    I often draw a second graph on the first but lower, to show that our aim is to get the pain down, at the same time as keeping going physically (see figures, section 13). This is an appropriate time to discuss the value of pain killers and that with nerve pain, reducing the pain is helping to 'cure' the problem, rather than what is commonly held – that pain killers just mask the problem and may leave you vulnerable to further harm.

16. The natural history of the disc may need discussing – more later...

For those contemplating surgery I use the following handout that I copied from The New England Journal of Medicine vol 356, p2245:

'If you have sciatica and find that rest and pain medication are not working to relieve your pain, should you consider surgery? Recent research provides the answer.

Sciatica refers to leg pain caused by a herniated disk in the spine that presses on the sciatic nerve. People with sciatica often experience intense pain that radiates into the buttocks, down the thighs, into the calves, and often into the feet.

Surgery can provide fast pain relief for sciatica, but you might do just as well without an operation, a study finds.

In this study, researchers randomly assigned 281 people with sciatica for at least six weeks to have surgery to decompress the nerve or to receive conservative treatments such as pain medication and exercise. On average people who had sciatica surgery felt their leg pain was better after four weeks while it took about 12 weeks for those who did not have surgery to note improvement. But within one year, 95% of the study participants said they felt significantly better, no matter what sciatica treatment they had.

Bottom line advice: *If you are experiencing searing pain or numbness in your leg from sciatica and conservative treatment is not working, then surgery may be right for you. On the other hand, if you feel you can handle the leg pain and are willing to postpone sciatica surgery, you just might find you don't need it.'*

Chapter NR 1.5

Nerve root mechanisms 3: to ectopia and beyond!

It seems that the cause and source of pain in sciatica, brachialgia or any other peripheral nerve related pain, at a beautifully reductionist level of investigation – is 'ectopia'! Sounds like a fantastic holiday destination!

Ectopia, let it be clear are invisible; they're tiny areas of axon membrane that have been 'remodelled' so that they become hyper-excitable. There is absolutely no means of clinically detecting ectopia with any modern technology. No x-ray, no scanner, no ultrasound machine, no blood test, nothing can visualise these incredibly pernicious sources of such nasty and crazy pain.

What's happened? What causes this state of affairs to happen? What's 'membrane remodelling'?

Devor's old diagram has it all (see figure NR 1.8). It's a cartoon of a myelinated sensory nerve fibre. On the left is the cell body, to the right, the axon. The gap in the axon indicates that it may be very long. At the right end of the axon is the cut axon, where it is swelling into a microneuroma with its axon sprouts starting to bud. Up in the cell body lies the nucleus and all those important protein building structures – you can see endoplasmic reticulum with the tiny circular dots, representing ribosomes for example. Marshall Devor has drawn lots of squares, circles and triangles to represent different ion channels and receptors – he's kept it pretty simple and focused in on sodium, potassium and calcium ion channels; alpha adrenoreceptors and mechanoreceptors (or 'stretch activated transducer channels' as he calls them). The reality is that there are many more varieties.

It is worth the reader reviewing the ion channel and peripheral sensitivity discussion in section 5 and the discussion of impulses and ion channels there too. The process

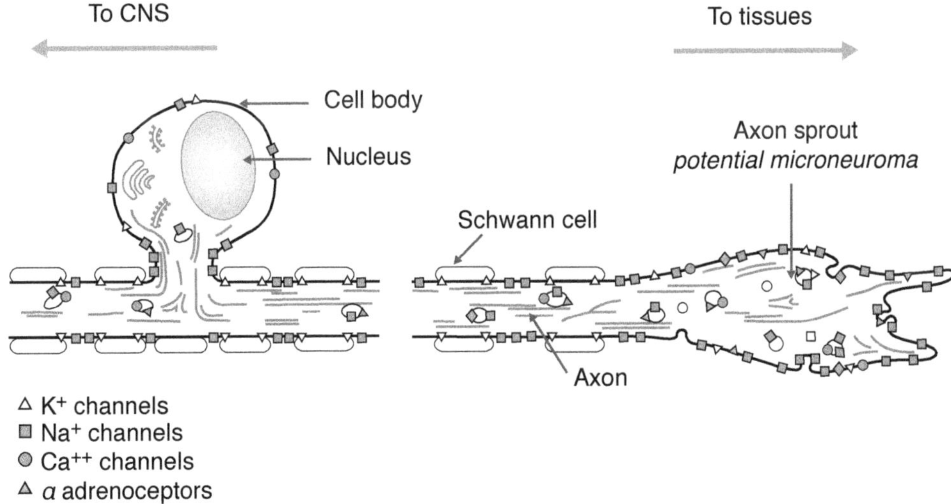

Figure NR 1.8 A myelinated sensory nerve fibre. Redrawn from Devor Textbook of Pain.

is similar here but madder! It's worth a quick review here, but with a slightly different and deeper spin on it perhaps.

Recall that it's the nerve fibre cell body, situated in the DRG way up in the nerve root area – where all these receptor and ion-channel products are manufactured. Devor calls the cell body 'a nutritive depot for the sensory axon', it's the protein factory, the scrutinising and responding centre for the individual fibre and does its best to provide for it.

A normal healthy nerve fibre ending has two functional zones: the transducer zone where a variety of stimuli are converted, or transduced, into an electrical signal or current and an 'encoding zone', where this mild electrical current is amplified to create the full impulse.

In order to 'transduce' there have to be receptors present specific to the stimulus being presented. Hence there are chemical and temperature receptors as well as mechanoreceptors, or stretch-activated receptors as they are also called. Further, in order for a stimulus to be converted or transduced to an 'electrical' impulse the receptor has to be functionally associated with an ion channel in some way. Thus receptors either have an ion channel as part of their structure, or they are very closely associated with them, they're 'nearby' if you like.

Recall that an ion channel is a protein structure, situated in the cell wall of the nerve fibre. When it 'opens', it changes its configuration to create a pore or channel for ions to flow through. The movement of ions across the cell membrane is what causes a change in 'voltage' or 'potential' and hence a mild electrical current. The main ions involved are sodium and potassium, but calcium ions may be involved too and thus specific channels for each of them must be present.

Ion channels are of two basic types, those directly associated with receptors as we've been discussing and those that are out on their own in isolation. They're often referred to as 'voltage' gated ion channels because they open when a voltage impacts on them.

Talking about ion channel opening and closing always makes me chuckle, because I'm reminded of the disc jockey/comedian Kenny Everett and his, 'in-the-best-possible-taste' sketches. Check it out on YouTube! The ridiculously cross-dressed, glamorously well-endowed but bearded Everett, heaps on all the clever sexual innuendo you can think of during a constant monologue of hilarious drivel about some situation he's been in or new show or film he's doing. All the while this is going on, he is constantly opening and closing his legs, revealing slinky underwear, stockings and suspender belts and always, at some point in the sketch he throws his legs up in the air, wide apart, revealing all! He then twirls them round each other, to end up in a rather entwined cross-legged position and as he does this he goes, 'And it's all done in the best paah-ssible taste.' You know it is coming and you always laugh when he does it. It's the wide open legs – ions in, followed by the entwined crossed legs, channel closed!

That wasn't funny I know. But go check it out on the internet and you'll see what I mean! It's a great vision to have and a great way of explaining how ion channels open and close!

So, a voltage gated ion channel as a protein structure that when zapped with an electrical charge can change its configuration – like Kenny Everett's legs unwinding, then winding up again, or, as I mentioned in the nociception chapter, the Boa Constrictor uncoiling to release its prey – to let a quick rush of ions into the cell.

A normal cell membrane sits at rest with an electrical charge – called the 'membrane potential'. Classically it sits at -70mV. Now, when sodium ion-channels open they let the ions into the cell from outside, whereas open potassium ion channels let these ions go from inside the cell to out. In the nerve fibre terminal zone, sodium ion channels, as just mentioned, are often built into and associated with specific receptors.

So for example, an 'alpha adrenoreceptor' may have a receptor protein structure specific to adrenaline or noradrenaline, which in turn is physically attached to a sodium ion channel. The adrenaline molecule locks into the receptor protein, the receptor protein then changes it's configuration and in so doing forces the adjacent ion channel to 'Kenny Everett', in go the sodium ions and very cleverly, 'chemical' (adrenaline) is transduced to electrical! Think about it, as we did with the story of Paul Bach-y-Rita at the end of chapter 19.6, it makes you realise that every form of stimulus ends up being 'electrical' in the form of impulses. That means sight is the same as sound, as touch as temperature, as taste, as inflammatory chemical and so forth – they are all just patterns of impulses. No wonder Bach-y-Rita had the imagination to realise that we could be trained to 'see' via our skin and later and more accurately, with our tongues!

These clever little receptor and ion channel friends are what lie at the heart of transduction and the formation of an impulse and hence, of feelings, like light touch or if the stimulus is intense and threatening, of discomfort, nastiness and pain.

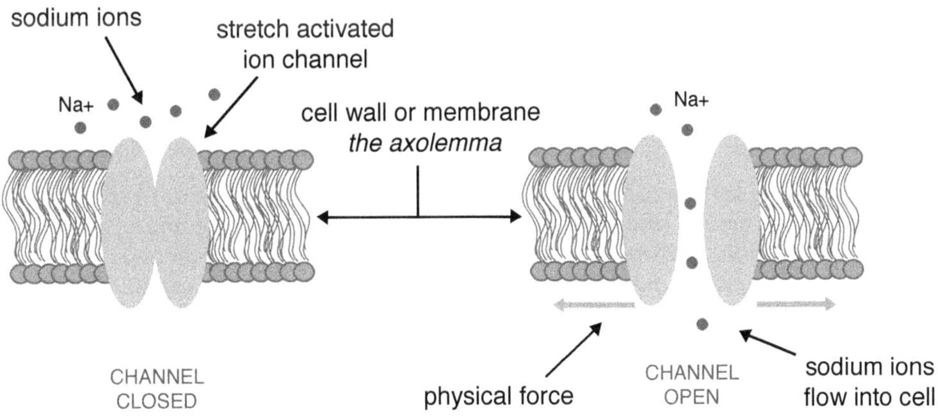

Figure NR 1.9 'Stretch activated' ion-channel/or mechanoreceptor showing sodium activity.

Clinically I am coming to an important bit: thinking of touch, pressure and movement; doing a physical examination and palpation; doing a neural tension test; awareness of a contracting muscle and any other 'mechanically' based input or test – means thinking that the cause of the sensation must involve 'stretch activated' ion-channels/or mechanoreceptors (see figure NR1.9). When a physical force reaches nerve fibre terminals containing these little units it will cause them to be virtually stretched open, thus allowing a flow of sodium ions through the cell membrane and hence, a change in membrane potential and the possibility of an impulse. At this 'transducer' stage, the voltage change is relatively minor and called a 'generator potential' or 'current' (see figure NR 1.10).

Right next door to the transducing zone is the 'encoding zone' or 'encoding compartment' of the nerve. It's packed with voltage gated sodium and potassium ion channels. This area takes the little currents from the transducer zone and converts, or amplifies them, into full-on impulses that smartly set-off down the axon to the CNS.

In impulse propagation down the length of the axon, the 'voltage-gated' sodium ion channels are first to open and a few ions flow from outside into the cell (figure NR 1.11). As they flow in it causes an increase in the number of positive charges on the inside compared to the outside of the cell wall. (Recall that sodium ions, like potassium, are positively charged 'anions'). This in turn causes the resting membrane potential to increase and if it reaches the critical 'threshold' level of -55mV, there's a sudden and massive opening of sodium ion channels and the voltage rapidly shots up to its peak at +40mV (see 'b' on lower graph in figure NR 1.11). This rise in voltage triggers the opening of the potassium ion channels and they then rush out of the cell, causing the charge imbalance to reduce and hence the voltage to drop rapidly back down again in the 'falling phase' of the impulse.

The result is a wave of activity flowing down the axon, as the voltage change in one part of the axon stimulates the ion channels to open in the next. The impulse travels like a falling column of dominoes, as far as the synapse in the CNS.

If you're thinking that the impulse leaves all the ions in the wrong place, the sodium being left on the inside, when they all started on the outside and vice versa for the potassium ions – you'd be right! How do they all get quickly back again? It's thanks to the sodium-potassium ion pump – a clever device of nature that grabs potassium ions on the outside and spits them out on the inside and the opposite for sodium.

The graph at the bottom of figure NR 1.11 shows the voltage variation of an action potential. You can see that voltage rapidly drops down before going up a little to very near threshold, before finally tailing off back to 'resting potential, which in the time frame here, is quite long. This little bounce upward is called a 'DAP' – a 'Depolarization After Potential' and leaves the nerve fibre in a heightened sensitivity state, very near it's 'critical threshold voltage' of -55mV. The effect of this is to increases its tendency to be able to fire again.

On the other hand, it also seems that the voltage sometimes 'hyperpolarizes' – it dips lower than the -70mV resting potential before gradually returning upwards again.

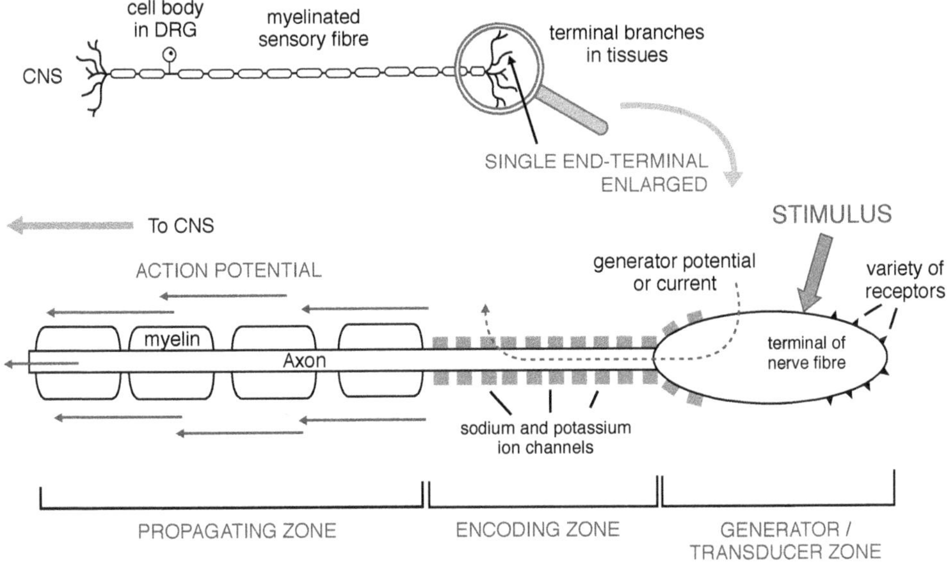

Figure NR 1.10 The 'transducer' stage of an impulse.

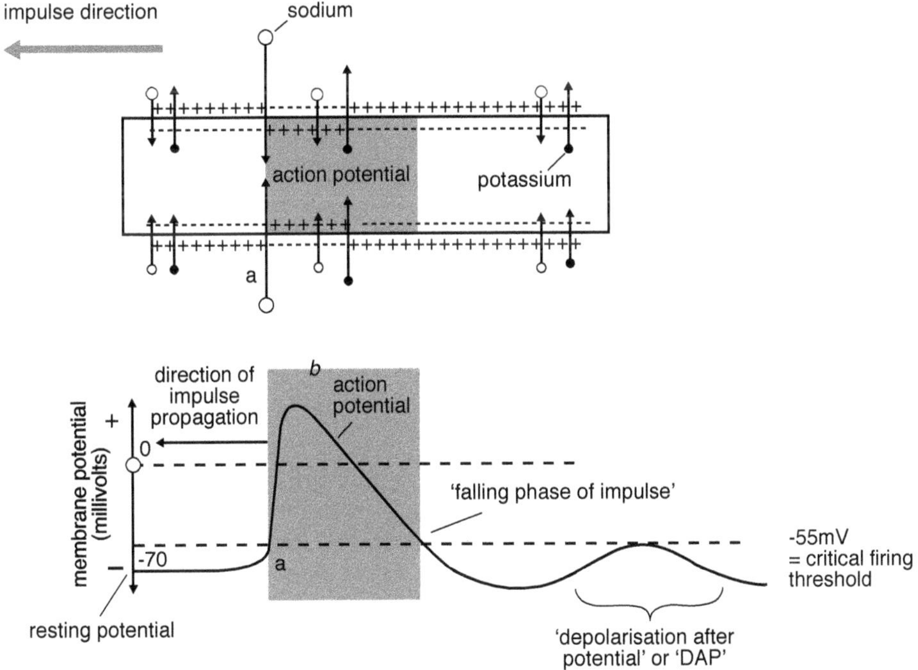

Figure NR 1.11 Impulse propagation down the length of the axon.

Simply and important for us clinically, if the voltage of a given nerve fibre is shifted lower, it becomes hyperpolarized – in other words, it becomes 'inhibited', or if it's shifted nearer the -55mV threshold it becomes 'sensitised'.

This is of major importance to having a better understanding of on-going increased sensitivity; another is understanding repetitive firing which helps our understanding of on-going pain.

It seems that some cells have a natural ability to keep firing on their own in normal conditions. Remember from Schmidt and Schiable's work, discussed in the nociception section 11, where they showed that around 35% of C and Aδ fibres were constantly popping impulses when the 'normal' joint was at rest?

It seems that some neurones exhibit what's called a 'sub-threshold sinusoidal current'! It actually imparts on the cell membrane 'intrinsic reverberatory properties'! This means that the neurones voltage is going up and down just under the 'critical-firing' threshold mark of - 55mV and not settling back to a more placid -70mV. When repetitive firing occurs – the voltage fluctuates up and down post impulse, but must at some stage hit the -55mV mark and, once the cell has readied itself, it then re-fires, settles back again, goes sinusoidal/reverberatory, hits the mark... of it goes again!

This is just like in the CNS, with our 'centrally' generated pain discussed in earlier chapters, yet another way in which nociception, in its broadest sense, can lead to pain for no pathological or physical reason whatsoever. The reason looks as if it's due to the contrite bloody mindedness of the nerve fibre, combined with a brain that's willing to process what it receives as pain!

Hurt with no harm. Pointless, maladaptive pain!

Now, you should be thinking, well if 35% of nociceptors are constantly signalling, doesn't that mean constant pain... in the normal? Well it could do, couldn't it? But remember that Aβ fibres are firing constantly too (albeit only 10% of them) and that in the normal state, impulses from these fibres reaching the dorsal horn are inhibitory. Also and as I discussed earlier, that constant 35% impulse-at-rest buzzing into the CNS may have an important function that's yet to be revealed. It may have an important trophic function for example, or it may be just the peripheral tissues way of saying, 'Hey, we're here and we're OK'. Who knows?

I hugely wonder whether this normal 35% input, could easily become pain in a vulnerability state? When you're healthy and 'up' – take no notice, when you're low and a bit down – the brain starts to listen to the body and 'lets' the incoming messages register as discomfort and pain?

That aside, the main reason for discussing repetitive firing or 'pacemaker' capability, is because it has been found to be a big part of nerve injury and the on-going ghastly pain that can follow. I'll return to this shortly, but first there's another cause of repetitive firing to acknowledge.

Most patients and clinicians would interpret constant firing of nerve fibres (i.e. constant pain) with constant stimulation – due to some 'constant' bad state of affairs in the tissues. Well of course; this is the other way of getting a repetitive firing process going and keeping it going. Patients and clinicians think: constant inflammation, constant adverse mechanical forces or stresses, or a constant high or low temperature, constant thing wrong or constant threat. The nerve fibres subserving the area are polarized by the stimulus, which then creates an action potential at the nerve end, which in turn initiates a series of action potentials that travel down the fibre as an impulse. Then there's a fall in voltage, followed be the DAP – the depolarizing after potential, leaving the generator zone extra ready to fire again; which it does, because the stimulating chemicals, forces, temperature etc. are still present and when ready, off it goes – constant firing due to constant stimulation and the potential for constant pain, if the brain wants to listen! In impulse 'speak' there's a 'persistent generator potential'.

We now have three potential mechanisms that can cause on-going symptoms from the 'periphery'. The first and biomedically logical, 'pain for a reason' – due to some constant stimulus causing the 'persistent generator potential'. The second, the 'pain for no reason' or out of all proportion to the triggering stimulus, 'self generated impulses' or 'pacemaker' capability. 'Self generated impulses' are likely to be 'set-off' by some triggering stimulus of course. This may be chemical, mechanical or thermal, or it may occur for no reason at all. A mechanical stimulus is most pertinent to any physical examination. The third mechanism is a combination of the two.

Let's now get back to symptoms derived from peripheral nerve fibres.

The word 'neuralgia' simply means pain (algia) derived from nerve (neur). Devor uses Trigeminal neuralgia as an example. Like post herpetic neuralgia (shingles), the slightest touch of the very normal looking skin in the affected area, gives rise to searing horrid pain that may go on and on for many minutes afterwards. The initiating brief 'touch', triggers a 'depolarizing generator potential' in the highly sensitised neurones in the area which then fire. After firing they enter a phase of sinusoidal voltage oscillation (the DAP), repeatedly going up just beyond threshold and back down, so that when the fibre is ready to fire again, another impulse will spontaneously occur. This may go on and on for many seconds, minutes or even longer. Think of your patients!

Using the clinical terms derived from pain science, it's allodynia combined with 'wind-up' – small, innocuous inputs, causing massive and on-going symptom responses in perfectly normal skin, that is out of proportion to any damage and totally useless.

For light touch to cause pain where there is no peripheral nerve involvement, there are two standard mechanisms described: the first is via central mechanisms – here, light touch stimulates normal Aβ fibres, which normally get processed in the CNS as an innocuous sensation, but when there's been some massive impulse barrage (section 5), the central cells and central nociception processing pathways plastically alter so that they respond to this Aβ input. Hence, causing light touch to be channelled into the nociception pathways and therefore the potential to be processed to produce pain. The other mechanism is for C and Aδ fibres to become highly sensitised in their peripheral terminals. Here, their firing threshold lowers so that they now behave like Aβ fibres. Light touch, which 'normally' has little effect on them, can now produce impulses and hence pain.

Out at the nerve terminals in the tissues of the body, small inputs causing a big reaction is all about the density of 'active' ion channels. Density, or numbers of ion channels is ultimately determined by gene activity. It's therefore about switching on the genes that are responsible for making their protein constituents.

The higher the density of active sodium ion channels, the lower the threshold for firing and the more likely the nerve fibre will become capable of spontaneously firing. Devor says that if the sodium ion density can be reduced, then the threshold for rhythmic firing will be reduced or even prevented.

If you've followed so far, it's a very simple step to flip back to the injured nerve and 'ectopia'. As I've said, the basic rule for a sensory fibre, coming from a tissue and going into the spinal cord, is that normal impulses start at the fibre terminals in the tissues and via the axon, are transmitted unhindered and fairly faithfully to the central synapse. When a nerve fibre has been injured, or severed, massive changes in the cell wall of the axon occur. In particular, changes in ion channel and receptor distribution, lead to areas that don't normally initiate impulses or aren't normally very sensitive, to become excessively so. As you can see in Devor's diagram earlier (figure NR1.8), the cell wall of the re-growing axon sprout is jam-packed with receptors and ion channels.

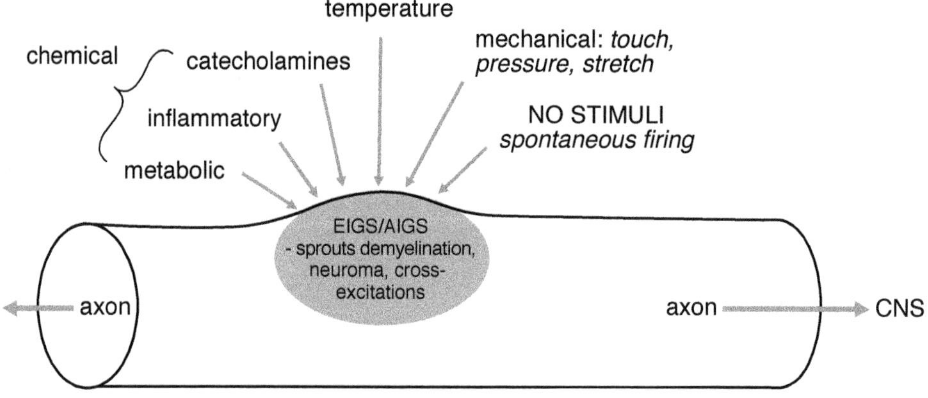

Figure NR 1.12 A schematic of an ectopic impulse generating site on an axon.

Figure NR 1.12 is a schematic of an ectopic impulse generating site on an axon, it could be at the regenerating end of a severed axon, or on regenerating sprouts along the axon, or anywhere along the axon (as here), even on the cell body itself. The figure has a list of stimulating agents on it:

- Metabolic, e.g.
    - a) agents from the immune system
    - b) agents of inflammatory and tissue breakdown
    - c) agents of tissue repair, healing and recovery
    - d) agents of hypoxia

- catecholamines
- temperature/thermal
- mechanical
- no stimuli!

Metabolic means chemical agents in the environment of the ectopic site. When a nerve fibre is injured there are plenty. A great many come from immune cells that become activated in the area, or are get attracted to it.

Here's a short list of agents that derive from immune cells:

- mast cells secrete tumour necrosis factor (TNF) and histamine
- neutrophils release prostaglandins and interleukins (IL)
- macrophages – TNF and prostaglandins
- schwann cells – TNF, ATP,IL's, nitric oxide(NO), and nerve growth factor (NGF).

If these immune inflammatory chemicals are to cause pain, then specific receptors for them must be present on the damaged nerve fibre.

In the UK, it's pretty standard for Drs to prescribe NSAIDs for nerve root pain and for years I've been observing very poor pain control with them, almost to the point of saying that I think they're a waste of time! Research project required! NSAID's and **acute** nerve root pain, please! Codeine and opiate derived analgesia seem to fair far better.

My favourite friend '**hypoxia' or 'ischaemia'** needs a mention. Recall from the nociception chapters that hypoxia leads to the release of several inflammatory chemicals, histamine and prostaglandins, for example. Later, in the nerve root physical testing section I'll discuss what I call 'ischaemic' tests. For now, you may have already noted, that some 'nerve root' problems actually come in with a very good range of movement and you're unable to provoke much of the pain with standard back or neck movements. I used to really puzzle over this until I noted that in some patients, if they maintained an end range position for some time, the symptoms gradually built up and spread and the longer the position was held, the worse the symptoms became – just like with Phalen's test for carpal tunnel syndrome! If you're wondering what Phalen's test is you need to study and read more! George Phalen was a hand surgeon famous for operating on carpal tunnel syndrome back in the 1950's. The eponymous test he campaigned simply involved sustained flexion of the wrist – which effectively reduced the size of the carpal tunnel and increased the pressure there. Increased pressure means decreased circulation and relative hypoxia. The longer the position is sustained, the greater the hypoxic conditions become. If the test produced 'nerve symptoms' in the hand the test was deemed positive and indicated that surgery was appropriate. The recommendation was that the test be sustained up to about sixty seconds and it's quite common for the test to do nothing to symptoms for quite a long time. Sometimes though, the pain comes instantly.

My observations are that it's the same for nerve root problems. Take a right sided vague arm pain. A quick overview of all neck movements reveals a bit of stiffness at end range but nothing more. Then sustain a movement towards the painful side – rotation, or side flexion, take it to comfy end range and wait , maybe ten seconds or a little more and the patient starts to tell you – vague scapular pain, now a little in triceps, ahh, there's the tingling in the thumb and then it's all building up, etc. Take another patient, same symptoms reported, but this time they turn to the side of pain and bang, the pain's there instantly.

I've never found anywhere in the literature that's discussed the possible mechanisms of this response, maybe I haven't looked hard enough? It seems obvious though, that the first, with the slow build up, is likely to relate to ischaemia – hence 'ischaemosensitivity' and the second, the quick onset of pain with movement, is likely to relate to simple 'mechanosensitivity'. I will discuss this further later when reviewing examination and diagnosis of nerve root problems. It is pleasing to note that Devor lists tissue ischaemia, hypoxia and changes in the level of blood gases, as known conditions that increase ectopic activity. Nice! Fits! Even increases in blood glucose can! Wow, have your patients ever reported feeling more pain after a 'Snicker' or Energy bar/drink?

Catecholamines are interesting because they include two major stress related chemicals: adrenaline and noradrenaline. So, if an ectopic site contains adrenoreceptors then there's the potential for adrenaline, hence stress, to cause pain. Catecholamines can arrive from the circulation, or be secreted as a result of sympathetic nerve fibre activity in the vicinity. It's worth making the distinction between feeling mentally stressed, which drives up catecholamines in the circulation and a physical stressor, like an injury or tissue inflammation, which drives them up by secreting directly into the tissues as well. Both may be enough to drive an ectopic site given the appropriate receptor availability.

Adrenaline driving ectopic sites on damaged nerve has been a major consideration underlying the mechanism of CRPS II. See Topical Issues in Pain 3 for a full discussion. The current state of research and thinking, has pretty much confirmed that it's **not an increase** in adrenaline/noradrenaline at all, the sympathetic system is innocent! In fact there's found to be a decrease in them – the key is that there's an increase in nociceptor sensitivity to adrenaline. Think of all those poor folk who've had their sympathetics ripped out by a surgeon? 'Yeah, but it worked!' When, in actual fact, outcome research shows that it didn't do that well at all... which is why the procedure is rarely done these days.

Temperature is interesting because C fibre ectopia calm down with warming and liven-up with cooling, whereas with Aδ fibres it's the opposite – they liven-up with warming and calm down with cooling. At a terribly reductionist level of reasoning and Devor mentions it, this could help explain the intolerance to cold of some chronic neuropathic pain states. I agree, but prefer to reason from the 'vulnerable organism' perspective which will be discussed in the Graded Exposure section.

Mechanical sensitivity of ectopic sites: I've already discussed this a little, but again, have you noticed the clear sciatic pain or arm pain patients where you think, this must be a nerve root problem; you perform all the standard physical tests and all the relevant neural tension tests and find very little. The symptoms are out of proportion to the degree of 'physical' and 'neural' tension test 'positivity'. This situation is very common, especially in the 'elderly'. One line of reasoning relevant here is that: no mechanoreceptors, or no 'active' mechanoreceptors equates to zero mechanosensitivity. Conversely, abundant 'active' mechanoreceptors present equates to increased mechanosensitivity and plenty of positive physical tests.

Thinking at this 'receptor' level helps the clinician to realise that sensitivity, because it relates to such a variety of cellular processes, is highly likely to be as unique and specific as the person who has the problem.

Another line of reasoning for the elderly sciatica who can happily and willingly move their back is this: that their lumbar spine, due to longstanding degenerative changes and stiffening, may have such limited movement around the irritable nerve that the movements they do, bring little physical force to bear on the areas of sensitivity. Many elderly folk can touch their toes – but it's all hip and zero lumbar movement, for example. Careful observation, during standard lumbar movement testing reveals little intervertebral movement in the low spine!

The moral here is that it's quite OK and quite explainable to have pain without having mechanically patterned responses to physical tests. A flexible elderly patient with raging nerve pain down their leg can often have a 100 degree SLR, just as the next sciatica's SLR may only be 20 degrees! Think 'receptors'!

No movement. This is all about spontaneous generation of impulse activity from the ectopic site. Presentations of constant on-going pain, pain for long periods for no reason, pain bursting on and off out-of-the-blue, or any combinations of these, can be accounted for in terms of 'spontaneous' impulse generation. Neuralgic pain has a mind of its own and because of this has often been viewed as crazy or 'impossible' pain. Many have felt that these unexplained pain behaviours must be generated in the mind of deceitful and malingering patients! Knowledge about peripheral (ectopic) and central processing mechanisms gives credibility to such pain, it is possible, it is real!

The 'proof' that pain derived from peripheral nerves is all about ion channels, is supported by the finding that nociceptive activity and pain, can be dramatically extinguished if known hyper-excitable areas of damaged nerve are injected with local anaesthetic. Lidocaine, the common local anaesthetic, works by blocking sodium ion channels in the neuron cell membrane. We've all experienced the deadening of a nerve at the dentist. It's a pity that lidocaine and other local anaesthetics are so short lasting and have such marked side effects if given systemically. The pain world uses the term 'membrane stabilizers' to describe any drug that blocks transmission or impulse formation at this ion-channel level. Anti-depressants, like amytriptiline and the anticonvulsant drugs used in the treatment of epilepsy, like gabapentin, have 'membrane stabilising' qualities and are often used to try and help neuropathic pain. Corticosteroids appear to have this capability too and it's mooted that epidural injections may produce their benefit by this mechanism.

For those of you who like a bit of biology you may remember the terms 'genotype' and 'phenotype' from your 'A' level biology courses at school. Genotype refers to a given individual's specific set of genes. We like to think of this as nicely fixed, but the reality is that mutations of genes and also 'epigenetic' changes, occur through life; and so the proteins produced and hence the makeup and features of the cells involved, may change somewhat. Think cancer for example, where mutations lead to abnormal cells with abnormal cell division biology.

Phenotype refers to the outward appearance of an individual. When you look at me, you see my phenotype. Likewise, when you investigate one of my C or Aδ fibres you will 'see' its phenotype, meaning, not only its outward appearance but also the details of its physical and chemical structure. All of which are ultimately dependent on the individual cell's gene activity – the activity that derives from the genotype! In pain biology the term 'phenotypic switching' often crops up – it simply means that for whatever reason, a cell changes its structure in some way and hence, changes its physiological characteristics. When a neurone is injured it changes dramatically – some genes get switched off and some on. The result is a massive change in 'protein-products' and therefore in its cell wall morphology and overall chemical footprint.

For example, if a C fibre is cut or 'axotomized', it reduces the production of the neurotransmitter substance P, but if Aδ fibres are, there's an increase in it. Both increase sodium ion channel production, but decrease the production of the ATP receptors ($P2X_3$) and the vanilloid receptor VR_1. The VR_1 receptor is best known for being responsible for transducing noxious heat, but also for detecting capsaicin (chemical in chilli peppers) and 'acid' conditions (i.e. protons, H^+) – all three of which, unsurprisingly, feel hot!

Now, if an afferent fibre is damaged but 'spared', meaning that there's no Wallerian degeneration and therefore that it's still 'in continuity' with its target tissues, the story is slightly different. Here, C fibres **increase** substance P as well as their VR_1 and $P2X_3$ receptors and both C and Aδ fibres increase their ion channels. That's the tip of a huge iceberg. The point is that changes in receptors and ion channels and their insertion, plus activation in 'novel' zones of the nerve fibre – change the structure, the phenotype, of the cell and hence change its function.

Enough chemicals! No, let's have more! Why? Because physiotherapy is overwhelmed with anatomy and biomechanics and unlike them, pain as well as psychology are ultimately electro-chemical. Sorry, you have to suffer a little more!

Chapter NR 1.6
Nerve root pain mechanisms 4

Inflammation now and to entice you on I'll then shift up a notch in the explanation hierarchy to discs!

I think that if we're going to adequately understand back pain and nerve root pain, we have to appreciate inflammation and chemicals a great deal more.

Pain researchers, using rats and mice, find that when they dribble 'inflammatory' cocktails on normal nerve they get a massive increase in mechanical sensitivity and in spontaneous firing. What's the cocktail? Do you remember our sexy lubricant carageenan, from the nociception chapters, which produced joint inflammation similar to that of arthritis? Well, there's another cocktail of chemicals used by pain researchers called 'complete freund's adjuvant' (CFA), which apparently is illegal to use in humans! It basically stimulates the immune system. So, inject it intradermally and you get skin ulceration and necrosis; in muscle, you get permanent lesions; and intravenously, you may get pulmonary emboli. Nice!

Inflammation in or around nerve fibres as observed in inflammatory neuropathies, like Guillian-Barre syndrome, results in massive demyelination. As we've seen, demyelination leaves the neurone very prone to developing ectopia and causing pain and other nerve related symptoms.

It's also observed that the very same thing happens when a loose ligament is tied round a nerve – the 'chronic constriction injury' model noted earlier. The constriction leads to oedema **and inflammation** forming. Bear this in mind for later when I discuss disc bulging and extrusion. If you think about it, a disc problem results in a similar state of affairs to the chronic constriction injury. The disc bulge or extrusion doesn't have to press directly on the nerve root, merely occupying more space than normal in a part of our back where there's not a lot of space to start with, is likely to create a compressive or 'constriction' effect and hence, oedema and inflammation. Degenerative enlargement of facet joints may have the same effect.

The point here is that changing space around nerve, such that there's increasing pressure on it, can lead to marked changes in the fluid and chemical environment. As noted, there can be massive demyelination, as well as the possibility of axon death (axotomy and then Wallerian degeneration) if physical forces and chemicals are sufficient. Wallerian degeneration means neuropathy, clinically the loss of nerve function – hence loss of sensation, loss of reflexes and muscle weakness if motor nerve fibres are involved. If these features present, then Wallerian degeneration must have occurred. This means the appearance of accompanying degeneration products, as the body deals with the dying cells and all the chemicals produced by the emergent immune cells and the various reactions that are caused.

Devor makes the point that this state of affairs in a nerve trunk, may lead to neighbouring intact and normal fibres developing ectopic firing capability. It's rather like being in a theatre with a load of happy, healthy, fit people but where there are just two or three inconsiderate patrons who are coughing and sneezing. Soon, happily fit neighbours start to succumb to the muck being spread around, or the premonition of the muck and they in turn start to play-up too!

Not only do normal neighbours 'catch' the ectopic capability, they may also start doing a bit of their own 'sprouting', being fertilized by the degenerative chemical soup. Normal neighbouring nerve fibre sprouting can be considered in two ways: firstly, as a rather altruistic behaviour in the sense of: 'That target tissue has lost its normal innervation. I'll wire up to it and see if I can help.' Or secondly, rather more like Burglar Bill, 'He's gone for a minute, I'll slip in here and have some of that.' Evolution would undoubtedly prefer the former! Intact neighbour sprouting is called 'collateral sprouting' and is considered to be yet another potential ectopic impulse generating site.

Think about this: injure a nerve root up in the lumbar intervertebral foramen. Local inflammation results and some nerve fibres will be damaged to the extent there's Wallerian degeneration. The distal degenerating axon may go a long way down the sciatic nerve, maybe all the way to the foot? That means there's the potential for further chemical insult to intact neighbours all the way down it. Injure a nerve in one place and you're very likely to upset another part of it somewhere along its length too. Clinically it means that a sciatica, or any nerve injury, can have foci of ectopia and hence mechanical sensitivity (positive neural tension tests, areas of sensitivity to touch, to palpate or to move, to muscle contraction), anywhere along the length of the nerve.

The common example that comes to mind, is the sciatic patient who finds they can't stand pressure of a chair on the back of their leg for long, they're much better sitting forward perching on the edge and so removing the pressure.

Now we know a mechanism for this sort of finding, we're able to explain it and make sense of it for the patient. We can 'normalise' it. What's weird is that if a patient reports this state of affairs you would expect to find significant tenderness on the back of the thigh, but quite often you can't! Even spending some time massaging it – it's frequently impossible to reproduce it or find anything much in the way of tenderness. Geoff Maitland used to say 'make features fit'. Well, in nerve pain 'features-not-fitting' is almost a diagnostic feature! So, 'features-not-fitting-makes-features-fit' is the phrase to adopt here. It's the typical inconsistency of nerve pain.

I can hear someone at the back going, 'Yeah Louis, but you've changed their posture from sitting to lying'. Yeah I did, but I've had many patients slide forward on the chair, get pain relief and then spend time palpating and massaging in this position and still not finding anything. Sometimes you can though. The key message is the 'features don't fit' one, plus, the fact that a nerve injury can occur in one spot and abnormality can spread others. Pain mechanisms move location and so can the sites of pain and tenderness. Don't forget that in most clinical situations it's probably impossible to tell whether a given area of pain or tender-spot is actually derived from tissues or nerve fibres in that area. Consideration must always be given to referred pain and tenderness as well as to secondary hyperalgesia, all of which relate to central mechanisms.

Right, so normal next-door neighbour nerve fibres can become abnormal or impaired too. They can also form abnormal synapses and areas where impulses can jump from one fibre to another. Thus, an impulse may start in an Aβ fibre and jump to a C, or any other combination. In the early 1940's it was noted that immediately when a nerve was cut the current would jump around from one fibre to the next, but it would very soon stop only to re-emerge again weeks later. The re-emergent 'coupling', as it was called then became very enduring. It all fits with the weird, sudden, out of the blue, ghastly and stubborn nature of nerve pain. It sometimes seems amazing that we don't hurt more!

There appear to be two types of impulse jumping, purely **electrical** – where myelin insulation has degenerated, which is called 'ephaptic cross-talk'; and **chemical**. Here, the repetitive firing of one neurone releases chemicals to such an extent that neighbours get sent into 'paroxsysms of self sustained firing'. Sounds very sexy, but the term 'crossed after discharge' for it, brings it back to mere 'smelly'. When I first found out about all this, I realised that at last we had explanations for sudden pains, sharp pains and on-going pains.

Over the years I have come to a bit of a conclusion. It's this: that a damaged nerve, in the process of trying to recover and rewire itself, may **in some people** produce pain and that **this pain is an unfortunate by-product of a very smart regenerative process**. Shut up or put up then? Maybe, but sadly the consequences of massive and crazy ectopic impulse activity can be massive and crazy central changes, at least in some people?

It seems that some of us may be more prone to getting painful ectopic activity than others. Could it be genetic? Well it could be that some of us are more predisposed to it, given the right environmental stimuli. That means genetics combined with environmental factors are likely to be operating. Let's have a look at 'genetic' or heritable aspects in rats.

It's well known to pain researchers that with experimental nerve injury, 'Lewis' strain rats show low levels of ectopic activity and hence low levels of 'autotomy' behaviour compared to 'Sabra' strain rats, where it is high. 'Autotomy' behaviour is the 'gnawing' and self-mutilation that many animals exhibit, in response to pain or loss/altered sensation. Pain scientists believe that this behaviour correlates well with levels of pain.

Devor and Raber 1990 actually took two strains of rat and observed the levels of 'autotomy' behaviour at seventy days after an operation that produced a 'standard' nerve injury. In other words the injury was the same in all rats every single time it was done. Note, seventy days! That's over two months since the injury – useful to know in terms of 'normalising' pain duration after nerve injury.

Take a look at the graph in figure NR 1.13 (following page).

The autotomy response in all of the rats varied a great deal. Note in the first generation of rats (that's generation zero on the horizontal axis): there is virtually zero autotomy behaviour in the 'Lewis' strain, yet for the 'Sabra' strain (upper graph) the autotomy score is very high.

Rats in each strain that showed exceptionally high or exceptionally low levels of autotomy they allowed to breed. When the brood were mature they repeated the nerve injury and then after seventy days picked-out the high pain/high autotomy and allowed them to breed and the same for the low ones. They did this over thirteen generations. As it's easy to see, the highs got higher and the lows lower and it neatly shows that breeding out for a pain and autotomy behaviour trait can be done. Don't

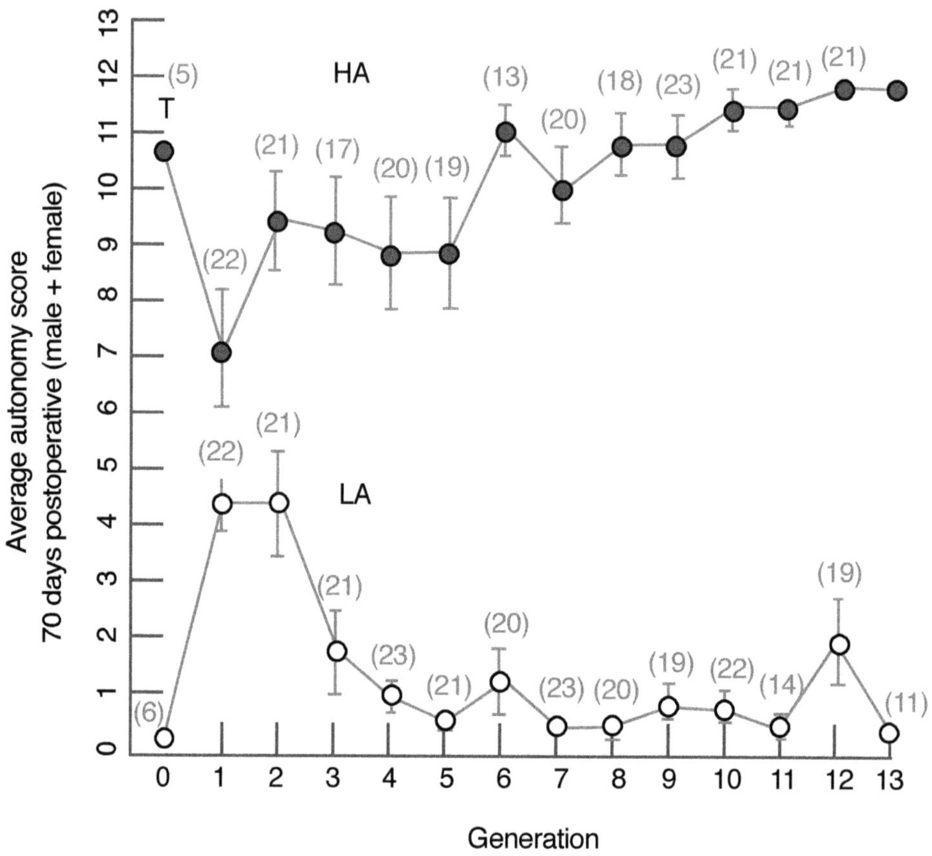

Figure NR 1.13 Genetic selection for rats with high(HA) versus low (LA) levels of autotomy. (Numbers in parentheses are the number of animals tested in each generation). Redrawn from Devor and Raber 1990.

forget that rats are brought up by parents and that environmental factors may still be in there! For us clinicians, it's enough to be able to say that some people are likely to be more prone to nerve pain than others.

As I've already discussed in the dorsal horn and central mechanisms chapters, the cause of central change is ultimately high impulse activity – the 'afferent barrage' arriving from the periphery via sensory afferents and most notably, from C and Aδ nociceptive fibres. The C fibre release of substance P is seen as vital to triggering and setting up the longer term heightened sensitivity of the second order cells. It's Shane's gift to Claudia and it ultimately triggers the up-regulation of gene activity, the production and installation of more receptors and ion channels and the fertilizer molecules that stimulate new synaptic growth and novel connectivity. In memory literature parlance it's called 'long term potentiation', or LTP and at this level of reasoning is at the heart of the problem of long term pain. Claudia's phenotype has switched – she changes, she's structurally not what she used to be and she's up for making-out with whoever's available. That's the story with central changes resulting from tissue injury and inflammation but it may be a little different with nerve injury though!

Devor reviews the impact of spinal nerve cutting experiments and sheds some new and interesting light on things. First of all, if a spinal nerve is cut (see figure NR 1.3), a massive increase in activity of the cut fibres is recorded, but interestingly, by far and away the most activity is from cut Aβ fibres – the large myelinated, low threshold 'light-touch' nice guys. Also, it seems that Aβ fibre ectopic activity weighs in far heavier than any from the C or Aδ fibres. Up to now, the mechanism for Aβ fibres causing pain has been put down to central sensitisation – a result of C fibre afferent barrages and the release of substance P with the ultimate formation of new and 'inappropriate' connections. Light touch and gentle non-noxious movement causing pain, was the result of Aβ fibre impulses impacting on a central processing change and it beautifully accounted for the phenomenon of allodynia and secondary hyperalgesia.

But, intriguingly, it was found that when C fibres were killed using 'neurotoxins' central changes still occurred! The only way to stop the central sensitisation was to stop the activity of the Aβ fibres! It seems that when Aβ fibres are cut, 'axotomised' – they phenotypically switch and start expressing substance P! An Aβ fibre turns into a C fibre!

It's time to move on to slightly easier mechanisms and reasoning.

In summary, a very clinically relevant issue is that when a peripheral nerve is injured it has the potential to create on-going nasty pain of many varieties and often weird in nature. Mad pain has a peripheral as well as a central explanation and those who suffer often need to be helped to understand this.

Section NR 1
Read what I've read

Adams A., Bogduk N., Burton K., Dolan P. (2012) The Biomechanics of back pain. (3ed). Churchill Livingstone. Edinburgh.

Butler, D. (1991) Mobilisation of the nervous system, Churchill Livingstone, Edinburgh.

Carpal Tunnel Refs:

Durkan J. A. (1991) A new diagnostic test for carpal tunnel syndrome. J Bone Joint Surg [Am] 73A(4): 535-538.

Gelberman R. H., Hergenroeder P.T., et al., (1981) The carpal tunnel syndrome-a study of carpal canal pressures. Journal of Bone and Joint Surgery 63A: 380-383.

Greening J., Smart S., et al., (1999) Reduced movement of median nerve in carpal tunnel during wrist flexion in patients with non-specific arm pain. The Lancet 354 (July 17th): 217-218.

LaBan M. M., MacKenzie J.R., et al., (1989) Anatomic observations in carpal tunnel syndrome as they relate to the tethered median nerve stress test. Arch Phys Med Rehabil 70: 44-46.

Lundborg G., Gelberman R.H., et al. (1982) Median nerve compression in the carpal tunnel - Functional response to experimentally induced controlled pressure. Journal of Hand Surgery 7: 252-259.

Werner, R. A., Bir C., et al., (1994) Reverse Phalen's maneuver as an aid in diagnosing carpal tunnel syndrome. Archives of Physical Medicine & Rehabilitation 75: 783-786.

Yoshioka, S., Okuda Y., et al., (1993) Changes in carpal tunnel shape during wrist joint motion. MRI evaluation of normal volunteers. J of Hand Surg 18B: 620-623.

Bove G. M. and Light A.R. (1997) The Nervi Nervorum. Missing link for neuropathic pain? Pain Forum 6(3): 181-190.

Devor M. and Raber (1990) Heritability of symptoms in an experimental model of neuropathic pain, Pain 42, 51-67.

Devor M. (1990) Sources of variability in the sensation of pain. Recent Advances in Restorative Neurology: 3 Altered Sensation and Pain. M. R. Dimitrijevic, P. D. Wall and V. Lindblom. Basel, Karger: 189-196.

Devor M. (1994) The pathophysiology of damaged peripheral nerves. In: Wall P.D., and Melzack R.(eds) The Textbook of Pain (3rd edn.) Churchill Livingstone, Edinburgh 79-100.

Devor M., Seltzer Z. (1999) Pathophysiology of damaged nerves in relation to chronic pain. In: Wall P.D., Melzack R.(eds) The Textbook of Pain (4th edn.) Churchill Livingstone, Edinburgh 129-164.

Devor M. (2005) Response of nerves to injury in relation to neuropathic pain. In: McMahon SB, Koltzenberg M (eds) The Textbook of Pain (5th edn.) Churchill Livingstone, Edinburgh 905-927.

Gifford L. S. (2013) Topical Issues in Pain 3. Sympathetic Nervous System and Pain. Pain Management. Clinical Effectiveness. CNS Press, Falmouth.

Wall P.D., Gutnick M. (1974) On-going activity in peripheral nerves: the physiology and pharmacology of impulses originating from a neuroma. Experimental Neurology 43:580-593.

Section NR 2

ROOTS, DISCS, STRANGULATION AND INFLAMMATION

Chapter NR 2.1
Roots, discs, strangulation and inflammation!

We're now going up a level from the previous discussions.

In my early days before I made some sense of 'pain', I really struggled to understand the relationship between discs, nerve roots and pain. I made that list at the beginning of the previous section. Back then all the explanations were mechanical, 'discs pressing on nerves' was about the only one. Yet the pain could be ghastly, on-going and sometimes hardly influenced by movement; or the patient just couldn't be still, they were constantly restless. Mechanics should mean simple on-off pain, but this seemed to be the exception rather than the rule. I was sure that inflammation was playing a part and later discovered literature to beautifully support this inkling.

Like Marshall Devor for the pain stuff here there was Kjeli Olmarker and Björn Rydevik's work through the 1990's and into the 2000's . They experimentally explored lumbar nerve root pathophysiology in pigs, dogs and rats. What they did was to take disc material, in particular nuclear material, out of the disc and then put it somewhere else in the animal's body, most notably in the epidural space around the cauda-equina and nerve roots. Because the material was taken from one area and effectively transplanted to another area in the same animal it was labelled 'autologous'. Hence articles titled, 'Autologous nucleus pulposus induces neurophysiologic and histologic changes in porcine cauda equina nerve roots'. It simply means, take a pig and transplant some nucleus pulposus from that pig's disc and put it next to one of its nerve roots. In the control animals they placed fatty tissue next to the nerve roots. They consistently noted that the nuclear material produced a clear inflammatory reaction as well as injuring the nerve and its nerve fibres within. To quote:

> *'Epidural application of autologous nucleus pulposus in pigs, without mechanical nerve root compression, induced a pronounced reduction in nerve conduction velocity in the cauda equina nerve roots after 1-7 days, compared to epidural application of retroperitoneal fat in control experiments. Histologically, the nerve fiber injury was more pronounced after application of nucleus pulposus than after control tissue application. The results demonstrate that nucleus pulposus may induce nerve tissue injury by mechanisms other than mechanical compression. Such mechanisms may be based on direct biochemical effects of nucleus pulposus components on nerve fiber structure and function and microvascular changes including inflammatory reactions in the nerve roots.'*
>
> From Omarker et al 1993 Autologous Nucleus Pulposus Induces Neurophysiologic and Histologic Changes in Porcine Cauda Equina Nerve Roots. Spine Volume 18 - Issue 11

Observations of these nerve roots shows intraneural oedema, reduced blood flow, inflammatory cells and ligands, nerve fibre damage with loss of myelin, intracellular oedema, expansion of Schwann cells, axon breakdown and loss of conduction. This may occur at one day after exposure, but note from above, may start as late as day seven. Clinically – there's a delay. This delay is so common in back injury. 'I felt a little sore or strained in my back, then I wasn't too bad, but four days later it went down my leg.'

'I went to see the manipulator, walked out looser, within three days I could hardly move and the pain was down my leg. The Dr told me that manipulation caused the problem.'

The really important thing about this research is that it shows how nerve root problems can arise with NO DIRECT MECHANICAL INSULT TO THE NERVE ROOT. In the reality of life we know that the annular material of discs can split and crack. These 'fissures' may occasionally breach the outer annular layer, to form a handy corridor for nucleus pulposus material to migrate down and thus escape into the surrounding environment. Regardless of the 'physical' effect of this material, thanks to Olmarker and Rydevik's work, we now have a paradigm to explain nerve root pain – via a chemical or inflammatory pathway. Remember also from Devor's work, that inflammation of a nerve is particularly malicious in causing nerve fibre damage, neuropathy and the production of ectopic sources of massive impulse activity.

Nucleus pulposus material is normally housed safely within the disc. Therefore it's never normally exposed to the environment outside and the ever-sampling, sniffing and checking immune system. So, when it does leak out of the annulus it appears to be viewed by the immune system as an 'alien' substance. If you can dare to think about the immune system as a learning system, which it very much is and therefore that it's task as we grow and mature is to get out there, do a bit of 'sampling', and get to know every last nook and cranny of its own body, (all its own smells!); then it's hardly surprising that it never comes across nucleus pulposus material because it's so well hidden away. It's isolated because there's zero circulation in the whole of the normal disc except the very outer annular layers. The end result is that if this deep dark fugitive called nucleus pulposus makes some kind of bid to escape into the outer world it causes an 'auto' immune reaction.

Chemicals in the nucleus that have been isolated and deemed responsible for immune recognition and subsequent inflammation include its specific glycoproteins and immunglobulins. The autoimmune response that's induced will then produce a cascade of chemical reactions resulting in a veritable minestrone soup, with its 'plethora' of inflammatory chemicals. Off it all goes!

Researchers knew about this way back in the 1960's!

Bobechko, W. P. and C. Hirsch (1965). "Autoimmune response to nucleus pulposus in the rabbit." Journal of Bone and Joint Surgery 47B: 574-580.

These guys took pulposus material from a rabbits' disc and injected into its ear! Seems an odd thing to do until you consider that it's much easier to observe and sample what happens in the ear, than deep in its spine. The reaction produced was maximal at around four days and persisted for three weeks. Think of onset and time course of our nerve root problems and you see a neat time parallel. The delayed onset and then that ghastly three weeks before it begins to slowly Toblerone down and recover!

Here's a great bit of work on natural history of dog disc herniation that again has parallels with human nerve roots. If you want more detail, read it yourself.

See: Otani, Koji MD et al. 1997 Experimental Disc Herniation: Evaluation of the Natural Course. Spine: Vol.22, 24: 2894-2899

So, there are twelve dogs, six in a 'sham' group and six in the full operation group.

They did laminectomies in both groups at the L6 level to expose the L7 nerve root and L6-7 disc. In the sham group they gently retracted the nerve root, let it go and then sewed the whole thing back up. Some sham!

In the operated group, they retracted the nerve root and then punctured the disc annulus and injected saline into the disc. This produces enough pressure to cause nuclear material to come squeegeeing out and thus leave a disc extrusion. They then sewed them up.

For two months they checked the roots nerve conduction and occasionally did MRI scans to see the state of the nerve/disc relationship. They continued the MRIs for six months post op.

They found:

- that conduction velocity was affected in the sham group!

  (Well, think about it, laminectomy equals remove one side of the back of the L6 lumbar vertebrae – quite an inflammatory mess! Oh if you're wondering, a dog has 7 Lumbar vertebrae and 13 thoracic. Thought you might like to know)

- that in the disc herniation dogs the conduction loss reached a maximum at seven days.

  (So injure today and you may not get signs of neuropathy for a day or two but no worse after that. In the clinic we often fear making a neuropathy worse. The message from here is that once it's happened, it's happened and that's it, plus...

- the good news: after two months, in all the dogs, there was full recovery of conduction

- Ah, but they noted that disc degeneration started at around seven days!

  (I'm going to discuss disc injury and degeneration further later on as it's so important)

- and there was no obvious sign of direct nerve compression in any of the dogs when observed on MRI scan. Again, nerve damage – neuropathy without direct physical nerve compression, plus with time, recovery.

There's plenty of good news in this research – the main one being that with chemical/inflammatory neuropathy there's a very high likelihood that neuropathy will recover. That's great stuff for the clinic. Do they teach that to undergraduates? Or any of this stuff?

I don't think so and it's a pity.

We're now coming to the point where 'mechanics' or physical forces come in to the equation! You know I don't feel right here, kidding! It's actually very interesting and revealing.

Let's start with the notion that mechanical forces can be brought to bear on nerves by pressure from fluid rather than via bony contact or a disc bulge or extrusion.

This 'fluid' thought should make us think of oedema and of course oedema is associated with the swelling of inflammation and, unless massive, is pretty much invisible on MRI scans. So, nuclear material leaks, there's an inflammatory response in and around the nerve root as it sits in the intervertebral foramen area and proximally, in the lateral recess of the lumbar spine. Inflammation builds and so does swelling, so there's an increase in pressure around the root. Now think what's around the nerve root in that space? The answer is that there's an extensive vascular network – nerves love and need blood like no other tissue. And depriving them of it by putting increased pressure on the vascular bed is detrimental, particularly to those high energy users – the fast and furious Aβ fibres and the motor fibres. They're big fast and highly metabolic compared to the lowly unmyelinated C fibres. Clinically it's the Aβ and large motor fibres that are first to suffer therefore. You lose sensation and the muscles go weak. Sensory loss may be quite subtle and that's why it's so important to have a tuning fork to test vibration sense in the clinic. Put one on your Christmas list.

Next, another form of indirect pressure: recall the 'chronic constriction injury' or 'self-strangulation' experiments from the last section where a loose ligature is placed round a spinal nerve and the effects monitored. Researchers noted that pain behaviours – protective postures, licking and autotomy, do not occur for 2-5 days and can last for up to two months. This neatly fits with the clinic observations again. It's a great pity that the researchers here don't give a spread of results. For example, do some rats recover in a week whereas others go on for three, four or more months? When the rats are 'harvested' (killed!) and the strangulated section of the nerve scrutinised, it is found to be swollen with clear damage and degeneration of A and C fibres. It seems that the ligature causes the nerve to markedly swell either side of it and that the swelling causes the pressure, which then leads to nerve fibre damage.

Now, I like to translate this process to the real world of the nerve root in its confined space. How do you bring about the equivalent of a chronic constriction situation? Here's my list:

1. Disc extrusion, protrusion, bulge, sequestration.

2. Degenerative bony and soft tissue encroachment – think osteophytes from the rim of the vertebral body and from degenerative facet joint thickening, think soft tissue from ligamentum flavum thickening (encroaches on radicular canal in lumbar spine).

3. Swelling due to inflammatory and immune responses.

4. Swelling of fresh disc material. Fresh disc material, due to osmosis, imbibes fluid and therefore swells. This means an early significant increase in the size of the material after the initial extrusion. This may be more relevant in the younger 'extrusion' material as the elderly nucleus pulposus becomes more annular-like and therefore less 'osmotic'.

5. Any prolonged posture, but, as I'll show later, lumbar extension is far more space limiting than flexion.

Key point, thinking about the constriction model, is that **there doesn't have to be direct compression of the nerve root to cause significant problems to the nerve**.

How do we survive?

If you think about all this we're really looking at a model that has a combination of inflammatory chemicals, plus ischaemia, caused by the increased pressure of these various physical elements. Clearly it could be one or the other, but for the most part I think one would have to consider both elements as playing a part.

This notion of ischemia has lead me over the years to make sure all my 'nerve root' patients (well all patients in fact) are doing regular cardio-vascular work of some kind and if at all possible. While horrid acute nerve pain makes cardio-vascular work the last thing on a patients' wish list, it's usually still very possible to do enough of a workout in another part of the body to get the CV system up and running. Think upper limb work for lumbar roots and lower limb for cervical roots. Pumping elastic 'therabands' for several minutes little and often through the day. Don't forget to give the patient a good understanding of why their doing cardio-vascular exercise for a nerve problem!

The other way of keeping circulation going in the area is to create pressure change right there simply by doing movement. Of course, it has to be tolerable/comfortable movement, which with a bit of ingenuity isn't usually too hard to find. By way of good rapport and simple experimenting with the patient it's usually very possible to find one or two standard back movements, for example done in supine lying or all fours, that don't cause too much pain or aren't too provoking. Keep the area squishing about – pressure up and down promotes circulation. The trouble is that if there's significant mechanosensitivity the nerve root is always going to want to scream a bit – whatever you do. But if you can find a way of moving the area, it's important. Hunter-gatherers who knew nothing of pathology just kept going the best they could and recovered (or expired!) regardless. We're designed to recover while we keep going the best we can. The best things are the simplest – I mean keep walking/moving.

I mentioned just now about the contents of the intervertebral foramen and I discussed the vascular network. In fact, the foramen contains not only the nerve root plus the vascular network it also contains varying amounts of adipose tissue. That's 'fat' and fat is pretty incompressible.

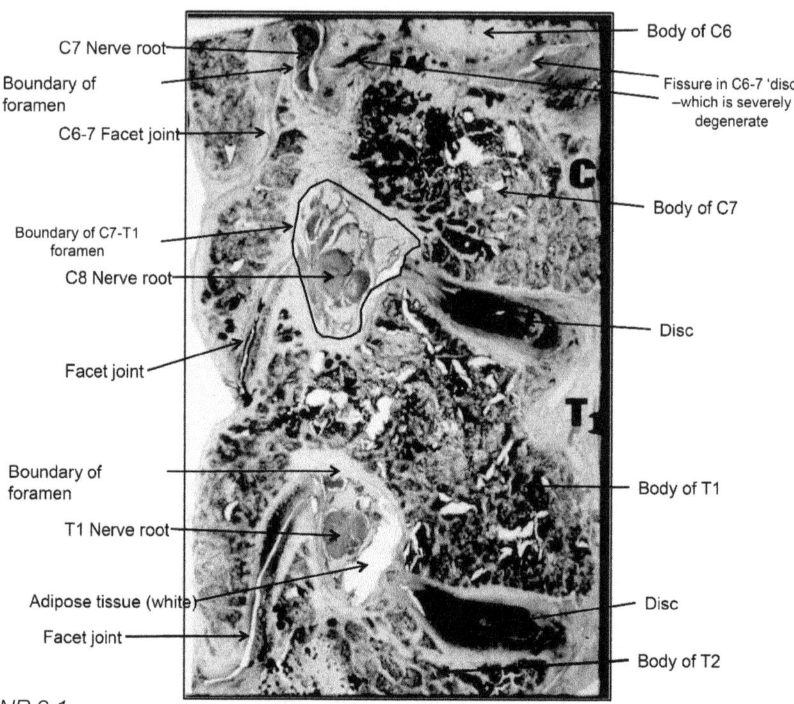

Figure NR 2.1 Sagittal section through the cervical/ thoracic spine -labelled

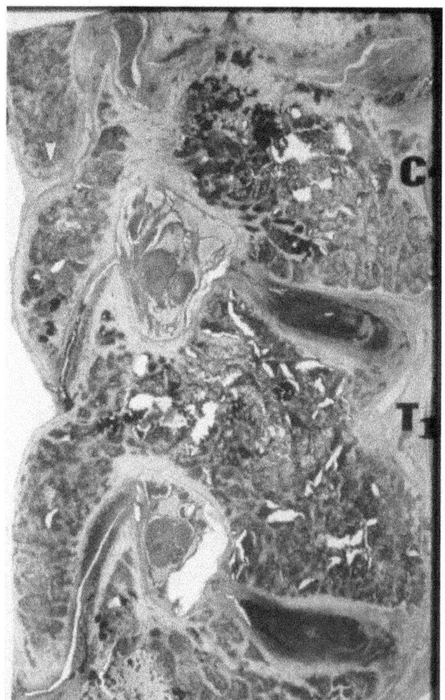

Figure NR 2.2 Sagittal section through the cervical/thoracic spine -not labelled

Take a look (concentrate!) at the sagittal section through the cervical spine (Figure NR 2.1 labelled and NR 2.2 not labelled):

1. The posterior aspect is to the left, anterior to the right. C6 vertebra is at the very top.

2. Remember that in the cervical spine the nerve root is numbered in relation to the designation of the vertebrae below: thus C7 root emerges through the intervertebral foramen made between the C7 vertebra below and the C6 vertebra above.

3. At the very top of the section you can see the C6-7 foramen is really narrowed compared to the C7-8 foramen below: this is due to the marked loss of disc height plus osteophytic 'beaking' which is clear to see; the disc as virtually gone and the situation is more or less 'bone-on-bone'; the C6-7 facet joint also 'beaks' into the foramen.

4. Note the C7 nerve root in the foramen is very squashed and there is little else there apart from some very meagre adipose tissues (white) that means a serious loss of vascular supply and plenty of compression to the nerve root.

5. Compare the above to the relatively massive size of the C7-T1 foramen!

   Here the C8 nerve root is very visible with its separate dorsal (sensory) and ventral (motor) roots. It is surrounded by adipose tissue and plenty of blood vessels.

6. The blood vessels are the ovals and circles that contain the darker blood – most obvious in the T1-2 foramen. The rest, the grey-white and white patches are adipose tissue.

Adipose tissue is not very compressible; so, if you can imagine extruded disc material pushing into the foraminal space, even a little bit, you should be able to easily see that pressure will come to bear on not only the blood vessels but also the nerve roots too. Any pressure on blood vessels, particularly veins, will tend to make them collapse and therefore restrict the flow of blood. Hence there being a huge potential for hypoxia and compression damage to the nerve fibres in the nerve root. I think it is easy to envisage a 'chronic constriction injury' type of situation with any disc bulge or extrusion, degenerative facet enlargement, osteophytic 'beaking', or degeneration related narrowing.

So, what of the person whose neck this is? Did they have problems? We don't know of course, but we do know that having 'pathology' like this doesn't necessarily mean the person has symptoms. However, I wouldn't mind betting that this person has a very stiff low cervical spine – due to the severe degeneration at C6-7; that they have poor triceps reflexes and some loss of muscle power in muscles supplied by the C7 root, for example, triceps. There may be some C7 sensory loss, for example in the tips of the index and middle fingers. Predicting pain however, is not possible, but I would have thought there is a fairly strong possibility of occasional stiff necks over the years and even of nerve root symptoms. The key point here is that slow changes around peripheral nerves gives them time to adapt and degenerative changes like those seen here, occur very slowly. On the other hand, disc extrusions and leakage of nuclear material via annular fissures, occurs on a much faster time scale and is more likely to give rise to symptoms in those who are vulnerable to ectopic sites forming and becoming active.

I would like to make a plea for someone to do some cadaver work on subjects with known 'pain' histories related to the spine examined versus those who haven't. A good neurological examination needs to have been done before they die! Thanks!

In the lumbar spine the nerve root normally occupies the upper pole of the foraminal space – very near the upper pedicle. In fact the vertebral body often has a groove on it where the root lies. The rest of the space is occupied by adipose tissue and the vascular bed, as in the rest of the spine. Anatomical studies show that some folk have massive nerves and others very small and also that there is great variability in foramen size (see Sato and Kikuchi 1993). For example, lumbar roots occupy a maximum of 35% of the foramen, 21% is the average and the smallest is as low as 2%! So, presumably it's best to have small nerves in a big space!

Olmarker and Rydevik's group with their pig experiments came to the conclusion that if you really want to mess up a nerve root then you need a combination of chemical, inflammation/swelling and physical displacement of the nerve root. Put them all together and the nerve really suffers. As already noted from the figure of the section earlier and I'll also discuss later the nerve root can suffer massive physical abuse!

Figure NR 2.3 is a summary figure. Up at the top are mechanical factors and down on the right 'antigenic/irritative' substances, referring to the leaking nuclear material for example. Note the dorsal root ganglion is one part of the nerve root/peripheral nerve that has been deemed to normally mechanically sensitive and therefore has the potential to produce instant pain when forces come to bear on it.

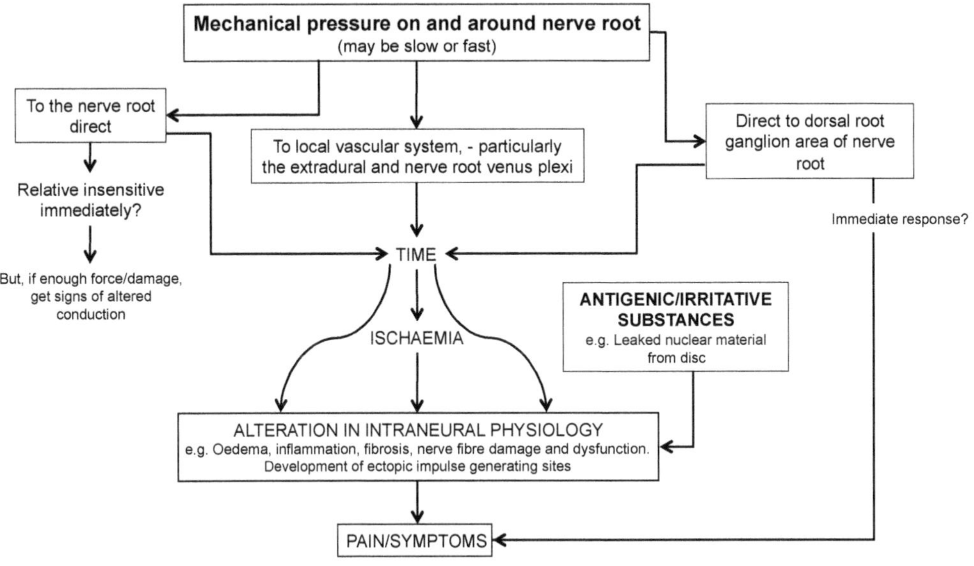

Figure NR 2.3 A summary. Up at the top are mechanical factors and down on the right 'antigenic/irritative' substances.

Section NR 2
Read what I've read

Farmer, J. C., Wisneski R. J. (1994) Cervical spine nerve root compression. An analysis of neuroforaminal pressures with varying head and arm positions. Spine 19(16): 1850-1855.

Ehni, B., Ehni G., et al., (1990) Extradural spinal cord and nerve root compression from benign lesions of the cervical area. Neurological Surgery. J. R. Youmans. Philadelphia, Saunders: 2878-2916.

Olmarker K. (1991) Spinal nerve root compression. Nutrition and function of the porcine cauda equina compressed in vivo. Acta Orthop Scand Suppl 242(27): 1-27.

Olmarker K., Blomquist J., et al., (1995) Inflammatogenic properties of nucleus pulposus. Spine 25(6): 665-669.

Olmarker K., Byrod G., et al., (1994) Effects of methyprednisolone on nucleus pulposus-induced nerve root injury. Spine 19(16): 1803-1808.

Olmarker K., Danielsen N., et al., (1991) Effects of chondroitinase ABC on intrathecal and peripheral nerve tissue. An in vivo experimental study on rabbits. Spine 16(1): 43-5.

Olmarker K., Holm S., et al., (1991) Experimental nerve root compression. A model of acute, graded compression of the porcine cauda equina and an analysis of neural and vascular anatomy. Spine 16(1): 61-9.

Olmarker K., Holm S., et al., (1991) Experimental nerve root compression. Presentation of a model for acute, graded compression of the porcine cauda equina, with analyses of neural and vascular anatomy. Spine 16: 61-69.

Olmarker K., Holm S., et al., (1990) Importance of compression onset rate for the degree of impairment of impulse propagation in experimental compression injury of the porcine cauda equina. Spine 15: 416-419.

Olmarker K., Holm S., et al., (1991) More pronounced effects of double level compression than single level compression on impulse propagation in the porcine cauda equina. Clinical Orthopaedics and Related Research.

Olmarker K. , Myers R.R. (1998) Pathogenesis of sciatic pain: role of herniated nucleus pulposus and deformation of spinal nerve root and dorsal root ganglion. Pain 78(2): 99-105.

Olmarker K., Rydevik R. (1991) Pathophysiology of Sciatica.Orthopaedic Clinics of North America 22(2): 223.

Olmarker K., Rydevik R. (1992) Single- versus double-level nerve root compression. An experimental study on the porcine cauda equina with analyses of nerve impulse conduction properties. Clin Orthop 279(9): 35-9.

Olmarker K., Rydevik R., et al., (1990) Compression-induced changes of the nutritional supply to the porcine cauda equina. Journal of Spinal Diseases 3: 25-29.

Olmarker K., Rydevik R., et al., (1989) Edema formation in spinal nerve roots induced by experimental, graded compression. An experimental study on the pig cauda equina with special reference to differences in effects between rapid and slow onset of compression. Spine 14: 559-563.

Olmarker K., Rydevik R., et al., (1989) Effects of experimental graded compression on blood flow in spinal nerve roots. A vital microscopic study on the porcine cauda equina. Journal of Orthopaedic Research 7: 817-823.

Olmarker K., Rydevik R., et al., (1993) Autologous nucleus pulposus induces neurophysiologic and histologic changes in porcine cauda equina nerve roots. Spine 18(11): 1425-32.

Rydevik B. (1993) Neurophysiology of cauda equina compression. Acta Orthop Scand (Suppl) 64: 52-55.

Rydevik B., Brown M. D., et al., (1984) Pathoanatomy and pathophysiology of nerve root compression. Spine 9(1): 7.

Rydevik B., Holm S., et al., (1990) Diffusion from the cerebrospinal fluid as a nutritional pathway for spinal nerve roots. Acta Physiologica Scandinavica 138: 247-248.

Rydevik B., Lundborg G., et al., (1981) Effects of graded compression on intraneural blood flow. Journal of Hand Surgery 6: 3-12.

Rydevik B., Olmarker K. (1992) Pathogenesis of nerve root damage. The Lumbar Spine and Back Pain. M. I. V. Jayson. Edinburgh, Churchill Livingstone: 89-100.

Rydevik B. L., Pedowitz R. A., et al., (1991) Effects of acute graded compression on spinal nerve root function and structure. An experimental study of the pig cauda equina. Spine 16(5): 487-493.

Sato, K., Kikuchi S. (1993) An anatomic study of foraminal nerve root lesions in the lumbar spine. Spine 18(15): 2246-2251.

Yoo, J. U., Zou D., et al., (1992) Effect of cervical spine motion on the neuroforaminal dimensions of human cervical spine. Spine 17(10): 1131.

Section NR 3

DISCS

Chapter NR 3.1

Discs, bulges, extrusions and protrusions–a short refresher

I wonder if you're where I used to be. Never being quite sure what all the 'disc' terms meant? What's the difference between a herniation, protrusion, extrusion, prolapse and a sequestrum?

According to Brock 1992 (see figure NR 3.1), the term '**herniation**' is the *general* term for a spectrum of disc disruptions that extends from simple '**protrusion**' meaning a *bulge* due to internal degenerative changes in the disc leading to the annular walls to bulge; to '**extrusion**' where end-plate material may dislodge or where the nucleus actually leaks out from damaged outer annular layers.

Brock's Classification

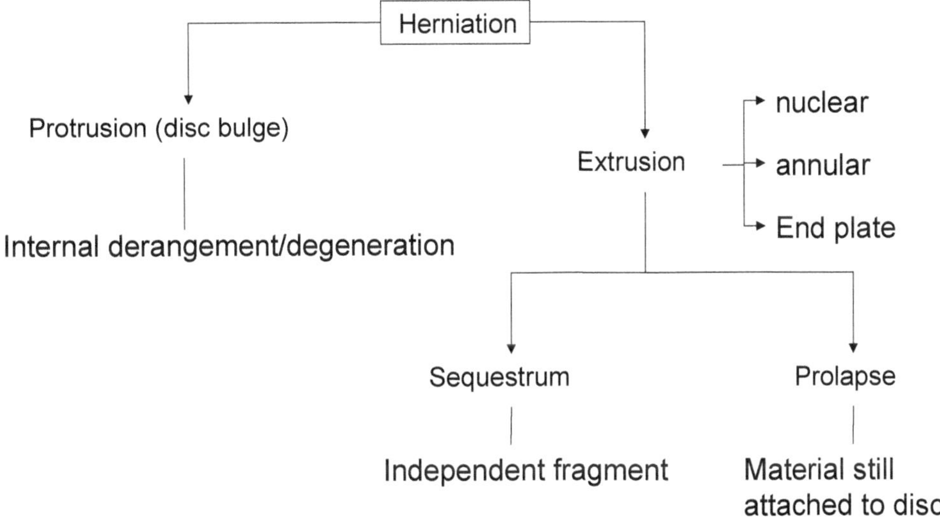

Figure NR 3.1 Brock's Classification

Extrusion crudely means insides moving to the outside and extruding. Extruded material still remains in continuity with the disc it came from. Brock uses the term '**sequestrum**' or '**extruded fragment**' to designate a distinct ('independent') fragment of disc. In other words it's become detached from the disc it came from. To add further slight confusion Brock defines a disc fragment that has extruded from the disc but is still continuous with the material of that disc as '**prolapsed**'.

Adams and Hutton, way back in 1982, used the term '**prolapsed**' to encompass '**nuclear extrusion**' as well as '**annular protrusion**'.

Figure NR 3.2 shows the three basic situations: bulge, extrusion, sequestrum.

Figure NR 3.3 shows an MRI scan of a massive disc **extrusion...**

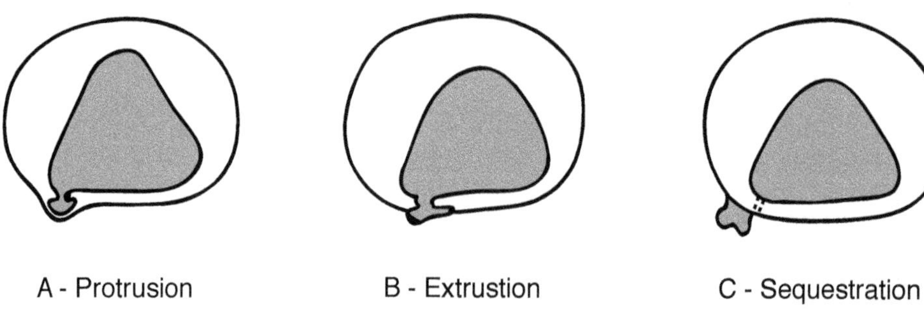

Figure NR 3.2 Disc bulge, extrusion and sequestrum

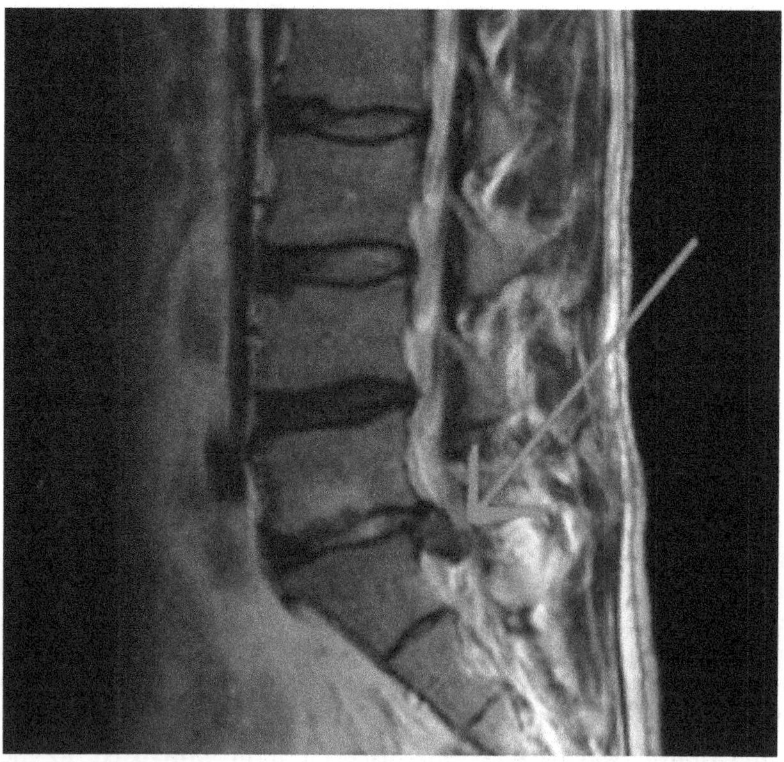

Figure NR 3.3 An MRI scan of a massive disc extrusion

There, simple if you stick with Brock!

For years I've been fascinated with and read tons of stuff on the disc, its biology, its injury mechanism and its recovery. What follows are what I feel are some useful clinical things:

1. I like to view disc prolapses, protrusions and sequestrations that come to intrude into the spinal canal, radicular canal (more later) or intervertebral foramina as space occupying lesions! This is material that is situated in places where it shouldn't be and it's usually quite firm; unless it's the more 'dribbly' nucleus pulposus of the young! Importantly, as we've seen, this material has the potential to physiologically and mechanically influence and upset adjacent tissue and structures; most notably nerve root tissue – the cauda equina in the lumbar spine and in the thoracic and cervical spine, the spinal cord. I also like to view this 'space occupying lesion' as a 'transient stenosis' situation. Stenosis is a general term used to mean 'narrowing' and is particularly well known when applied to blood vessels and the lumbar spine of the elderly. I believe we can learn a great deal about the 'mechanics' of back pain by reflecting on what is known about lumbar stenosis and I will devote more space to this in a later chapter.

2. Amazingly the body has an inherent capacity for clearing away extruded disc material. For example in a group of 69 patients diagnosed by MRI (magnetic resonance imaging) as having lumbar disc herniations (remember that's the 'general' term for all types), 31, which is just less than half of them, showed a reduction in the size of the herniation of at least 70% when re-evaluated between 6 and 15 months later. 36% of the subjects there was a decrease in size of between 50 and 75% (Bazzao et al 1992). The patients were conservatively managed, in other words, the outcome, the diminishing size of the herniation, was the result of that persons own biology. Here's another study...

3. Ellenberg et al 1992 documented that patients with CT evidence of herniated discs and EMG evidence of radiculopathy had a 78% rate of disc reduction. And another study...

4. Matsubara et al 1995 found that medical care involving medication, physiotherapy, traction and epidural steroid injections resulted in disc regression in 60% of the cases... and another...!

5. Bush et al 1992 scanned and later re-scanned, 111 non-operated patients, who had presented with sciatica due to lumbo-sacral nerve root compromise and reported that 64 or the 84 herniated/sequestrated intervertebral discs showed a degree of, or complete, resolution at one year! That's 76%! They also noted that only 7 of 27 patients showed any resolution where the discs were 'bulging' (i.e. in correct terminology – 'protruding'). It seems that the body is good at clearing away the exuding stuff that comes out of a disc, but not so good at doing anything too smart with a bulge. Considering the incredibly sluggish metabolism and virtually non-existent capacity for the

disc to heal I find it quite surprising that 7 of the bulges were recorded as resolving – however much. I guess a reasonable way of reasoning this would be if the disc responded by degenerating and then stiffening? (Discussed later). Stiffening should be seen as a very adaptive way of securing a bad situation is likely to be seen as a bit of an anathema to manual therapy, that likes to keep individual spinal joints moving well! The phrase 'move-better = better-off', while generally admirable, isn't always the biological reality. All the spines that I've observed over the years stiffen with age. It may well be with good reason as far as the protection of the nervous system is concerned? On the other hand, keeping as much movement as long as possible has got to be an overarching and worthy principle of any therapy, if not in life! If the surrounding nerves and tissues can manage to adapt to bulges and being compressed a bit during movement, without any long term detrimental effects on conduction and more importantly, function, why not keep things moving? The key in management is the timing of appropriate movement.

6. In the Bush et al study, the authors noted that a large percentage of all patients re-scanned showed improvement in their levels of pain and all patients were able to work and follow their usual leisure activities. Further, of the 74 patients who had neurological signs on presentation, 70 had made a partial or complete recovery.

7. Other studies, and there are probably plenty more with the very same message, show similar findings in lumbar and cervical discs. They all note that changes in the size of the disc extrusions over time, frequently parallel the clinical improvement in signs and symptoms of patients managed conservatively. (See research by the Saal brothers)

8. Kimori et al 1996 reported that the most rapid improvement in symptoms occurred in the first 3 months of observation.

9. Most important of all is the finding that regardless of what happens to the disc, radicular pain can still improve – even if the bulge or extruded material remains. Nerves can adapt! It may be worth reviewing the squashed C7 nerve root in the C6-7 intervertebral foramen that is shown in figures NR 2.1 and 2.2. Consider the process that arrived at the situation shown as taking a long time, possibly many years and also consider that as the space diminished priority was given to preserving the nerves above all other structures. As you can see, there is no evidence of blood vessels or adipose tissue, just the lonely squashed nerve root, still doing its best to function!

From the patient's point of view and for us who communicate with them it's encouraging to know: firstly, that the likelihood of improvement is very good *whatever happens.* Secondly, that there is a very strong possibility that any disc or end plate material that has extruded will be cleared away.

Fascinatingly, it seems that mechanical or anatomical factors that originally caused the problem for the nerve, do slowly resolve in quite a high proportion of individuals.

Thus, disc extrusions get nibbled away, thanks to the various chemicals and cells of the recovery and immune systems. One clinically interesting thing to note is that osmotically swollen freshly escaped disc material gradually deflates – presumably as its chemical make-up changes and it becomes a less osmotic structure. Think of it as 'dehydrating' or drying up and shrivelling up perhaps.

As an aside, it's interesting how researchers view situations – all those algogens and immune cells amassing round the newly extruded nuclear material are seen as the problem – as the problem causing the pain, as the pathology. To biologist me, I would prefer them to be viewed as part of a wonderfully positive process that clears the mess up, but with the unfortunate side effect for some of us – pain! From this perspective the plea is to be patient; give your biology time, it is clearing up the mess in a much better way than the spinal surgeon's scalpel. I have to admit though, that here in Cornwall we have a very good spinal surgeon and that I occasionally refer patients to him. These patients invariably have clear cut nerve root presentations related to disc extrusions and they do very well with his microdiscectomies. I would like to think my 'top-down' preparation of these patients and my follow up rehabilitation is a big factor in them doing well too? That means a massive consideration of 'shopping basket' components, especially the yellow flags.

Further clinical points (some of which can occasionally be used for discussing and explaining with the patient):

1. Extrusion of disc material is not a disaster – it is highly likely that the material will diminish in size and may even be cleared away completely. The studies discussed have also demonstrated significant decreases in neural tissue displacement and swelling and lack of evidence of any residual perithecal (around the dura) or perineural (around the nerve root) scarring and fibrosis (Saal 1996).

2. The literature that I've read strongly suggests that there is far less of a need for surgery than was previously thought. Even those with clear and even quite marked neurological signs have a favourable prognosis (Saal & Saal 1989; Saal 1996).

3. Even if the protrusion or extrusion remains there is a strong possibility of recovery. It is commonly stated that 20-30% of the population have asymptomatic herniated lumbar discs. The message is that the body has very favourable adaptational capability. The key to recovery is finding the best means of management to get there. Support for 'active' rehabilitation rather than passive fix and surgery has been mounting for years (e.g. Saal 1996).

4. The main thing that's needed in the clinic is belief in this process: then good pain control and management, plenty of time and patience and return of function and movement when appropriate to the presentation.

5. A big thought relates to the type of material extruded: I can happily imagine the immune system chemically breaking down, absorbing and removing the 'softer' nucleus pulposus material, but less so the tough old degenerate

annulus, end-plate material or bony material – all of which can go to make up extruded material.

6. Over the years though, I have observed a great many lumbar problems with sciatica come and go and come again and go again. Longitudinal studies of the natural history of back and sciatic pain following sciatica and disc disruption would be invaluable. My observation is that a great many are never the same again. Their backs have a certain vulnerability, they have varying degrees of recurrence of both back and the nerve related symptoms and back- nagging is never very far away, even in care-free, get on with life individuals. Let's face it, once a disc has prolapsed and extruded it's never the same again, the motion segment relationships alter, therefore altering the biomechanics and the relationship of the structural anatomy that surrounds the nerve root. More later!

7. If you're at the beginning of your career and are going to stay put in your practice for a good long time, how about setting up a good quality longitudinal study for post-sciatica – whether operated on or not and make it as long as you can?

I feel that it has always been my duty to the patient to give them as accurate a natural history as possible for their problem. In effect this is a 'normalising' process, where the patient needs to accept how the condition they have 'normally' behaves and recovers and how long it may take.

Chapter NR 3.2
Dirty discs to discuss 1: fluid movement and 'discogenic' symptoms

I think it's very instructive to look at and discuss some pictures of discs in a variety of states. I was given the pictures in the following chapters by Trish Dolan, who is well known with her husband Mike Adams for a massive amount of research on disc injury and degeneration. Together with Nik Bogduk and Kim Burton they wrote the book 'The Biomechanics of Back Pain' now into its recent third edition. To me it's essential reading on biomechanics and back pain that we should all study and know.

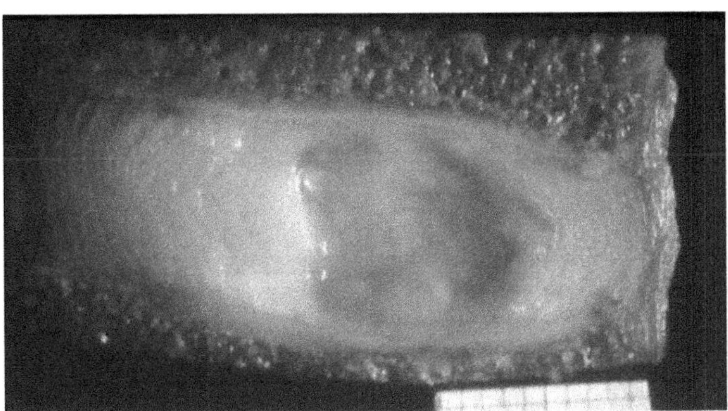

Figure NR 3.4 'In 20's – grade I disc degeneration'

The first figure NR 3.4 is titled 'In 20's – grade I disc degeneration'. Forget the 'degeneration' bit for a moment, what this lumbar disc section shows is a nicely defined nucleus and you can see that it's a bit 'mushy', 'liquidy' and 'toothpasty' in there. You can also see the annular rings beautifully, anterior to the left and posterior to the right. Posterior is towards the spinal canal and intervertebral foramen of course. Note that the nucleus is nearer this posterior side. There's a beautiful bone to end-plate to disc differentiation and the whole thing produces a healthy separation of the vertebrae above and below. There's no bulging or evidence of any fissures and I think most of us would be pleased to have discs like this one. It's classified as 'Grade 1' degeneration because of the distortion of the annular rings – most notably posteriorly. This disc is 'typical' in anyone between the ages of 15-40 years old. I'd like you to look at it, especially those who follow the 'McKenzie' type doctrine to discs and the derangement model used to explain symptom behaviour, see that the nuclear zone is very much contained within the very firm walls of the annulus. This nucleus and the material it contains cannot move its location when the disc is in this state. The only way nuclear material moves is when a radial crack or fissure forms from the annular-nucleus boundary into the annulus, thus allowing the possibility of nuclear material to track along it.

Mike Adams along with co-collaborator Billy Hutton, were experimentally producing cracks and fissures in discs way back in the early 1980's. For example, they'd dissect out a neat vertebrae-disc-vertebrae motion segment from the lower spine of a formerly healthy youngster, who'd usually just died in some road accident. The motion segment would be mounted above and below in cups of dental plaster to fix it in place and then it was compression loaded repeatedly, while maintaining it in full flexion. Typical compression loading quoted was forty cycles per minute for six hours! Nice! While it's not really reality it does show what may happen to a healthy disc when it takes heavy forces in flexion day in day out. They started out with low-ish loading and gradually built it up. What they noted was that water was expelled during the early loading cycles and that as a result the range of flexion increased. This was due to simple tissue 'creep' occurring.

If you take a bit of collagenous material, like tendon or ligament, attach one end to a clamp and the other end to a weight and then watch and wait: you'll notice that fluid oozes out of it and that it gradually elongates, fast at first and slower as time goes on. All collagenous material has this 'creep' property and a good deal of money is made out of it. All clinicians have to do to improve range is take a bit of time and hold the joint, muscle, tendon, nerve, whatever, at end range. It can also be done by repeating the movement over and over again for a while, 'I've improved your range, that'll be fifty dollars thanks.' I like to give my patients the 'do-it-yourself-kit' though, it saves them time and money and I can go to sleep happier at night.

Clinically, creep also equates to repeated movement increasing range. Even easy repeated movement away from end range squishes and squashes the tissues and fluid will move out. Remember, if a tissue is injured or inflamed in any way it will contain more fluid than normal. This, in part, is due to osmotic forces sucking fluid in. (Inflammation means more chemicals, therefore a higher osmotic pressure gradient and therefore a greater tendency to imbibe fluid than usual). Repeated movement of damaged tissue, think of a cut finger a couple of days old, tends to hurt quite a bit to start with, but gradually eases as movement goes on and increases, often allowing a pretty much full range fairly quickly. If the movements are repeated in a relaxed early range and pain free way, and then the range to pain reviewed, the general feeling and range are often much better too. Think for example of easy pendular exercises for a sub acute shoulder problem with limited range, or lumbar crook rotations for an acute low back problem. Regular movement of a swollen healing tissue is what we often do naturally. Remember – pain tells us to move quite often!

My point is that repeated movement improves range and a 'tissue' based explanation may well be related to fluid movement and decreased pressure in the tissues.

'You're a 'creep' my dear fellow!'

Fluid returns during rest of course and the whole thing stiffens up again. TELL THE PATIENT THIS IS NORMAL! In my old manual therapy days I'd do some rotation mobilisations to a low back problem, reassess their bending etc. and invariably the range felt more relaxed and improved in range – great, ego fulfilled, I fixed you, you're grateful to me, I'm a clever fellow. The trouble was the patient would come back the next time and report:

'Louis, felt great for a few hours, sat in the chair later on, couldn't get out of it. Worst I've felt since the whole thing started.'

'Oh, ah, right, well, hello and it's very nice of you to come back again...'

I now avoid all this by normalising the stiffness pattern – freer with movement, stiffer with rest and to expect it. That's usually sufficient, but for one or two patients I may tell them how movement shifts fluid out, which leaves the tissues more pliable and creepy. But if they stop and rest, the fluid will flow back in, the tissues will tighten up a bit, even shorten and they'll then stiffen up again and that they should expect it.

'Don' blame me – it's NORMAL and as you get better it gets less and less.'

Use the cut finger analogy, 'It frees the more you move it and use it, but stiffens up again when you rest, same in your back. As it heals and gets stronger so it gets less stiff and frees more easily...'

The other clinical observation I'd noticed way back in my career, was that for spinal problems, especially acute and sub-acute lumbar ones, which may well have some 'fluid' movement/inflammation (tissue) mechanism going on, was that if I put them prone and did some Maitland type postero-anterior pressures on their spine for several minutes, I'd find on reassessment that while extension would greatly improve, flexion would be massively stiffened! You can achieve the same result by leaving them prone and putting on some fancy electrotherapy machine for ten minutes. Sometimes they can hardly get off the treatment couch. It's also a pretty normal part of the ageing spine for some of us! If I stay prone for more than ten minutes I'm very 'stiff to bend' getting back up. It gets amplified when there's a back pain problem though:

'Arghhh... what've you done Louis..?' I remember a patient screaming at me. And then, I rather witheringly tried to alleviate the situation by doing more of the same, in the hope it would all magically get better. It never did and quite a few disgruntled acute low back pain patients crawled out of the clinic. Chiropractors and other five minute treatment folk never notice it, the less you do, the more quickly you get on with it and get them out of your rooms – the less time they have to stiffen-up!

These days though, it's no sweat. I tend to avoid this happening, by not doing prone and p-a's for long on acute, sub-acute or 'degenerate' type backs in a bit of a flare-up, especially where extension appears limited and painful. If you put the patient on their side and do the same pressures, or even do an electrotherapy treatment for half an hour, there's no such reaction. Or hands-off, just get the patient to do easy, mid range movements in any direction that's comfortable. My reasoning is just like a nasty shoulder problem – work with big active or passive movements and/or accessory movements (pushing in the back with your thumbs) nicely, comfortably and pain free, in nice parts of the mid-range. Prone, for a great many backs, is actually end of range extension plus a bit more for the low lumbar joints.

Now, if I do get a stuck or stiffened-up flexion response it doesn't faze me. All I do is get the patient on their back and do repeated flexion – passively if I'm energetic, or they can do it actively by grabbing one leg and then the other and pulling towards them – it's 'grab a knee', which is actually hip and lumbar flexion. If doing it with one leg at a time becomes easy, I then get them to do it grabbing both legs and pulling. It's simple McKenzie flexion in lying (FIL)! I'm not guided by any 'centralisation' rules here – if extension is free, but flexion's gone stiff just do some easy flexion – 'fearlessly'! Patients often venture that they actually do this in bed, or they go to all fours and curl up. I call this all-four-curl-up, the 'Mecca' position i.e. flexed hips, flexed knees and spine to be done four times a day towards Mecca... sorry, no offence, no cartoons, don't come after me, small joke, that's all.

While talking about fluid movement, please also note that normal discs imbibe fluid all the time if they can, but most when you're horizontal, weight-off in bed. There's a 'diurnal' (24 hour) variation in our height as a result – we're taller in the morning than at the end of the day. In the young this can be as much as 25mm, the average is 19mm and in astronauts as much as 100mm growth occurs due to weightlessness – that's four inches taller! You can increase you're height overnight by 2% when you're young and on planet earth, but it's only 0.5% when you're old. If you want to be taller stick to the high heels or 'platforms, because this isn't really a big enough deal to be noticeable. 'You know I feel sexy in the morning!' 'Maybe it's because you're taller darling!' Another small joke, maybe I should move on?

So, that's normal disc, it has clear osmotic behaviour – stop moving and it sucks fluid in, gets turgid and goes stiff! This is especially evident in the morning. In the internally injured disc the whole fluid thing is probably amplified – there's a stronger pulling pressure! You've all had patients whose movements feel free and good, who then go and spend an hour or two in front of the TV and can't get out of the chair. If you sit slumped, as most do, you won't be able to straighten up easily – you'll be flexed when you stand. Stiffness after not moving is a normal part of life and morning stiffness is, well, obvious. If you ask over 50 year olds whether they feel stiff in the morning you'll find that 65% say yes! I like the quote from Bywaters (1982) who did the survey to get that figure. He said, '... man starts as a jelly and ends as a stiff. The stiffness of old age is merely built in obsolescence...'

Collagneous tissues suck in fluid and therefore mechanically stiffen, if they're injured and inflamed they do it even more, that's muscle, ligament, tendon, cartilage, discs and even nerve itself. Some of us are far more aware of stiffness than others and some of us vary in flexibility far more too. For example, for the Graduate Diploma in Manipulative Therapy I did, back in 1985, my research project was titled 'Circadian variation in human flexibility and grip strength'. I measured various ranges of movement in volunteers every 2 hours over a 24 hour period (see Gifford 1987, 1994, 1995). It was a kind of scientific 24 hour group bonding session if the truth be known. One of the measures was fingertip to floor. The results showed greatest stiffness in the early morning hours and rapidly increasing flexibility through the day and once up and about. The average variation in range over the 24 hour period was around 14.4cms, but it ranged from 26.2cms (10 inches) to 5.5cms (2 inches). The variation in fingertip to floor bending was reflected in the lumbar intervertebral measurement assessed using goniometry.

Some of us vary more than others. The one who varied by 10 inches could only just reach his knees first thing in the morning, but within an hour he could reach his ankles comfortably. He reported that the restriction feeling was mainly in the backs of his legs – including the calf. In other words, not just the hamstrings and not the lumbar spine either! Was that due to the disc? Or the nerve, or the muscles of the back of the leg? Who knows?

The overall message here is that the disc is the largest single dollop of collagenous material found in the body. Its mechanical properties, as well as those of all other tissues of the musculoskeletal system, are hugely influenced by fluid movement. Movement of fluid in and out of collagen, due to changes of posture and movement is, probably the single most rapid change that can occur in those tissues. So, when looking for a 'tissue' explanation for a rapid change in 'feelings', 'symptoms' or range of movement, to me the major consideration has to be fluid movement in collagenous tissue. Think about the patient who one minute can hardly bend forward and touch the tops of their knees. You get them to lie down and do some nice rotation mobilisations to their lumbar spine, or you get them to do simple crook rotation exercises followed by easy pelvic rocking. Then, you get them to stand them up and they now reach forward to the tops of their ankles. How do you explain that?

1. Pure tissue explanation says – fluid movement...
   ... nothing else changes so rapidly in the tissues.
2. Changes in muscle tone – ah, but this involves processing!
3. Changes in pain – ah, processing again.
4. Less fearful/more confident/ because of what you might have said...
   e.g. 'Up you come and try that bend forward again, you should be
   a lot freer this time'... Ah, processing again...
5. And so on.
6. Sudden change in mechanics? Come on, pull the other one!

As I've said, injured collagen has a higher osmotic fluid 'suction' potential – it therefore clamours to be swollen. Think acute joint, muscle or back injuries and you'll often see the pattern of stiff from not moving, freer once gets moving and this gets a good deal less as it all settles. For this pattern, think osteoarthritis too, but rheumatoid arthritis and ankylosing spondylitis fit the pattern big time, – they're the mothers-of-all joint inflammations and one of the key diagnostic criteria for them is lengthy morning stiffness – one to three hours when really inflamed. In our practice, about once or twice a year, a misdiagnosed 'polymyalgia rheumatica' turns up. It's the same story, massive and long lasting morning stiffness in the shoulders/back/hips. They can hardly move and of course they respond fantastically well to steroid treatment, which quells the inflammation – it's almost magical in its effectiveness.

In common-or-garden wear and tear/degeneration/OA and joint or muscle injuries the pattern is often the same (though there are always plenty of exceptions) but it's less severe and for far less time than those grand-masters of inflammatory arthropathy. Improvement of morning stiffness is an important element of treatment and management monitoring. Quite often this pattern responds very rapidly to simple NSAIDs. The clinician's job is decide whether the stiffness is adaptive or maladaptive, as it may make a difference to management strategies. For example: take the tabs, quell it and get moving, or accept it, normalise it and get going at a pace that is commiserate with the recovery pathway. Overall though, if you adopt a graded exposure approach, the notion of adaptive vs maladaptive may not matter one jot!

Patient explanation note:

If acute sprain/strain/muscle/joint/spinal pain patients come in with this pattern of morning struggling and stiffness I normalise it, unless it's very significant (1-2 hours or more). In which case, it's a red flag and further diagnostic tests plus medical review that are required. I often use the tight stiff cut finger example as I've already mentioned. I tell them that the stiffness lessens as it heals and that the reaction is a NORMAL HEALING PATTERN. What's going on in their back/shoulder/knee/sprained muscle is a smart, 'please move and warm me up slowly' request. Thus, it's good to do nice easy movements to get it free and that doing this regularly through the day is good too. But, warn them to expect it to be stiff after resting/sitting, and that when it happens all they have to do is do.

MOVE BEFORE YOU MOVE...!

For example, for a low back patient who has been sitting for a while, before they get up, I show them and get them to do movements like: simple flex forward and back, gently up into a little extension, repeat 5-10-15 times depending on what's needed. They can also do, easy rotation, grab a knee, side bending, hip hitching, whatever feels easy to do. It's all the directions you can, the easier ones the better.

In my practice we give simple 'move before you move' exercises for all tissues and joints when appropriate. It's pretty obvious, but here are some examples of common ones:

- shoulder = variations of pendular standing or leaning forward
- knee = sitting on table with legs dangling and swinging
- hip = stand on opposite leg or on a book, lean forward a bit holding onto a chair and swing.

Traction disasters!

I used to call this water movement 'fluid ooze'! In the bad old days we used to use traction a fair bit, these days due to a few less than enthusiastic outcome studies for it, it's largely been abandoned in favour of a computer generated sheet with pathetic little exercises, ten reps three times a day and no follow-up!

Some patients seem to do well by being tied up tight and put on a rack!

A traction disaster is when a patient with horrid low back pain comes in, can hardly move, is doubled up and may even have some pain radiating down the leg. You've fiddled about with everything you can think of and got absolutely nowhere, the patient's getting rather tetchy with the lack of progress and things are feeling heavily pressured. Then you suddenly think of traction, (yep, 'that's impressive, let's go for it) and proceed to belt them up and leave them for twenty minutes while you go do the next patient because you're already running late. When you come back after eight minutes or so, they're either very comfortable or have gone to sleep for the first time for many days. The timer goes off, they wake up and as the traction eases down you can see the relaxation go from their face and a look of slight alarm and tension. Oh, Oh... OK... Oh... OK ... Oh. They're moaning now and clenched up. You feel slightly sickened by what you're witnessing, then the swearing starts with the uh, uh...uh... uh... God... oh... and you're thinking, 'I wish he'd bloody shut up, the patient next door's going to be shitting themselves, how the hell am I going to get them up and out of here? Bugger it, I wish I worked in an office.'

They can't move an inch, they go to lift their head and bang... 'Arghhhh' and so on. The gasping 'What have you done to me Louis?' comment usually comes next. It takes you half an hour to get them off the couch, dressed and out the door. The place pongs with sweat and you're muttering something like, 'Make an appointment for tomorrow, you're actually a lot worse than I thought. Oh, don't forget to do that little exercise I showed you.' You've now got a stack of three patients wound-up and checking the time every two minutes and this moaning person walks past them in the waiting room. You're wishing you had a back door exit or a trap-door to a basement that turns failed patients into meat pies!

The patients either end up with sciatica, or they come back a lot better after a really bad time for 12-24 hours. Or, you never see them again. Or, they go to the local chiropractor who sorts them out in one go!

Quite often they've been referred to you by your best friend or your neighbour, or some important celebrity and now you are doomed. It seems pretty obvious that tying someone up and stretching them is a bit, well, inquisition-medievalist-goth-new-age-fantasy stuff. So it's hardly surprising that by doing this you receive a free ticket to the traction-therapists-disaster-underworld-special-interest-group with a special all-inclusive eternal meeting with Hades!

I still put patients on traction from time to time, but they no longer suffer this sort of disaster. There is certainly a fairly regular category of cervical nerve root presentation that gets a degree of relief from modest traction. Responsive lumbar roots seem to be less common. The key thing in the history is significant morning stiffness or stiffness after resting – be it lying or sitting. If this is the case, avoiding traction is probably wise. Or, do it very lightly to start with and not for long and have it on intermittent so the pull goes on and off. Or, be more relaxed when it comes off, expect increased discomfort and stiffening, but go with it. When you're cool with it, you quietly explain to the patient that as the traction is released they may get a little more discomfort and that's normal. Tell them to try and stay as relaxed as possible and follow your instructions as you release the belts and gently bring their legs down off the leg supporting stool. Get them to do easy small movements, like pelvic-rocking into flexion, then into flexion-extension as it eases – the aim is to build the movement range and speed gradually as the stiffness settles. I also use 'grab-a-knee' or 'crook-rotation' – whichever one feels the freest to do. The thoughts in my head now are, traction can hardly have 'blown the disc' – sure it's turgid and full, but that means that lots of repeated movement will force a bit of fluid out and slacken things down a bit (move before you move). You don't let them get up in one hit. You get them to roll onto their side and up... 'Breathe slowly, stay nice and relaxed, smoothly, up you come' and so forth. Traction disasters are a thing of the past, and it may well be down to my confidence with 'fluid ooze' and turgidity. It's nice to see some consistency of a reaction with musculoskeletal pain conditions from time to time and this stiffening scenario is one of them.

So, from a tissue perspective, my attitude to traction is that it very quickly mimics the overnight inward fluid 'ooze' which stiffens the disc and more than likely the whole of the sensitised segment. So, if the disc has an un-breached outer annular wall it will still have its hydrostatic properties, when fluid is imbibed, it becomes more turgid, there's more pressure in it. Traction, by helping this mechanism to occur quickly is bound to make the segment stiffer and if the segment is mechanically sensitised, it'll make it hurt more too!

If a fissure is about to breach could traction be the little last straw that tips it? The answer is probably, yes, but it's rare.

Chapter NR 3.3
Dirty discs to discuss 2

I now return to the early laboratory work of Mike Adams and Billy Hutton introduced in the last chapter.

Cyclical compressive loading in flexion for hour after hour of young healthy discs, leads to radial fissuring (see figure NR 3.5). The annulus gradually deforms into a 'bell' shape, pushing and stretching the annular rings to bulge and then tear posterior-laterally. Eventually the fissure reaches the surface and ruptures through the outer annular wall. Once the fissure has reached the surface, extrusion of material from the nucleus and annulus can occur. Remember that the posterior longitudinal ligament overlies the back of the disc and may prevent egress of material, if the breach is posterior rather than lateral.

Not all the discs in the experiments extruded material, indeed some sustained vertebral body fractures or remained undamaged, but a great many showed the 'bell' shaped distortions of the annulus often with incomplete radial fissures.

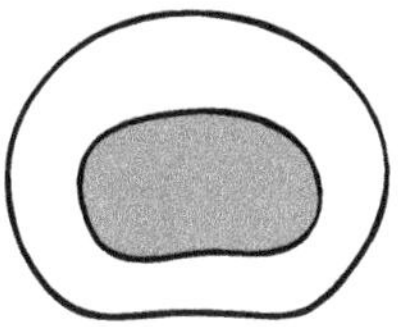
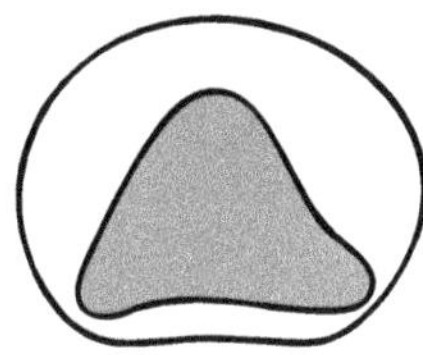
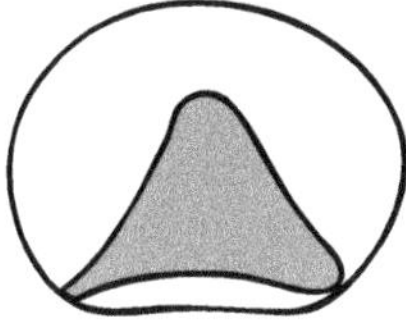

Figure NR 3.5 Schematic disc showing bell shape annulus after many hours of compressive loading

This incomplete radial type fissure is illustrated in 'B' in the next figure NR 3.6. It is a typical 'degenerative' pattern for discs through life, as are 'A' (concentric clefts) and 'C' (peripheral rim lesions). So, what Adams and Hutton managed to do to a normal disc in a few hours of flexion loading can happen to discs over long periods of time in normal life. It's called 'fatigue-failure'. It clearly makes discs more vulnerable to extrusion/bulging/prolapse/herniation and also, once a radial fissure breaches the outer annulus, to the loss of the 'normal' fluid movement mechanisms discussed in the last chapter.

The degenerative changes shown in figure NR 3.6 'C' are called 'peripheral rim lesions'. These can lead to bulging and even avulsions of the peripheral annulus and end-plate material. What's neat is that to counter this disc bulge, the body does a bit of strengthening by producing osteophytes – as you can see in the sagittal section of 'C'. Osteophytes are an attempt to reinforce the outer annular wall and prevent excessive bulging. The adjacent bone of the vertebral body also does its bit via 'sclerotic hardening'. Viewed by a radiologist or doctor making a diagnosis, osteophytes and sclerotic bone are evidence of 'degenerative' pathology or disease. Viewed from a biological perspective it's a clever adaptive mechanisms to help stiffen, strengthen and stabilise the weakened disc! What follows is a real life example of this.

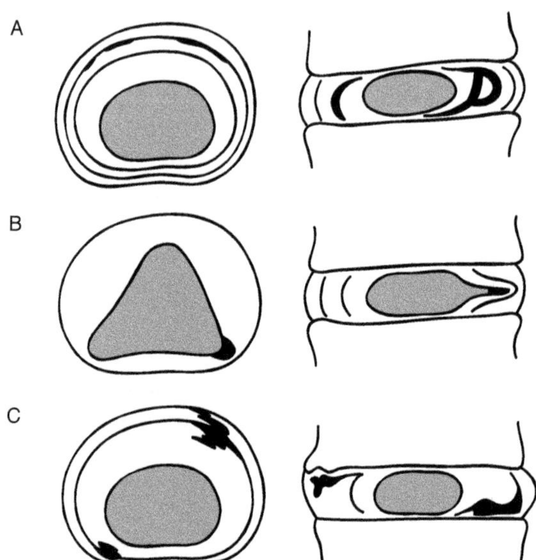

Figure NR 3.6 Typical 'degenerative' pattern for discs through life, 'A'(concentric clefts) 'B' incomplete radial type fissure and 'C' (peripheral rim lesions)

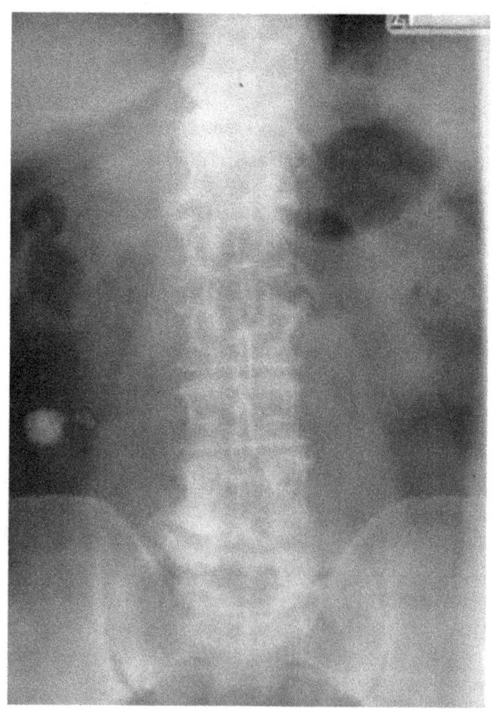

Figure NR 3.7 X-ray showing massive osteophytes to the left of L4-5 and to the right of L1-2, but also global narrowing between vertebrae and osteophytes of the rest of the spine too

The x-ray in figure NR 3.7 shows massive osteophytes to the left of L4-5 and to the right of L1-2, but also global narrowing between vertebrae and osteophytes of the rest of the spine too. The fellow, who the x-ray came from, is shown in figure NR 3.8 and 3.9 (when he was around 90% better!). As you can see he has a marked and fixed flexion deformity of the lumbar spine. In the picture the posture is 'straight' for him. He worked as a Cornish 'hedge' builder. A Cornish 'hedge' is like a dry stone wall – there being no mortar and a great many very large stones! He told me that he had spent the best part of thirty years hedging, and therefore, bending picking up and moving the stone. Not surprisingly he'd suffered back pain from

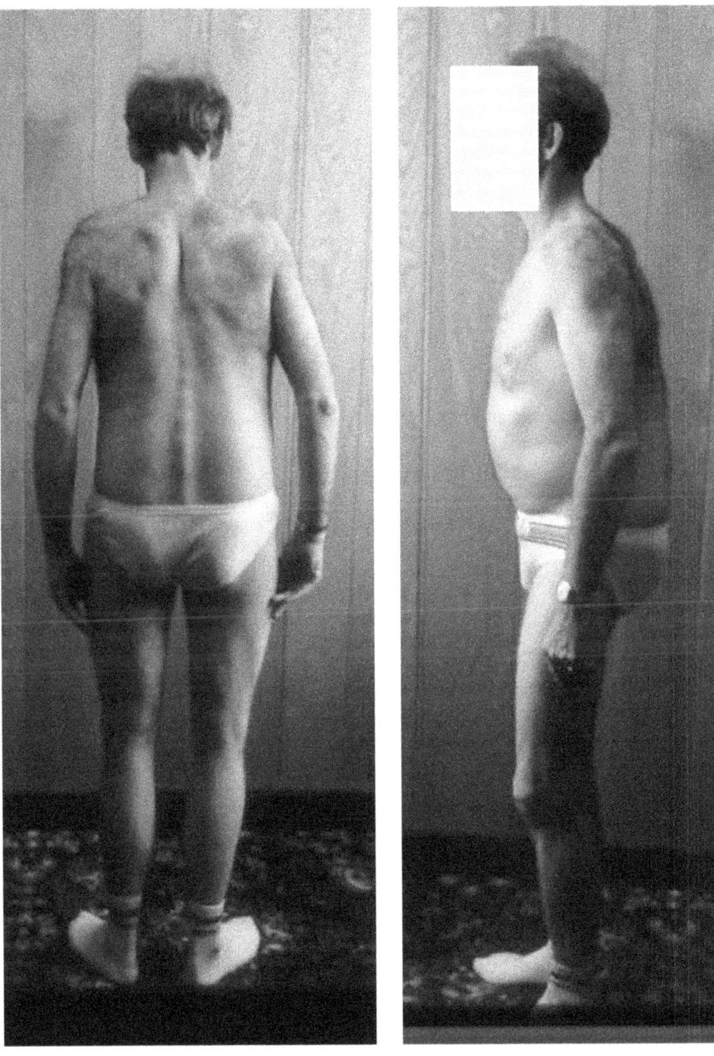

Figure NR 3.8 and 3.9 The 'owner' of the lumbar spine in figure 3.7. A Cornish 'hedge' or wall builder

time to time and occasionally sciatica but he always carried on working and it always got better. From time to time he said he found traction helpful and this was why he had come to see me! His old therapist had retired and he'd struggled to find any therapist who had a traction machine. He's a great example of a functioning but severely degenerate back which has adapted to it by stiffening in flexion (more as to why flexion later) and osteophyte formation. As you can imagine, there was zero intervertebral movement in all directions. However, thanks to good hips and long hamstrings, he could touch his toes easily. He certainly couldn't lie on his stomach!

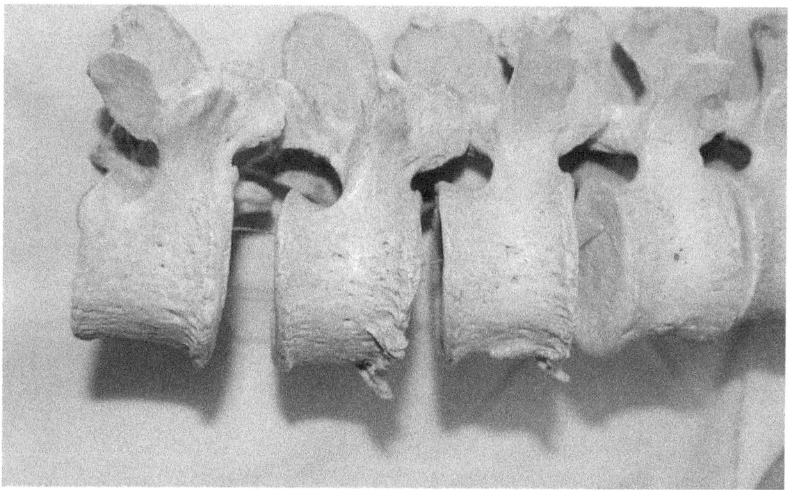

Figure NR 3.10 Large osteophytes on the lower spine vertebral bodies of a skeleton

Figure NR 3.10 is a real skeleton and as you can see, the lower spine vertebral bodies have plenty of large osteophytes on their anterior margins. There are none posteriorly or postero-laterally adjacent to where neural tissue resides. As far as the neural contents of the spine are concerned this is a blessing! There are twice as many disc rim lesions anteriorly and antero-laterally than posteriorly. Osteophytes, if they are putting pressure on neural tissue are not such good news.

Disc forces and dangers?

In their review of the 'activities that could cause disc prolapse' (in the light of all the experiments on cadavers they did) Adams et al (2012) listed the following:

- manual handling that heavily loads all at once in bending, lateral bending and compression

- on-going excessive bending and loading, or on-going excessive bending, then high load – as in a lift with the spine in flexion following a long period of working in a flexed posture

The term, 'sagging on your ligaments' which I remember Robin McKenzie using is apt here. Meaning, there's danger in lifting with the spine sagging and stretching unphysiologically at end range flexion; especially if it's been 'sagging' at end of range bad posture for a long time prior to the lift! If you've got weak back muscles you're not going to be strong enough to hold your back away from end range for long either. 'Sagging on your ligaments' is 'lazy-lifting' but it's also the normal way most people bend forward too. So, make sure your patients learn to be able to lift with a strong, but not over-tense, straight back. Not lordotic, but neutral straight, so there's even loading as far as is possible through the vertebral body-disc-vertebral body of the low lumbar spine. In my experience most patients (and many physios that I've taught on my courses) are hopelessly uncoordinated at this, plus they've got weak legs/ quads – so they can't lift with bent legs and close to the object either.

- falling on your buttocks with legs straight out in front
- lunging to catch a heavy object that's falling or slipping out of your grasp
- any event involving the trunk being dragged forwards into flexion: strong muscle contraction adds to the compressive effect
- heavy flexion exertion first thing in the morning, 'when the discs are swollen with water'
- a heavy lift after the spine has been allowed to 'creep' into excessive flexion.

Let's now take a look at the actual forces involved. In the experiments that Mike Adams, Billy Hutton and Trish Dolan did they used between 2.5 and 4.5kN of force to produce disc disruption and sometimes disc extrusions. It seems that many manual handling tasks generate peak compressive forces that are greater than this. To quote them (Adams et al 2002):

> *'It appears therefore that discs could prolapse in-vivo whenever the number of loading cycles per day is sufficiently high that fatigue damage accumulates faster than the discs' adaptive remodelling response can deal with it. It is difficult to predict when this might occur, because it depends on the age, health and work experience of the individual as well as the work environment.'*

I've always found it difficult to relate the forces used in the experiments to real life. I assume the reader does too and so I'm going to dedicate the next few minutes to putting it all in a better perspective.

Professor Alf Nachemson was the original guy here, a spinal surgeon and researcher who devoted his life to trying to figure out back pain. He was disarmingly honest too. I remember listening to a keynote lecture he gave at a manual therapy conference in Holland in the late 1990's. He started by saying, 'I've been studying and researching the causes of back pain my whole life, we didn't have a clue about it when I started and we still don't have a clue!' Alf sadly died in 2006, but he will be most remembered for his work measuring pressure in discs.

He measured 'in vivo' intradiscal pressures on volunteers in a variety of positions. His original work was back in the 1960's and revised in the early 1980's.

What follows are some of his findings given in kilo-Newtons (kN). What does 1kN mean? 1kN is the force exerted by gravity of a mass of approximately 100kg. That's round about 225lbs. If I stand on you you'll feel a force of around 0.7kN or my weight, 70kg, or around 157lbs (11 stone and 3 lbs)

(If you want to convert kN to kilos multiply by 100: if you want to convert to pounds, multiply by 225.)

Here are some of Nachemson's figures from real live individuals in different positions:

- lying: 0.150kN-0.250kN (34-56lbs, say about one third of my body weight)
- standing: 0.500kN-0.800kN (112-180lbs, about my body weight)
- sitting erect:0.700-1.0 kN (157-225lbs, my body weight plus a couple of bags of coal)
- stooping to lift a 10Kg weight: 1.9kN (427lbs or two and two-thirds of me!)

Now you can see what the potentially disc damaging forces of 2.5-4.5kN (562-1012lbs) mentioned above means relative to your or my actual weight! It's roughly between three and a half and six and a half times my weight going through the one disc over and over again for six hours before it leads to fatigue failure! To me that's a big force for a long time!

Here are some more 'calculated' figures for the lifting forces that might go through a healthy young man's low lumbar disc when he lifts (from Adams et al 2002):

4.0kN (900lbs) when lifting a 14Kg weight (that's 5.7 lots of my weight on one disc!)

5.5kN (1236lbs) when lifting a 29Kg weight (that's 7.8 of me!)

I hope you can see why it's so very hard to break a fresh cadaver, even one from a frail old fella'!

Here's a neat quote to make you think... (p 100, Adams et al 2002):

> *'Antagonistic contraction of the abdominal muscles (sometimes called co-contraction) increases the stability of the trunk but at the cost of increasing spinal compression by up to 45% during simulated lifting movements.'*

Here's another (p.101):

... *'Lifting with the knees bent increased the compressive force by approximately 5% compared to straight-leg (stoop) lifts.'*

Oh, that's not supposed to happen, we were always told to bend the knees! Well this is just one bit of evidence but it shows you how shaky the evidence is for what we do and tell our patients. Look it's only 5%... and the following needs to be taken into consideration....

> *'Increasing the distance of a 10kg weight from the feet, from 0cm to 60cm (2 feet) increased the peak compressive force from 2.8kN to 5.2kN and lifting 10kg quickly (in 1 second) increased the peak compressive force to 5.3kN compared to 3.2kN when the lift was performed more slowly.'*

Adams et al (2002) also reassure us (p 101):

> *'Values of peak compressive forces measured in these studies are approximately 50-70% of the ultimate compressive strength of cadaveric lumbar spines of similar age and gender so they would not be expected to cause injury. However, repetitive loading can damage cadaveric specimens at 40-50% of their ultimate compressive strength so compressive fatigue damage might be expected to accumulate at forces above 4kN in a typical young man.'*

(That's 5.7 times more force than the weight of me)

How strong is the spine then? ...p 134 ...

> *'The compressive strength of the lumbar spine ranges between 2kN and 14kN, depending on the sex, age and bodymass of the individual, with a typical value for a young man being 6-10kN. The high and low extremes refer to male athletes, and old women with osteoporosis, respectively.'*

Disc prolapse by sudden loading, requires an average of 5.4kN with a range from 2.8 – 13.0kN and the average flexion angle was 15.8 degrees with a range from 9-21 degrees.

It seems to me that the best message regarding lifting is:

1. Try not to lift too suddenly. Think about it before you do it and plan the most efficient way of doing it.
2. Try a little test lift to get the 'feel' of what you're lifting.
3. Keep your back straight or a little flexed when you lift as far as you can – not too flexed and not lordotic either. You need the 'Goldilocks' position – that's 'just-right' somewhere in between! This needs practice, most people haven't a clue where this is, but some fall into it naturally.
4. Try not to 'sag' on your ligaments – meaning lift with the spine at end range flexion. If you're not strong enough to lift the object in question without doing this – then get training and get stronger by doing the posture plus a graded lifting programme.
5. Try and be as smooth and relaxed as you can, try not to over-tense your back and abdominal muscles.

6. Keep the object as close to you as you can. If you have strong legs this is made easier to do if you bend your knees. I don't think I'd ever tell anyone to lift a heavy weight with straight legs – using your legs enables you to get closer to the object.
7. While carrying a heavy object stay relaxed, be smooth and don't get alarmed! Apparently peak spinal compression during manual handling increases by between 30 and 70% when subjects are alarmed!
8. If you can't manage to maintain a lift and feel you're going into a lot of flexion – drop it! If more than one of you are lifting a single object agree a 'drop-it' routine, so you don't injure the others when you let go. Best is to get the right number of 'lifters' for the object.
9. The figure 4kN equates to lifting a 14kg weight from the floor. Don't do this day in and day out.

While on this topic it's worth flipping to another perspective, that of the epidemiologist! Thanks to a review by Bernard (1997) the following activities have been identified which may lead to or aggravate low back pain:

- heavy physical work (strong evidence)
- lifting and forceful movements (strong evidence)
- bending and twisting (postures)
- whole body vibration (strong evidence)
- static work postures
- combination of these factors.

Devereux et al (2004) examined the role of work stress and psychological factors in the development of musculoskeletal disorders in the 'Stress and MSD study'.

Physical work risk factors causing or contributing to low back pain are:

- lifting 6-16kg greater than 10 times per hour or lifting greater than 16kg at all and always/often working with the back in an awkward position
- pushing and pulling objects combined with tasks requiring lifting.

But...

- this report further identified that workers highly exposed to psychosocial work risk factors and not physical factors were 1.7 times more likely to report low-back complaints compared to workers with low exposure to them
- the greatest risk was when the two combined – high psychological work risk factors plus high physical work risk factors. These folk are four times more likely to report problems when compared to workers exposed to neither set of factors.

It seems amazing that the physical work factors are almost identical to the psychological work factors! Put in the context of knowledge about pain processing and the brain, it's perhaps much more easy to understand. The 'Vulnerable Organism' is a good way of looking at and reasoning these sorts of issues (see later).

I would advise readers to review this chapter in Topical Issues in Pain 5:

Hunter, N 2013 Evidenced based management of low back pain in occupational health. Topical Issues in Pain 5. Gifford LS (Ed) CNS Press, Falmouth.

Some thoughts and summarising from the shop-floor...

1. Some folk have strong discs and some don't and amongst our day to day patients the reality is, we've no idea who is who.

2. It is highly likely that those who lead active and athletic lives from an early age have stronger discs/musculoskeletal systems.

3. As we get older some of us are highly likely to have plenty of annular defects. Some may be radial fissures and some may be very near breaching the outer annular wall leading to a disc prolapse. So, while the disc is a very strong structure, the likelihood of a herniation or extrusion occurring under even modest forces may, in some people, be quite high.

    - Most clinicians have come across patients who ended up with sciatica after something simple... 'I just bent down to tie up my shoe lace.' 'I sneezed a couple of times on the third that was it.' 'I didn't see the bottom step/the curb/I tripped/the car went over a big bump/I was blowing up a balloon.' Etc.

    - In my lectures I used to ask the participants to raise their hand if they'd ever had patients come to them who blamed a strong manipulation or forceful technique/therapist or exercise on their sciatica and always a very large percentage put their hands up. It is always my belief that while we get messed-up patients from 'them' – they must also get them from us!

4. Easy repeated movement in any direction moves fluid about. It may even cause a decrease in pressure within the collagen being moved and increase the tissues 'creep' and therefore range of movement. Decreased pressure on sensitised tissues means less pressure on the sensitised nociceptors there and therefore pain relief.

5. Where 'swelling' is near the surface and obvious, for example sprained knee or ankle ligaments – massaging the swelling away feels good and quite often frees the movement. You may recall from the nociception chapters earlier, the positive or 'adaptive' nature of swelling – it dilutes the inflammatory chemicals produced by the injury and healing mechanism. Instinctive massaging, moving and squeezing the swelling away helps to remove the metabolic by products via lymphatic return. Deeper avascular tissues clearly can't be massaged and so require regular movement. Ten repetitions isn't

likely to do much to the fluid in the disc, but it is often enough to make things feel a bit freer.

6. What's good about the McKenzie system? Answer, regular movement. What's bad? Answer, to me it's the fixation with just moving in one direction ('movement preference' being taken too literally and rigidly, which can create fear of movement too) and often going too far and too hard into that range. Saying 'we do it because it works' is not good enough. Look, I get the same results as you by going with regular easy movement in all directions, big relaxed movements in directions that are easy and smaller relaxed movements in those that are more sensitive and limited or feared. As time progresses and the problem settles all movements are taken further, repetitions increased and functional loading and stresses re-introduced. I call it the graded exposure 'twisted ankle approach' to back pain. It's easy, its natural, its risk free and it doesn't involve any questionable theories about disc derangement and correction.

7. Wise action is to start easy and build slowly, just as you would for a twisted ankle. Forcing and demanding movement in one direction and demanding that the patient doesn't waiver from some enforced posture, I would propose, is at loggerheads with rational biology and somewhat risky. Just as you wouldn't do an end range high velocity manipulation to a freshly twisted ankle, nor should you push a movement repeatedly to end range just because the pain is going where you want it to.

8. As we'll see in the next chapter the notion that discs can rapidly change in parallel with symptom resolution has to be reviewed (I really want to say, is a joke!). If a 'McKenzie derangement 3' is better in two days it's certainly not because of some rapid change in the disc. And it's certainly not because the fluid or nucleus has moved and stayed in a more stable position. The only answer is that a 'change of processing' must have occurred.

9. If there are fissures in discs, particularly radial fissures, then fluid and nuclear material can be forced down them by movement. Otherwise for fluid movement, think of the normal disc as having very sluggish sponge like qualities. If you squeeze and let go a sponge in a watery environment – some fluid gets squeezed out and some sucked in. The more you move, the more the fluid moves out relative to what's going in. The result is a less turgid and slacker disc which will now go further in the direction that it's being moved in. When the movement and pressures stop the water quietly gets sucked back in again and the disc stiffens. There is a clear parallel with what many of us feel after rest and after movement; which gets amplified in the patient with their sensitised back tissue.

10. If a disc is internally injured, as must happen in all of us through our lives, it may have the potential to cause pain or swell more due to increasing concentrations of 'inflammatory' or 'breakdown' molecules.

11. Think about the amount of physical stress you put through your back – fatigue-failure may be being speeded up!

12. If your disc is going to go, it'll go and I don't think there's an awful lot you can do about it. I tell my patient's this. Just like I tell them is the case for a tendo-achilles problem. TA's can have a degenerate core; neither the patient, nor you know about it. The result is it's a weakened structure and presumably more likely to give or tear. If it's going to go, it'll go and then you'll either walk and run flat-footed for the rest of your life or get it surgically fixed.

13. You may think I'm paranoid but I now view every simple acute back pain as a potential sciatica! That doesn't mean I avoid treating and rehabilitating them up to a high level of functional confidence? As time goes on and the problem improves, so my confidence parallels this and my instruction that discs and backs are incredibly strong structures meshes with progress.

14. Looking at the psychosocial evidence, in relation to the heavy bias of these chapters to tissues is almost a relief. How come a psychosocially stressed worker is almost equally likely to get low back pain as one who's exposed to high physical risk factors? My answer is the vulnerable organism, which I'll discuss later. For now, it's simply 'when you are low you hurt more easily'.

Section NR 3
Read what I've read

Adams A., Bogduk N., Burton K., Dolan P. (2012) The Biomechanics of back pain. (3ed). Churchill Livingstone. Edinburgh.

Bernard B.P. (1997) Musculskeletal disorders and workplace factors: A critical review of epidemiologic evidence for work-related musculoskeletal disorders of the neck, upper extremity, and low back. Department of Health and Human Services, National Institute for Occupational Safety and health, Cincinnati. OH.

Bozzao, A., Gallucci M., et al., (1992) Lumbar disk herniation: MR imaging assessment of natural history in patients treated without surgery. Radiology 185(1): 135-141.

Bush, K., Cowan N., et al., (1992) The Natural History of Sciatica Associated with Disc Pathology. Spine: 17(10): 1205-1212.

Bush, K., Chaudhuri R., et al., (1997) The pathomorphologic changes that accompany the resolution of cervical radiculopathy. A prospective study with repeat magnetic resonance imaging. Spine: 22(2): 183-187.

Bywaters E. G. L. (1982) Mobility with rigidity: a view of the Spine:. Annals of the Rheumatic Diseases 41: 210-214.

Ellenberg, M. R., Ross M. L., et al., (1992) Prospective evaluation of the course of disc herniations in patients with proven radiculopathy. Archives of Physical medicine and Rehabilitation: 74: 3-8.

Devereux J., et al., (2004) The role of work stress and psycholgical factors in the development of musculoskeletal disorders. The stress and MSD study. Robens Centre for health Ergonomicw, University of Surrey HSE Research report no 273

Gifford L. S. (1987) Circadian variation in human flexibility and grip strength. Aust J Physio 33(1): 3-9.

Gifford L. S. (1994) The influence of circadian variation on spinal examination. In Boyling J. and Palastanga N. (Eds) Grieve's Modern Manual Therapy. J. Boyling and N. Palastanga. Edinburgh, Churchill Livingstone.

Gifford L. S. (1995) Fluid Movement may partially account for the behaviour of symptoms associated with nociception in disc injury and disease. In Shacklock M.O. (Ed) Moving in on Pain. Chatswood, Butterworth-Heinemann Australia.

Hunter N. (2013) Evidenced based management of low back pain in occupational health. Topical Issues in Pain 5. Gifford LS (Ed) CNS Press, Falmouth.

Kimori, H., Shinomiya K., et al., (1996) The natural history of herniated nucleus pulposus with radiculopathy. Spine: 21(2): 225-229.

Gifford L. S. (1995) Fluid Movement may partially account for the behaviour of symptoms associated with nociception in disc injury and disease. In Shacklock M.O. (Ed) Moving in on Pain. Chatswood, Butterworth-Heinemann Australia.

Hunter N. (2013) Evidenced based management of low back pain in occupational health. Topical Issues in Pain 5. Gifford LS (Ed) CNS Press, Falmouth.

Kimori, H., Shinomiya K., et al., (1996) The natural history of herniated nucleus pulposus with radiculopathy. Spine: 21(2): 225-229.

Komori H. (1996) Natural history of herniated nucleus pulposus with radiculopathy.Spine: 21(2):225-229

Maigne J.Y. (1994) CT follow-up study of 21 cases of nonoperatively treated cervical soft disc herniation. Spine: 19(2):189-191.

Matsubara Kato Y.F., et al., (1995) Serial changes on MRI in Lumbar disc herniations treated conservatively. Neuroradiology 37: 278-383.

Mochida K. (1998) Regression of cervical disc herniation observed on MRI. Spine: 23(9):990-997

Saal J. (1996) Nonoperative management of cervical herniated disc with radiculopathy. Spine: 21(16):1877-83

Saal, J. A. (1996) Natural history and nonoperative treatment of lumbar disc herniation. Spine: 21(24S): 2S-9S.

Saal, J. A., Saal J. S. (1989) Nonoperative treatment of herniated lumbar intervertebral disc with radiculopathy. An outcome study. Spine: 14(4): 431-437.

Saal, J. A., Saal J. S., et al., (1990) The natural history of lumbar disc extrusions treated non-operatively. Spine: 15(7): 683-686.

Section NR 4

ANATOMY AND BIOMECHANICS OF NERVE ROOTS

Chapter 4.1
Anatomy and biomechanics of nerve roots - compression

The great majority of nerve root related pain problems present with a greater or lesser degree of mechanically patterned pain. For example, the leg pain of sciatica gets worse when the sufferer bends forwards or backwards, or it may get better if they curl up on their side, or when they slump in a chair and put their feet up on a stool.

This section sets out to explain the common 'mechanically patterned' pains that I have observed over the years in my clinical practice. I am going to start with an overview of nerve compression anatomy and biomechanics and later briefly review nerve elongation factors. I wish this material had been taught when I was a student.

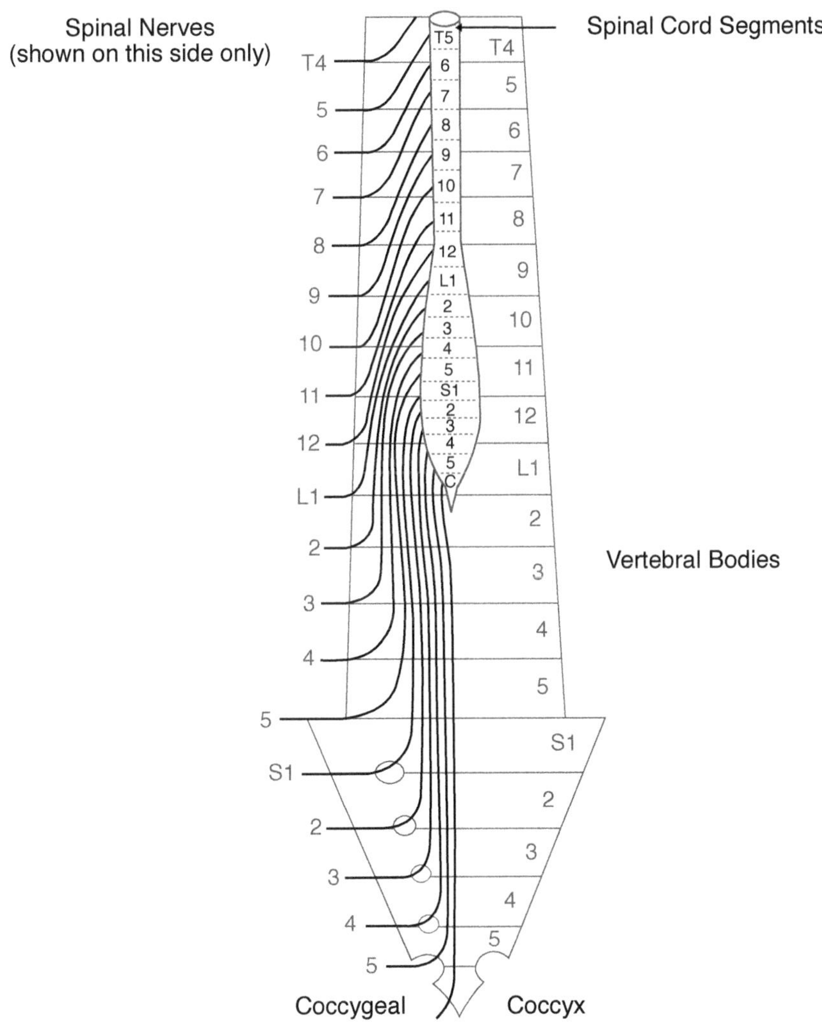

Figure NR 4.1 The relationship of the cord and the nerve roots to the vertebral bodies

Lumbar nerve root compression with movement: required anatomy and biomechanics

As you should know and should appreciate that many patients do not know, the spinal cord ends at around the L1-2 vertebral level. That means there is no spinal cord below this point, just a thick dural tube containing all the nerve roots neatly packed together and bathed in cerebrospinal fluid – the 'cauda equina'. Figure NR 4.1 clearly illustrates the relationship of the cord and the nerve roots to the vertebral bodies. It does not illustrate the dural sac.

Let's take a common example that we deal with every day in the clinic, the root of S1. S1 nerve root leaves the spinal cord way up at the level of the T11 vertebral body. It then courses downwards in the dural sac towards its destination, the exit foramina at S1-2 of the sacrum. That's approximately 16 cms long.

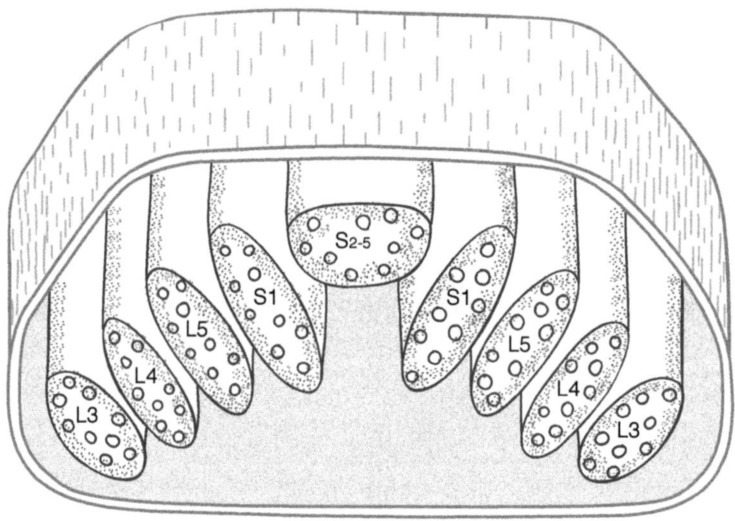

Figure NR 4.2 The dural sac containing nerve roots

The illustration in figure NR 4.2 shows the dural sac containing nerve roots. Note that the roots are duplicated on either side. In my lectures I used to ask the participants if they could work out what vertebral level this 'section' through the dura and cauda equina was taken from. You need to use figure NR 4.1. The key things to note are that all the nerve roots from L3 and below are present and L2 is absent, plus, there's no spinal cord. No spinal cord means that the section must be below the level of L2 vertebra. Since L2 root leaves the dural sac, somewhere around the junction of L1 and L2 vertebrae, the section must be somewhere below that and above the point where L3 leaves. Thus the section must have come from somewhere between the vertebral bodies of L2 and L3!

An important feature of all nerve roots is that once they leave the spinal cord they all take a downward and lateral course. The lower the nerve root, the more downward and longer the course has to be. Look at the T4 nerve root at the top of figure NR4.1. It's downward angle is quite a shallow gradient, compared to the lumbar and sacral roots and it's also a much shorter root too. Even the cervical roots have a slight downward angulation after leaving the cord.

The next important thing is the shape of the spinal canal in the lumbar spine. It is well worth having a full vertebral column to hand.

Figure NR 4.3 though rather complex is well worth taking time over to understand. Illustration 'c' in the bottom right of the figure shows a horizontal section through the bony body and arch of L5 vertebra. You can follow the arrow up to illustration 'a' to see exactly where the section was taken. If you're wondering what 'a' is – it's looking down on the back of lumbar vertebrae L4 and L5 with the back of the vertebrae removed to reveal the dural tube (3) and the exiting nerve roots of L4 and L5 (4, 5) on either side. The four pedicles (2) have been cut through and the neural arch, the facets, the transverse processes and the spinous processes have all been removed. Imagine a massive laminectomy! The discs between L4 and L5 and L5-S1 are clearly shown.

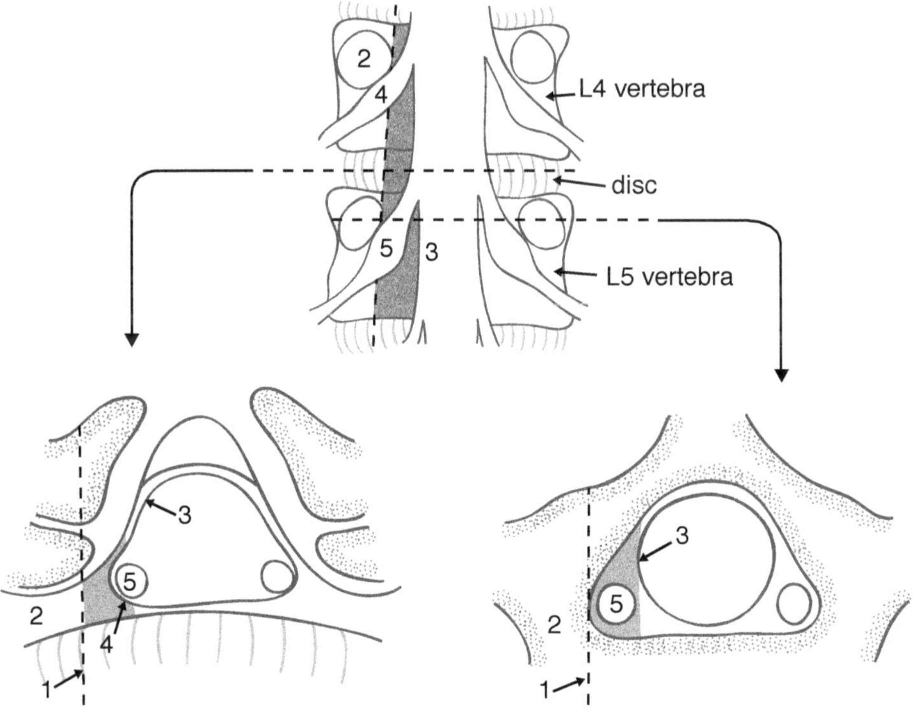

Figure NR 4.3 (opposite) Showing the radicular canal of the L4 and L5 vertebrae (dark shaded). Note where the L5 nerve root (5) leaves the dural sac to enter the radicular canal – it's at the disc/pedicle level above its exit foramen

One important thing to note from 'c' is the triangular shape of the bony spinal canal. If you have a skeleton handy I recommend you look at the shape and relative size of the bony canal at the lumbar and then higher levels for comparison. For example, at T12, or even L1, the canal shape is nearly circular and remains so way up to around T1-2 level. From C7 or T1 up to about C3 the canal shape is triangular again. Note that as you go up the vertebral column, the diameter of the bony canal gets larger and larger. At C1 and C2 the canal diameter is very large – which it has to be in order to accommodate the massive size of the spinal cord. As the cord descends from the brain, the number of neurones it contains gets less and less and so its size diminishes. If you think of the spinal cord at the atlas level, it contains the motor, sensory and sympathetic neurones for the whole of the body and all the limbs. But, by the time the cord reaches the upper lumbar levels it only carries those involved in communicating to and fro with the lower abdomen and legs.

Now imagine being able to shrink down in size and to then find yourself inside the dural sac where the L5 nerve root emerges from the spinal cord (see figure NR 4.1). You're surrounded by cerebrospinal fluid (CSF) and you're actually standing on the floor of the dural sac that's adjacent to the mid part of the body of T11 vertebra. Your assignment is to follow the course of the left L5 root to its exit intervertebral foramina at L5/S1. Before starting you look around and see that the space you're in is packed with other nerve roots and the lower end of the spinal cord. Immediately next to you laterally is the L4 root and then L3, all the way out to T12 which is just about to leave; piercing the dural sac and then going on its way to the intervertebral foramen between T11 and 12 vertebrae. Medially are the sacral roots and the lower end of the spinal cord; then towards the right side of the canal, if you peer over the top of the cord, are all the other paired roots that go to form the cauda equina on that side. If you can imagine you're 'walking' down inside the dural tube with L5 and all the other neighbouring roots you'll notice that at every vertebral level, a nerve root leaves the confines of the dural sac and you're then able to shift a little more laterally. After L4 root leaves, you're now the outermost root and are hard up against the lateral wall of the dural sac. You're now standing on L4-5 disc, right at the section illustrated as 'a' and 'b' in figure NR 4.3. As you can see from 'a' one step more and you'll be leaving the dural tube on your way to the intervertebral foramina between L5 and S1 vertebrae.

Before going on imagine again that the dural sac is transparent, so that as you've gone down you've been able to see the outside structures. Above your head and to your sides is an archway – sometimes bony, consisting of the pedicles to the sides, the bony neural arch above but also medial aspects of the facet joints and sometimes soft tissue; there's the ligamentum flavum and the retrodural fat pad. To simplify it, think that when you're standing on a **vertebrae** the archway that surrounds you is bony, but when you are standing on a **disc** the archway is bony to the sides – the facet joints; but soft tissue above – being the retrodural fat pad as well as ligamentum flavum. This distinction between the two positions is important, as I'll explain in more detail. At the level of the disc, the size of the spinal canal can change significantly with movement, yet, when on a vertebra, the canal size is fixed and therefore can't change with movement. Section 'c' in the illustration shows the 'fixed' nature of the wholly bony canal, but section 'b', the level of the disc, is where a great deal of change in dimension can occur.

One thing that was never explained properly to me was why S1 nerve root was the most common nerve root injured or responsible for sciatica? L5 certainly wasn't uncommon, but L4 and L3 certainly were. Think about S1 and you should think 'Why is it a root that exits the spinal canal between S1 and S2 – a wholly bony area and one whose dimensions are pretty much fixed and un-alterable throughout life, so commonly injured?' The answer is that it's the level above that's the important danger area – especially for roots S1 and L5.

Let me explain a little more and it will become clear.

If you look at 'a' in figure NR 4.3 and note the point where I left you standing with L5 root. You're on the L4-5 disc, you're inside the dural sac but over in the left corner. You're standing at '5' in the section 'b'. Your exit from the dural sac occurs just distally to where you're standing on the L4-5 disc. By the time you step onto L5 vertebra and are adjacent to the pedicles, you will already be out of the dural sac – see section 'c' now. You're '5' in this diagram, on your own and alone in an area called the 'radicular canal' or 'lateral recess' of the lumbar spine. The left lateral recess is the shaded zone in all three illustrations, it is bounded by the lateral wall of the dural sac medially and a vertical line joining the medial borders of the pedicles (indicated as '1' in all three illustrations). Thus the lateral border goes, bony pedicle, then 'window' of intervertebral foramen, then pedicle and so forth all the way down. If you look at a lumbar vertebra you'll see how this lateral corner of the triangle of the spinal canal is very tight and quite sharply angulated, hence the term 'lateral recess'. Now, the zone where the radicular canal is bordered laterally by the foramina is actually partially bony posteriorly/dorsally, it being the medial border of the anterior rim of the superior facet of the vertebra below! You need to look at a lumbar spine/sacrum to follow this or note it in 'b' of the figure. This area 'under' the facet joints is often referred to as the 'sub-articular' zone.

Figure NR 4.4 should clarify and simplify. This figure is all about the relationship of the nerve roots after they have left the dural sac to the discs above their exit foraminal level. So, note that S1 root leaves the dural sac above the L5-S1 disc, travels across it in the radicular canal (facet joint overhead!) then onto the sacrum and out of S1-2 foramina. L5 root leaves the dural sac at the level above its exit foramina, actually on the L4-5 disc before travelling down in the radicular canal and out. But look at L4 root – its exit from the dural sac is below the disc above! Its only danger is at the foramen it exits in – where it goes over the L4-5disc. But note the nerve root exits in the superior part of the foramen – where it's actually on bone rather than the disc. If you look at real lumbar vertebrae you'll note a 'groove' in the bone that the root lies in, just inferior to the pedicle on the vertebral body. This means that direct compression or pinching is unlikely but the effects of indirect compression as we've already discussed must be taken into account.

Figure NR 4.5 illustrates the impact of disc bulging, extrusion or narrowing in relation to the dural sac and nerve roots. Note the L3-4 disc extrusion is less likely to have any direct impact on a nerve root than those at the lower two levels.

In the mid 1990's I came across a paper by Lance Penning:

Penning L. (1992) Functional pathology of lumbar spinal stenosis (review). Clinical Biomechanics 7(1):3-17.

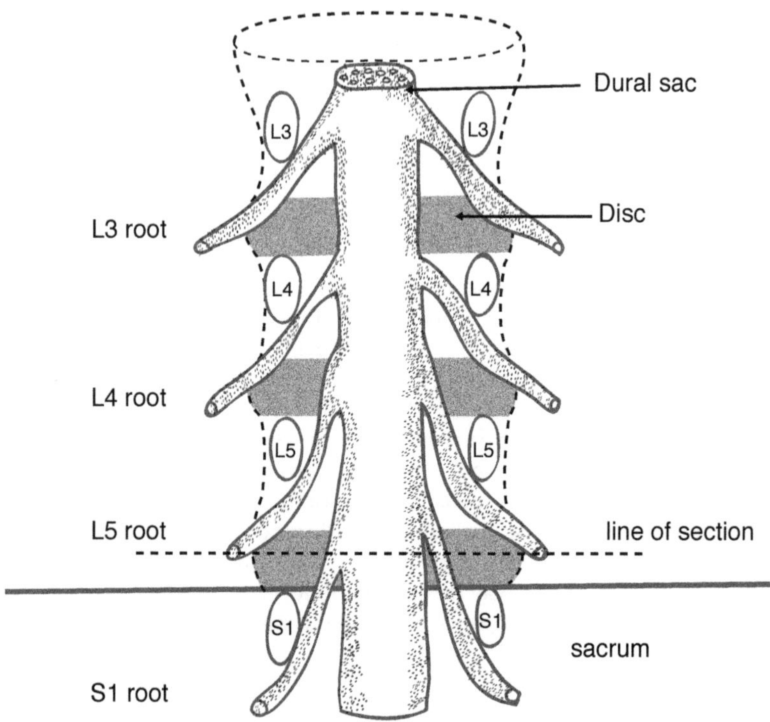

Figure NR 4.4 The relationship of the nerve roots after they have left the dural sac to the discs above their exit foraminal level. Redrawn from: Sato K. and Kikuchi S. (1993) An anatomic study of foraminal nerve root lesions in the lumbar spine. Spine 18(15): 2246-2251.

For me, unravelling the details of this paper in relation to the mechanically patterned pain behaviour of day to day back and nerve root pain was one of the most helpful things that I have ever done. Back then I found the paper to be quite complicated and required a great deal of study. I'm going to summarise what I found useful from it, especially in relation to clinical presentations; and you'll see why I like to view all disc extrusions and protrusions as being part of a 'stenotic' scenario or presentation, and often as 'transient'. The other thing to note is that at the time, the world was awash with the Mckenzie system and 'extension' principles were the order of the day for the majority of back pains. The notion that extension reduced derangements of the disc and that flexion tended to worsen them was a significant issue. My problem was that the vast majority of acute low back pain and sciatic presentations I was dealing with found varying degrees of flexion relieving. They came in stooped, sometimes shifted to one side; they reported getting most comfort slumped, curled up in bed on their side or in full flexion curled up on their legs. Coming upright, going into extension or lying prone just made it all worse and really aggravated any leg pain that was already there. I have never seen, in all my clinical years of treating acute low back pain, a patient come in who is 'stuck' in extension or finds massive relief in extension. They're either 'stuck' straight, or the majority, as I said, are flexed to varying degrees.

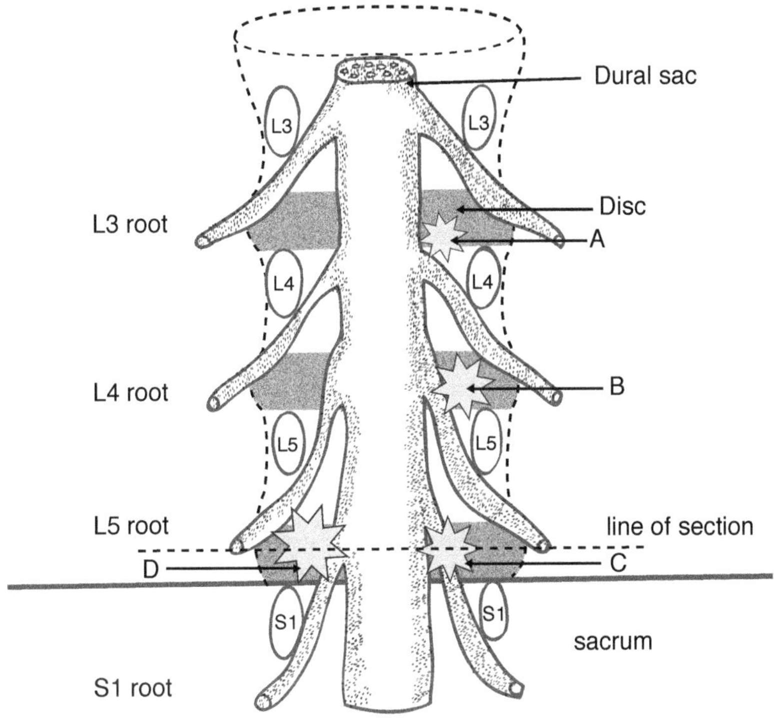

Figure NR 4.5 The impact of disc bulging, extrusion or narrowing in relation to the dural sac and nerve roots.

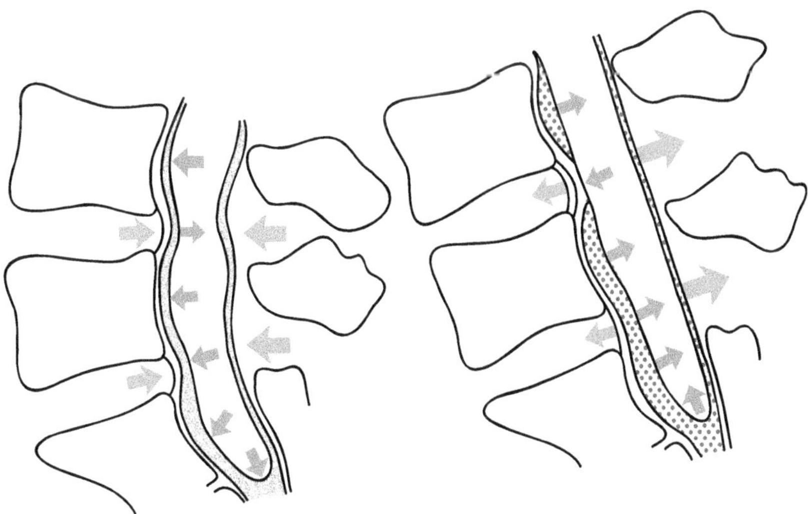

Figure NR 4.6 Demonstrating the relation of the dural sac and spinal canal effect going from full flexion on the right to full extension on the left. Redrawn from: Lance Penning's paper.

For years researchers of spinal stenosis focused on the dimensions of the **bony** canal, but Lance Penning uncovered a 1942 paper written in German by Knutsson. The paper demonstrated that, **at the level of the disc the cross sectional area of the spinal canal increases in flexion and decreases in extension.** The decrease was due to the **disc bulging backwards and the flaval ligaments bulging forwards**.

Work done on **normal** spines found that at the disc level the cross-sectional area of the spinal canal decreases: by $40mm^2$ when the spine goes from full flexion to full extension; and by $50mm^2$ when going from lying to standing. To put that in the context of the size of the spinal canal, that's a decrease of approximately one third – in normals! The change of the **canal** by around **one third** in size impacts the **dural sac** which gets reduced in diameter by **9%**. Figure NR 4.6 is redrawn from Lance Penning's paper and admirably demonstrates the effect of going from full flexion on the right, to full extension on the left. On the left, as the spine extends the posterior annulus of the discs bulge backwards into the spinal canal. At the same time the ligamentum flavum (large arrows to the right) folds and buckles thus pushing forwards into the canal. Further compressive effects occur via the retrodural fat pad (more on this later). As can be seen the effect is to reduce the dimensions of the canal at the 'disc' level. The heavy shading represents a plexus of 'anterodural veins' which clearly get compressed. The dural sac as a whole is compressed but also shifts in an anterior direction, as indicated by the arrows. In flexion the reverse happens: the posterior annulus flattens, the ligamentum flavum flattens and retracts and the whole dural sac moves posteriorly. The anterodural venous plexus expands in size.

Clinical points here: no wonder if we stand or keep a strong lordosis for any length of time we intermittently like to flex! Flexion is a compression relieving movement – taking pressure off not only the venous plexus, but all the neural elements in the spinal and radicular canal too. No wonder that 'disc' related pain presentations tend to be more comfortable in flexion and that extension is provocative. This will be amplified if any of the tissues in the confines of the spinal and radicular canals are sensitised in some way.

My postural advice is: yes, to stand in lordosis is fine and healthy for compression loading purposes, but to maintain lordosis for long periods doesn't make sense – in terms of compression of structures, as well as in terms of any potential ischaemic consequences. The best advice is to never stay still for long periods. Your back actually tells you what it wants you to do!

Let's now look at situations where the spinal canal gets narrowed – spinal stenosis. Lance Penning describes:

'The Rule of Progressive Narrowing', *'The more the canal is structurally narrowed by a stenosing process, the more it will be functionally narrowed by additional extension.'*

This means that in severe grades of stenosis, even the slightest extension motion, or the slightest increase in axial loading, may lead to compression of nervous elements.

As we've already seen in normals when going from flexion to extension – while decreasing the size of the canal at the disc level by around a third, actually decreases the dural sac by a mere 9%.

Penning gave these figures for the dural sac:

Group I = normals = 9% narrowing of dural sac in extension.

Group II = mild stenosis = 32% narrowing.

Group III= moderate stenosis= 45% narrowing.

Group IV=severe stenosis=67% narrowing.

Penning highlighted the importance of what he called 'lateral squashing of the dural sac', that was due to thickening of the flaval ligaments and enlargement and encroachment of degenerative facet joints.

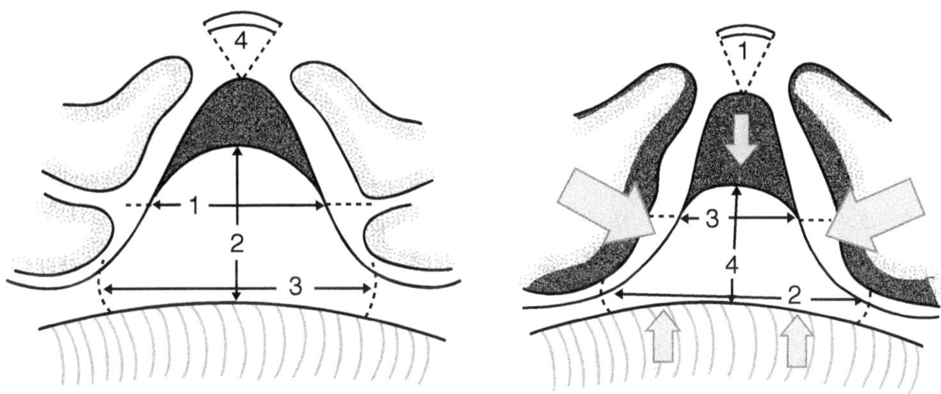

Figure NR 4.7 Two sections through the low lumbar spine at disc level.

Figure NR 4.7 shows two sections through the low lumbar spine at disc level. On the left is a normal spine, on the right a markedly degenerate and hence stenotic spine. The stenosis is caused by the disc bulging (see the smaller arrows) and the thickening of the facet joints (dark shading) note the larger arrows and the changed shape of the dural sac.

In the normal canal on the left, note (the numbers here refer to those on the left hand figure):

1. Equals normal 'interflaval' or transverse diameter of the dural sac.
2. Equals normal antero-posterior diameter of the dural sac.
3. Equals normal interpedicular diameter, which doesn't change, see '2' in the right hand figure.
4. Equals normal 'interflaval' angle.

The dark area above the dural sac is the 'retrodural fat pad' and therefore being fat is incompressible.

Note in the very 'stenotic' canal on the right:

1. Equals reduced interflaval angle.
2. Equals interpedicular diameter, which is unchanged.
3. Equals interflaval diameter, which is markedly reduced.
4. Equals the antero-posterior diameter, which is also markedly reduced.

As mentioned above, the two arrows below indicate the bulging of the disc.

As is clear, the dural sac gets squashed from the sides by the flaval ligament and the thickening of the facet joints, the compressed retrodural fat pad forces the dural sac anteriorly and the bulging disc posteriorly.

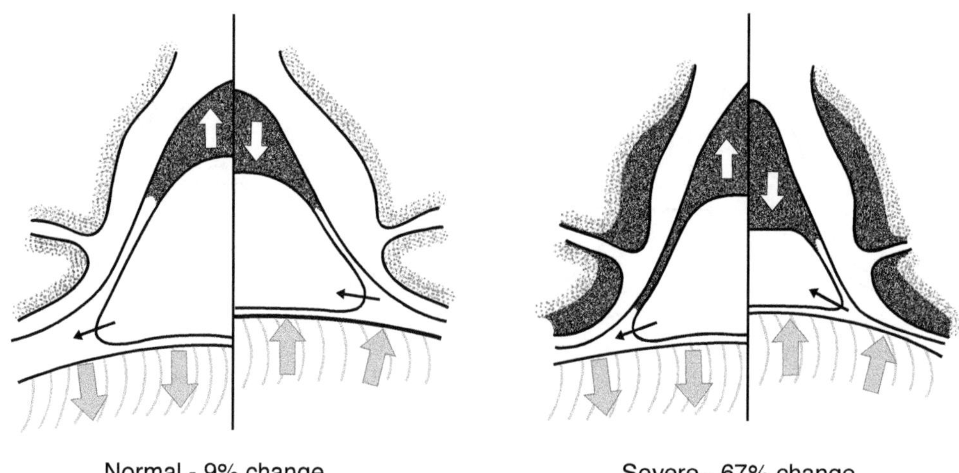

Figure NR 4.8 Summarises the effects of flexion (left half) and extension (right half) on the normal spinal canal (left diagram) and the stenotic canal (right diagram)

Figure NR 4.8 summarises the effects of flexion (left half) and extension (right half) on the normal spinal canal (left diagram) and the stenotic canal (right diagram).

In the normal extension, note the arrows indicating the disc bulging posteriorly and the effects of compression of the fat pad, by the buckling of the flaval ligaments, pushing the sac in an anterior direction. The slight difference in size of the dural sac is indicated. The marked increase in dimensional changes is clearly shown in the right diagram.

The next sequence of figures NR 4.9, 4.10 and 4.11 may help to visualise the effects of flexion/extension on, not only the dural sac, but also the root in the lateral recess – here S1, as it traverses the L5-S1 disc. To appreciate what you are looking at, you have to imagine that you are looking up from below at L5 vertebral arch and pedicles, but that the facets on either side are the superior facets from S1. The facets from L5 have been left out.

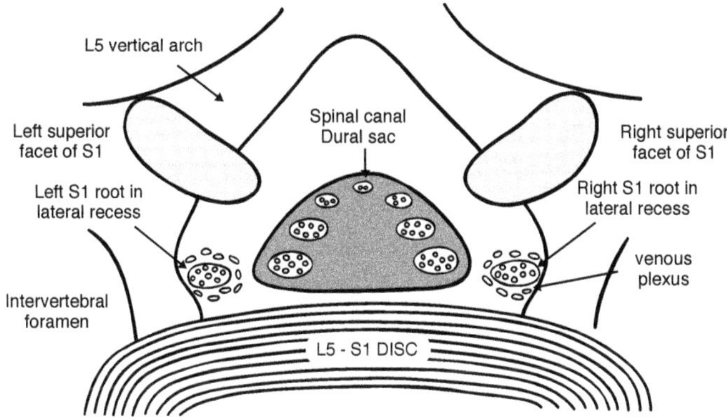

Figure NR 4.9 Shows the normal canal in flexion.

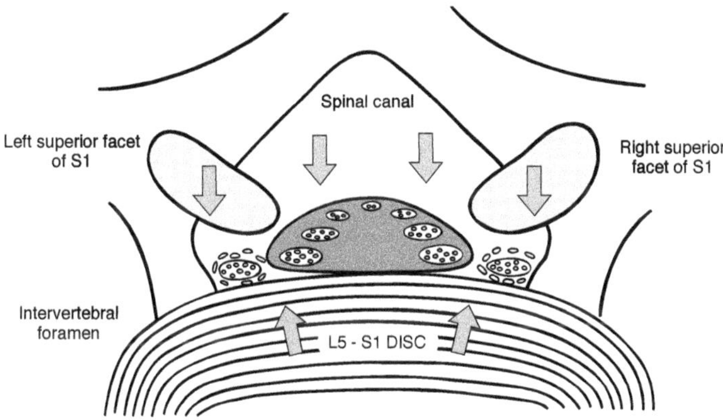

Figure NR 4.10 Shows the normal canal in extension.

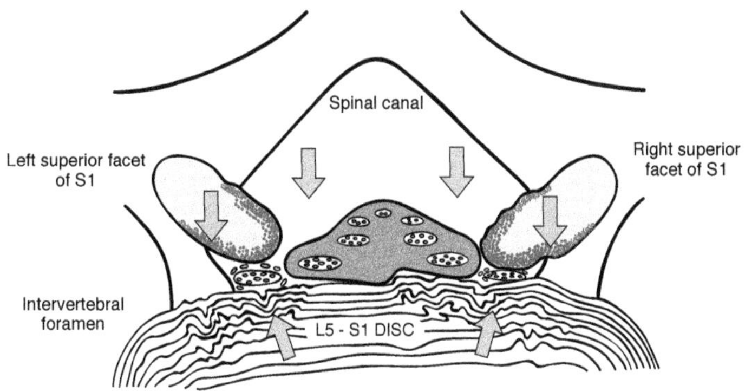

Figure NR 4.11 Shows the degenerative spine in extension.

Figure NR 4.9 shows the normal canal in flexion. As can be seen, there's plenty of room for the dural sac and the S1 roots in the lateral recesses. Figure NR 4.10 shows what happens in extension. The superior facets of S1 go downwards, making the lateral recess smaller; the dural sac moves downwards, due to compression by the folding ligamentum flavum and the compression of the epidural fat pad via the mechanisms already discussed. The L5-S1 also bulges backwards.

Figure NR 4.11 shows what happens in the degenerative spine in extension. As you can see the degenerate and enlarged facets now directly compress the roots in the lateral recess, as does the bulging and degenerate disc. The nerve roots do actually get flattened!

Figure NR 4.12 shows a nerve root ('1') being compressed in extension in two places. Superiorly by the facet ('2') as it moves forwards into the lateral recess and inferiorly, by the bulging disc. Apparently it is not uncommon to find actual 'dents' or impressions in the L5 and S1 nerve roots where this pinching and compression is occurring.

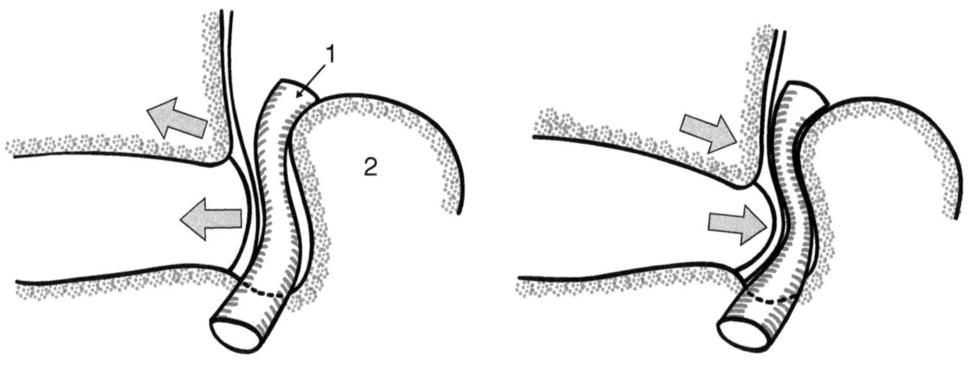

Figure NR 4.12 A nerve root ('1') being compressed in extension in two places.

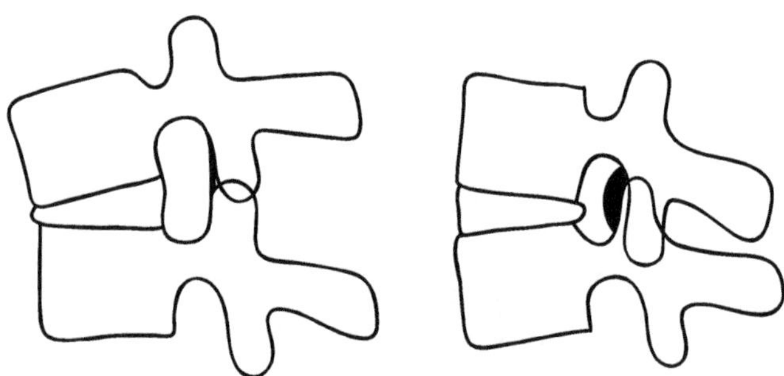

Figure NR 4.13 Shows the forward facet movement and the backward bulging of the disc into the intervertebral foramen and the radicular canal.

The simple side-on diagram in figure NR 4.13 neatly shows the forward facet movement and the backward bulging of the disc into the intervertebral foramen and the radicular canal. Note how much smaller the intervertebral foramen gets in extension.

I hope that it's now clear to the reader that a bulging or extruded disc will amplify, or have the same effect on the neural contents, as space occupying changes caused by much slower to occur degenerative processes. That is the degenerative processes that cause thickening of the facet joints, their ligaments and the adjacent ligamentum flavum, as well as those that lead to degenerative changes in the disc.

To me a disc bulge or extrusion can be viewed as a 'space occupying lesion', with the one good proviso, that any extruded material has the potential to be removed, or at least to be significantly reduced in size. Hence, the neat descriptive label 'transient stenotic effect' which I feel is appropriate.

It is well known that the nervous system is capable of adapting to change, so long as the changes are reasonably slow. I vaguely remember, therefore cannot recall the source, a cadaver study of the low lumbar nerve roots that showed in some individuals; roots with massive dents; some that were 'flattened to ribbons', due to the loss of space in the radicular canal, the spinal canal and the intervertebral foramen. The researchers also found, that in a large number of those with the 'flattened' nerve roots, there was no evidence of any complaint of back pain or sciatica when their medical notes were examined!

I was recently made aware of some research work that had MRI scanned living subjects' lumbar spines in different positions:

Jinkins JR, Dworkin J, 2002 Upright, weight-bearing, dynamic—kinetic MRI of the spine: pMRI/kMRI. In: Kaech DL, Jinkins JR. Spinal Restabilization Procedures: Diagnostic and therapeutic aspects of intervertebral fusion cages, artificial discs and mobile implants. Elsevier, Amsterdam.

These researchers took MRI scans of patients in: the standard recumbent position (rMRI); in upright neutral position (pMRI) and in upright flexion and extension positions – which they called 'dynamic-kinetic acquisitions' (kMRI). Figure NR 4.14 shows one of their typical results, which were also done on cervical spines too. The letters (a)-(d) here correspond to those in the figure.

(a) Is a scan in the recumbent position and therefore non-weight-bearing. In other words, this is the standard MRI position that most of our patients get scanned in. It shows: '... mild generalised spondylosis and minor narrowing of the central spinal canal inferiorly.'

(b) Is with the patient in upright neutral, they're adopting their normal standing posture. It shows, though not that clearly to me, '... mild worsening of the central spinal canal stenosis inferiorly.'

(c) Is with the patient in upright extension and showing a good range of movement l feel. The effect is pretty self-evident: '... severe worsening of the central spinal canal stenosis inferiorly.' You can easily see this. It's at the disc/ facet level of both the L5-S1 and L4-5 discs.

(d) Is with the patient in upright full forward flexion. The contrast to (c) is marked: '...demonstrates complete reduction of the central spinal canal stenosis at every lumbar level.'

I hope I have now made my point: that the neural elements of the spinal column at all levels, are relatively compressed in extension and relieved of that compression when the spine is flexed. Further, that when there is any form of wear and tear/ degenerative change or disc bulging/protrusion/extrusion – this feature is amplified. The patient doesn't have to be 'old' and spondylotic; a young spine with a disc extrusion or protrusion is going to have their spinal canal significantly narrowed by extension.

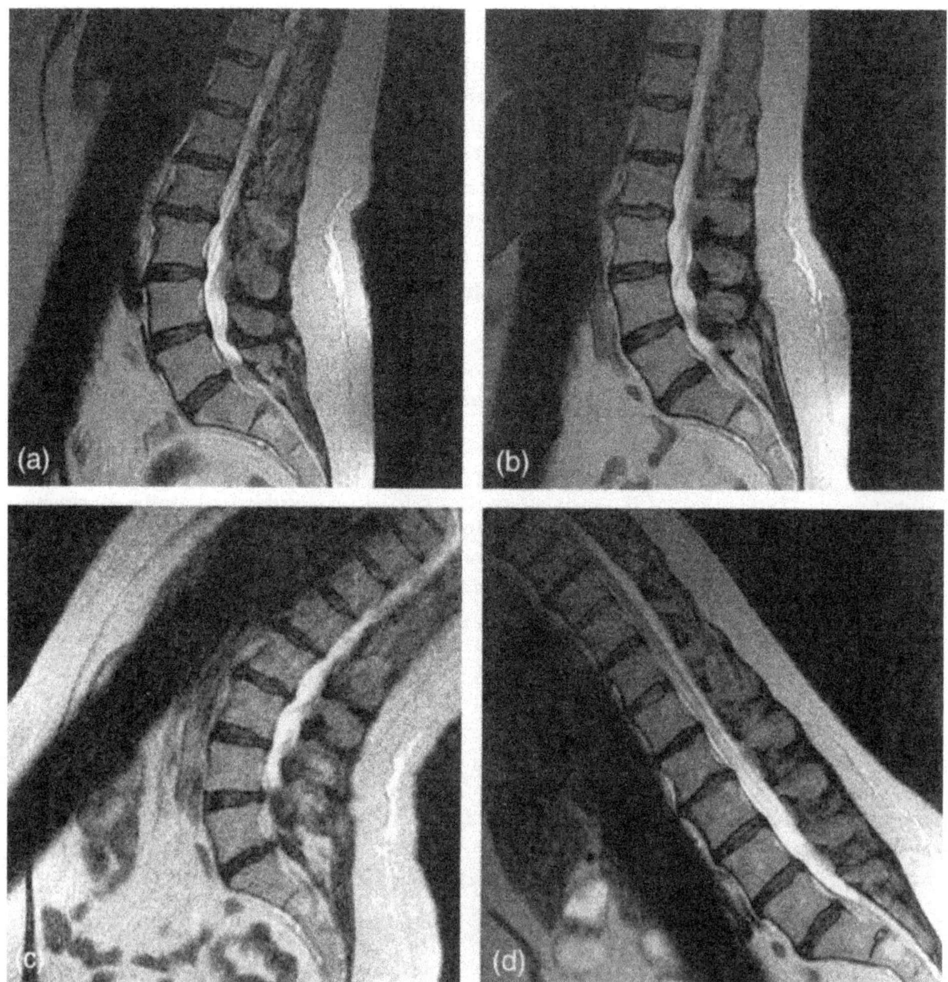

Figure NR 4.14 MRI scan results- see text.

Here are some important clinical points:

1. No wonder a great many spinal pain problems prefer to be flexed, or flexed and deviated away from the painful side.

2. No wonder that as the spine degenerates with age, the spine tends to lose extension range and particularly the lumbar spine, its lordosis.

3. No wonder lying prone often makes acute and sub-acute low back pain worse and often leads to the radiation of pain into the leg. This may be straight away ('mechanosensitivity') or delayed with a gradual increase and spread ('ischaemosenstivity').

4. Some classic acute sciatic and simple back pain problems often find it hard to lie supine with legs out straight; they get instant relief if they flex their legs up into crook lying. If they can lie supine with legs straight, gentle pelvic rocking into extension often makes the pain worse.

5. No wonder flexion, sitting slumped and on all fours curled up or curled up on the side so often eases things up.

6. This may help explain why sciatic pain or referred nerve pain down the leg can frequently (consistently and repeatedly in my experience) be made worse by extension.

7. This may help explain why a great many of the elderly lose their calf reflexes and often have relatively weak calf and other L5/S1 related muscles.

8. Extension is a nerve compression movement; the same applies in the cervical and thoracic regions of the spine. The more degenerate the spine the more compression is likely to be occurring.

9. My observation over the years indicates that forcing extension quickly and rapidly in acute and sub-acute low back pain patients often leads to worsening of the condition, possible sciatica and not that infrequently, neurological deficit. This does not fit at all with McKenzie therapists teaching and experience and needs researching in an unbiased way.

10. My recommendation for best management of acute and sub-acute low back pain, as will be demonstrated in the 'graded exposure' section of the book, is to use what I call a 'the twisted ankle' approach. The key features are 'gradual' and 'all directions' when possible. Using rapid changes in pain to help decide on 'directional preference' is, to me, not wise action. Changes in pain can happen quickly, given the rapidity of gating and inhibitory neural currents. That damage, injury or insult may be occurring while pain lessens is perfectly possible, given our knowledge of the incredible

potency of central sensory modulation. Remember, the rate of response of neurones to physical damage can be hours, often days or even weeks after insult. Just because the pain improved while the patient was with you, doesn't mean their nerves haven't been injured!

11. The same rationale applies to the cervical spine but here there is no radicular canal. I will give further clinical details in chapter NR 5. For now is your observation like mine, that as we all age, the triceps reflex gets harder and harder to get? Just like the ankle jerk mentioned above. This simple observation of S1/C7 reflex loss with age would be very easy to quantify and make a beautiful research project! I've been asking for years but no one's done it yet. Come on!

Chapter 4.2
Anatomy and biomechanics of nerve roots – elongation

As well as compressing nerve roots, spinal and limb movements also stretch and elongate them. This topic has been covered, reported and reviewed at length elsewhere (see 'Read what I've read'). I have already made the point that, although I was very much a part of the 'Adverse Mechanical Tension' (AMT) of the nervous system movement (see Butler and Gifford 1989 1989a)[1] in the late 1980's and early 90's, I was never enamoured by the treatment side of things, more especially, when treatment techniques were developed in the early 1990's that can only be described as bizarre. For example, the so-called 'sliders' and 'tensioners' and stuff like 'In: slump knee extension left... Do: upper limb tension test 2b.

Thankfully, I was never in a position where I had to teach these 'combinations' and the reality was that they made me feel embarrassed and awkward. I didn't really want to have anything to do with them. Those techniques, to me, were akin to doing connective tissue massage (CTM) on a patient with frozen shoulder or arm pain, or even neck pain. CTM is a skin pulling manipulation done in a very specific way – starting over the buttocks and moving up over the torso towards the symptomatic area. The patient is treated in sitting, with their trolleys (trousers!) pulled down to expose half their buttocks and the therapist works from behind them. So, imagine what you say to your patient with a frozen shoulder? 'Sit up here dear, pull your trolleys down and I'm going to start work on your buttock zones, which have to be cleared before I go any further.... What on earth might the patient be thinking? 'Whoa... Did I hear that right...?

An aside: my Mum Jean Gifford, a physiotherapist for many years, treated lots of her patients with CTM. She had become friends with Maria Ebner, the author of 'Connective Tissue Massage Theory and Therapeutic Application' (1975, New York). Maria used to visit Cornwall for her holidays. Mum learnt the techniques and even taught some CTM courses. Her patients accepted the treatment and came back for more! Maybe patients accept pretty much everything that is offered to them therapeutically when they have a problem and are seeking help! I'm thinking all the alternative therapies now, like reflexology or all the '... ologies' out there for example!

I was very unhappy teaching material that I didn't actually feel comfortable with, or do with my patients and thankfully when I stopped teaching the very popular neurodynamic courses, in the late 90's, it was with great relief. However, what I've never abandoned is doing all the useful basic tests really well and from there making the findings make sense in the light of pain science and sensitivity states. That is why I continued to teach them in the context of nerve root problems on my 'Nerve Root' courses and that is the context I will relate to them here.

Even though it was written in 1997, my chapter 'Neurodynamics' in the book 'Rehabilitation of Movement' by Judith Pitt-Brooke is still a great reflection of my perspective on the topic of neurodynamics today. You can download it from the blog[2]. My advice to readers is to learn the techniques really well; the handling –

1 - Butler and Gifford 1989, 1989a papers: http://giffordsachesandpains.files.wordpress.com/2013/07/amt-pt1-and-2-butler-giff.pdf

2 - Gifford LS Neurodynamics chapter in 'Rehabilitation of Movement by Pitt Brooke http://giffordsachesandpains.files.wordpress.com/2013/07/neurodynamics-p-b-2.pdf

practice it like no tomorrow until it becomes second nature. Then really focus on practicing the communication as you do the handling. I say this because when I taught the tests the number of clinicians I observed who were really good at handling the tests and communicating with the subject at the same time was sadly very, very, low. I have to say that if the operator is at all sloppy with the handling and/or the communication – there's a very strong likelihood of getting inappropriate conclusions. On my nerve root courses I used to demonstrate how I would teach the patient to do the tests actively in front of me rather than passively; the trick was good communication and the results, I believe, were far more accurate than passive handling. In fact I would completely reverse the way the tests are currently taught – if I were to teach them today. My neurodynamic courses would all start with doing active tests and perfecting them. Then get the course participants to do the active tests first, in all the patient examinations where they were deemed necessary. The passive tests I would reserve for uncertain conclusions and clarification only. So, for the great majority of patients – no hands-on required. It's much better to do them actively and much more accurate. I will give a couple of illustrations of this later.

Now, some points about nerve tension/elongation!

Nerves are beautifully adapted to move and elongate. In cadaver studies, during SLR, the sciatic nerve in the sciatic notch has been shown to move when the heel is only 5 cms above the horizontal. By thirty-five degrees, nerve roots begin sliding then elongating. Observers of this cadaver work should always be alert to the fact that exposure of the nerve frequently severs the connective tissues, that may naturally tether and restrict the nerve's movement. We may be seeing more movement than there actually is.

Everyone has different movement and elongation capabilities in all collagenous tissues, this includes nerve tissue. For example, I can't bend forward and touch my toes – the classic reason given for this is 'tight hamstrings'. Listen further though, when I keep my legs locked straight and bend forward I reach a point where tightness builds and I get a nasty deep pulling feeling. That feeling is in the back of my thigh, across the back of my knee, down my calf and often into the foot. If I then bend forward, with my knees bent about 20-25 degrees, I can touch the floor – I still get a tightening and pulling feeling, but this time the pulling feeling is pleasant and only and very definitely in my hamstring muscles. There is nothing across my knee and down my calf and the feeling is quite different. The straight leg bend forward is 'nerve'; the bent-knee forward bend tension is 'hamstring'. Note how 'definite' I am! I've done this test on many hundreds of patients and many with sciatica – the response 'That's my nerve pain' versus 'That feels muscle pull in my hamstrings' is very consistent. It is my belief that tight hamstrings protect a tight or short sciatic nerve. Those of you who are good at touching your toes won't understand what I'm on about. Now, if I want to improve my flexibility, I can soon get to touch my toes by repeating forward bending with flexed knees and getting that 'nice' hamstring stretch. Let's say I do 10-15 repetitions and then come back up and re-test toe-touching with straight knees. This time I can go about 30 cms further and just touch my toes with far less 'nasty nerve pulling discomfort.'

Now, the reason I'm relating this is that I believe strong nerve mobilising is a risky thing to do. You may remember 'Trevor's slump' from chapter 2.3? The forces we used were ghastly. Giving someone a neuropathy is bad practice. OK, the system may be very strong but if a clinician gave me a neuropathy I would be very, very, angry – nerve injury can lead to a lifetime of pain and loss of nerve function. I have given three patients neuropathies and they were all caused by strong upper limb tension test end range 'mobilising' techniques. In fact, when we were practicing the test on each other in Adelaide in 1985, one of the students practiced on me and gave me a numb thumb that lasted for three weeks. I have never witnessed any **sciatic** neuropathies caused by strong 'elongation' techniques (slump, SLR); I have witnessed a lot caused by over-zealous lumbar extension – yes, McKenzie related, but also combined movement into extension related too and a great many, following forceful lumbar rotation manipulation.

The cool thing about slump and SLR testing/techniques, is that the lumbar spine is free to flex and this may be a kind of 'safety valve' I believe. You may be puzzling about what I'm on about and getting too! All will be clear shortly...

Try this: lie on your back and do, an active straight leg raise to end of range (this only works if you are 'tight' in SLR, like me) – make sure you keep the knee locked straight and keep the leg up so that you can feel a decent amount of pulling in your leg. Hold that exactly, now, do a pelvic rocking movement into low lumbar extension and note what happens. For most with tight SLR's even the smallest movement into extension can increase the pain dramatically. Pelvic rock into flexion relieves the pulling symptoms dramatically too. There are two parallel aspects of this. First, is that the extension compresses the already tense nerve root. Second, is that the pelvis rotates so as to increase the length of the hamstrings/pull in the leg of the sciatic nerve. Also, if you think about the course of the lumbosacral plexus from the nerve roots into the pelvis, you can see that lumbar extension will tend to have an elongating effect there.

Now, the overall point I'm trying to make is about being safe with neural elongation. In the lumbar spine and with sciatic nerve root related problems, it is common for the SLR to be limited and this can be addressed in the management process. It's a finding of note for 'diagnosis' and also a physical impairment that gets put into the 'impairment' compartment of the 'Shopping Basket' (see chapter GE 4.11 and 4.12).

Having witnessed such massive amounts of force in manual therapy and suffered some awful results if not 'disasters', I now see these approaches as un-biological and unnecessary, even a form of mal-practice. I will now use a typically 'stuck' SLR in a patient, who has had sciatica for about six months, to illustrate how I tackle the problem safely. It has 'graded exposure' approach written all over it.

Don is around about 40, male and has left leg sciatica. There's no calf reflex and the calf and foot evertors are grade 4 power-wise. The SLR is about 40 degrees and the slump is positive at knee extension – 45 degrees, increased by neck flexion. When he bends forward standing the left knee tends to flex and he deviates towards the left. The right SLR is about 70 degrees and produces a little left leg pain. He reaches to about his kneecaps.

Let's use SLR. I bring it up to 40 degrees and the pain goes down the leg. If I slightly adduct the leg the pain markedly increases, abduction it reduces very rapidly. Medial rotation increases lateral decreases. The goal is to see if I can find a way of safely getting the SLR range improved without exacerbating symptoms or putting the nerve in danger of further damage.

The symptoms are clearly mechanically patterned, pain-on with increased range, pain-off very quickly with release. But, like all these sorts of problems, there's an on-going background leg 'toothache' type pain too.

The process here is good old Maitland style, test-do-and re-test, to find the best movement or stretch to do and then turn it into a home exercise. I'm doing it this way because it explains some of the principles more clearly, but in practice I usually get the patient doing it all – no hands on.

So, my first goal with this fellow is to get some kind of stretch going, with the feeling being hamstring and not nerve. I'm going in search of hamstring stretch feeling.

I do the SLR to 40 degrees his pain comes on and I ask him to remember the feeling – exactly, the quality and the location. It's a horrid, nervy, dragging feeling from his mid buttock to his foot.

I then flex his hip to beyond 90 degrees flexion, hold it there and then slowly start extending the knee, I watch the hamstring tension building and he soon goes, 'That's the leg pain coming back.' I ease the knee extension slightly and take the hip into a little abduction and lateral rotation; I repeat the knee extension...

'It's going tight'...

'Where do you feel it?' He points to his hamstrings...

'Is it like the sciatica pain?'

'No... it's pulling my hamstrings.'

'Nasty? Or, can I go a bit more firmly?'

'It's fine, push on if you want...'

So, now I can do knee extension in this position, or I can hold knee extension and flex the hip further; I can adjust hip rotation and ab/adduction all the while searching for a reasonable 'hamstring' stretch. In most sciatica's it's pretty easy to find. Mostly, you end up in a degree of abduction and lateral rotation. The key is to keep the importance of 'nice hamstring stretch' in the mind of the patient. If I've got that, I usually spend about four or five minutes doing some on-off stretching and come right back and re-test the SLR. Then get them up and look at forward bending range. The range can often improve by several inches.

When you've read the Graded Exposure and Case History sections of the book and understood 'make it easy' (see Clara's acute whiplash chapter CH 02 for example) you'll see that that, is what this, is all about. It's simply finding the easiest way of getting the most out of something, in the least painful/painless and safest way possible (it's fire-apart-depart too!). I don't want to spoon feed you too much, but I hope you can see that with the patient in supine with me doing 'In: hip flexion, plus abduction, plus lateral rotation... Do: knee extension... There are a few more options possible, if it's proving hard, to not get the leg nerve symptoms. For example, you can play with side flexion and flexion/extension of the lumbar spine... Simply move the trunk or raise and lower the end of the treatment couch.

The next trick is to find a way for the patient to do this at home and it's usually very easy to achieve the same, 'pull' without the 'nerve' symptoms by doing it all sitting on the edge of a chair.

Don easily finds he can get a good hamstring stretch going with legs wide apart, left leg slightly extended from right angles and then flexing forward towards the floor between the legs. With sitting, what I usually do is start with sitting at the edge of the chair, knees more or less together and getting the patient to simply flex the trunk forward onto the thighs. Don could do this fine. The next steps are to slowly extend the good leg, keeping the heel on the floor and testing, by coming forward with the trunk. Don could do this easily and all he got, as the heel moved further forward, was pulling in the right hamstrings until the leg was fully straight, when he got a behind knee pull – just like I do. With the left leg, he moved the foot forward about six inches and immediately got the sciatica. I then got him to move the left leg into more and more abduction and repeat the forward flexion test. When he got into full abduction he could manage a good hamstring stretch and that's the position he started in. The key rule was to always make sure he felt the hamstring, not the leg pain. Sometimes it is easier to do it on the side of the bed. At this stage Don was unable to do it here.

All it involves is simply sitting parallel to the edge of the bed (use treatment couch) facing either the foot or the head end i.e. one leg on the floor the other up on the bed. The leg on the bed is the painful leg; good leg/foot is on the floor. It's simply, crook leg in long sitting but with only one leg up! The foot on the couch is kept flexed and trunk flexion is explored in different positions of leg extension and abduction. Another way of course, is simply putting the one leg up on another chair, but make sure the knee's flexed! Don't forget, if the starting position is already causing pain you can get the patient to rest back on their hands to extend a bit. If this is the case though, I'd go back to edge of chair sitting.

Right, so the trick from all these starting positions is to be able to progress and I hope you can see how easily that can be done. For example, by extending the leg a little further, by bringing the leg from abduction towards neutral, foot movements can be included etc. Other 'progressions' can include, going further into discomfort, using longer more sustained stretches and even going into the 'nerve' pain – which is essential, if you're reasoning 'desensitise, which you should as things settle and progress. Remember to educate the patient about desensitisation, as well as the unpredictable nature of nerve pain and reactivity. It's common for a patient to be pushing into the nerve pain related 'stretch' and feel really flexible after, but then to find that some hours later the whole thing has flared up. Make sure you 'normalise' this reaction and that if it's too much for the patient you adjust the stretching plan to bring it down. The trouble is, one day it can be great, another it can be awful – NORMALISE!

Last thing that's popped into my head is – I use simple standing and bending forward a lot for this sort of problem, with legs apart, knees bent, legs in lateral rotation... and then progress from there. So, do you bounce or do you sustain your stretches! With me, it's no rule whatsoever. I don't care what the theory says; it's what the patient says they feel best doing. I personally find sustained stretch of anything in the limbs not that nice, but easy bouncing pressure on/off is great. Spinal sustained stretches seem OK. Anyway, think about what you like/dislike. I get my patients to try both and choose whichever one they want. If they're getting somewhere without doing any damage, that's fine by me.

So that brings the next question up! What's 'blocking' the movement in a 'stuck' SLR? For that matter, what 'blocks' the movement in any limited SLR? The term, Adverse Mechanical Tension in the nervous system, made us all think that the answer was a stuck nerve; like one of the nerve roots was stuck and tethered down in the intervertebral foramen somehow. Well fine, but it's hard to imagine the loss of only a small amount of movement there, causing a loss of thirty, forty or more degrees of SLR. The answer is surely more likely to be muscle tightness/tone related to pain and sensitivity. A mechanically sensitised nerve root, which may actually be in danger of further damage from elongation forces, cleverly includes 'elongation' protection mechanisms in its presentation. In early acute sciatica with markedly limited SLR the pain invariably stops further movement and the resistance encountered, if one heartlessly tries to explore further, **is muscle tension**. I am pretty sure Toby Hall, Max Zusman and Bob Elvey showed this back in the late 1990's. Good on them, it makes complete sense that a nerve, vulnerable to damage by elongation, includes increased reflex tonal increases in those muscles that can protect it. That's mainly the hamstrings. You may remember all the 'muscle' 'factoids' back in chapter 13.3. Like, when a muscle is rested in a shortened position, the sarcomeres reduce in number and that, if the muscle isn't used, there's a progressive increase in fibrous tissue – which in turn replaces the dwindling contractile tissue. Length changes can occur very quickly.

It's my opinion that a 'stuck' SLR, as we're describing for 'Don' here is actually the result of a shortened, weakened and fibrotic hamstring muscle. Note, that there are many sciatic presentations with a 5-6 month plus history who do have very limited SLR's, but they're not 'stuck' in that solid 'physical' way like Don's. I hope you clinicians know what I mean? My point is – that if you put one under anaesthetic and did an SLR it would be full but the 'stuck' one would remain limited. Think 'Trevor' too (chapter 2.3). Given this, I hope you can see the logic of maintaining **hamstring** extensibility in all sciaticas with limited SLR's. Stretching, without provoking the nerve, as I've shown can start almost straight away. It's also important to keep the muscle working too – from as early on in management as possible (more on this in chapter NR 5). Encourage walking and moving, use all the muscles... Sod the posture, just move!

Now let's think about 'stuck' upper limb tension tests? I have to say I have never come across one in relation to a nerve root problem. All the significantly positive and limited nerve root related ULTT's I've seen had soft 'end feels'. The pain response and muscle tone increase were the key limiting features. I expect this has been investigated but I haven't reviewed the literature here for a while. I've also never seen a 'stuck' femoral nerve.

So, the truly nerve root related 'stuck' nerve may be a myth; the clinically 'stuck' nerve is most likely due to physically shortened muscle and may only be a feature of the sciatic nerve. That's my opinion. Now, I'm certainly not saying that nerves don't become tethered in the tunnels and canals they run in. I've certainly seen many nasty limb injuries where significant scar tissue must have curtailed normal nerve sliding and elongation movement, I can think of many medial elbow fractures for example. Tethering in the intervertebral foramen and even of the dura inside the spinal canal –one tends to feel is likely to be well compensated for by the length of the peripheral nerve and its natural elasticity. Clinically the most common issue is sensitivity and where movement is affected, mechanosensitivity.

Next, a topic I like: **features not appearing to fit**, particularly areas of pain provocation while performing a neurodynamic test. For example: a patient with radiating pain down the inside of their forearm and paraesthesia in the vague area of the medial hand/hypothenar eminence/medial fingers:

- being made worse by upper limb tension test 1 (ULTT1)
  – which is taught as biasing towards the median nerve...

- being unaffected by upper limb tension test 3 (ULTT3)
  – which is taught as biasing towards the ulnar nerve,
  whose distribution is the medial forearm, where these symptoms are.

Remember, when there's a nerve <u>root</u> problem a test that's biased to the ulnar, median or radial <u>nerve</u> won't bias the forces of these tests to any particular <u>root</u>. Try this: go online to say Wikipedia or open Gray's anatomy and bring up a diagram of the brachial plexus. Now, while looking at the illustration imagine taking any one of the three major arm nerves (which actually start roughly in your axilla) and giving them a pull while observing the brachial plexus; you should be able to envisage the pulling forces being beautifully shared and dissipated across all the various cords, divisions and trunks to a greater or lesser extent. You should also be able to easily see why the tension test bias to a particular ***'peripheral nerve'*** just cannot bias to a particular nerve root and why tugging on the median nerve, via ULTT1, can easily put tension on the lower cervical nerve roots. And hence produce symptoms in the distribution of those roots i.e. the medial forearm into the hand.

A big clinical issue is that nerve root referred symptoms are usually only rarely, very 'roughly' in the so-called 'dermatome' and symptoms are anatomically very vague, compared to frank peripheral nerve injury. If you injure the ulnar nerve and have loss of sensation, that loss is likely to be in a very precise area – the ulnar nerve's cutaneous innervation field (have the Gray's anatomy limb cutaneous innervation field illustration always to hand in the clinic!). Typically, it's the whole of the little finger and only the medial half of the ring finger. It's incredibly precise. Sometimes the nerve pain distribution is too. With nerve root problems you just do not get that sort of precision – especially with pain distribution. With numbness and with paraesthesia, because they are more 'skin' related symptoms, sometimes the symptoms can just about fit the distal dermatome! But they don't often. Tip: if you see a nerve root case history in a journal where the pain symptoms are in a typical dermatome... be sceptical, be very sceptical!

In my clinical practice over the years, dealing with frank '***peripheral nerve injury***' is relatively rare. Damage to an ulnar nerve for example, usually involves severe injury or fracture to the medial elbow, or maybe some kind of traction injury and this is where ULTT3 is very clearly positive. In fact, you hardly need to do the test, as mere elbow flexion or even a bit of forearm pronation is often enough to cause massive cascades of paraesthesia and nerve related pain. Adding scapular depression (actively) just adds to the festive sizzle and the more you do it the worse it all gets.

What I'm really saying is that the high focus on the various 'ulnar,' 'median' and 'radial' nerve 'biased' upper limb tension tests, for analysis of peripheral nerve mechanosensitivity, may be a little out of balance with the actual shop floor levels of utility. The simple 'active' ULTT, which I do with most of my nerve root problems, is all I generally need (see chapter NR 5). I may back that up with doing the standard passive ULTT1 occasionally, but that's it. The other tests, the ULTT2a (median) and b (radial) and 3 (ulnar) – I must have usefully used for analysis probably half a dozen times in the last five to ten years. I hear the screams of dissent. And my answer is that those tests are hugely positive in a great many 'sensitised states', but they are not positive in terms of anything significantly 'wrong' with the nerve under test. Their sensitivity, in the great majority of musculoskeletal pain states, most likely relates to *secondary hyperalgesia* rather than any ***significant*** pathology (primary hyperalgesia). I'm thinking of sub acute, sub chronic and chronic conditions that often have pain and other dysaesthesias[1] in the upper limb – typically post whiplash and any overuse syndrome like RSI. Differentiating shoulder related referral from ULTT related mechanosensitivity can be prone to massive errors in my experience.

If the reader has the time and inclination it is well worth getting illustrations of the lumbo-sacral plexus and doing the same sort of 'imaginary' exercise. The main thing to note is that the sciatic nerve pulling from below is likely to cause a massive dispersion of forces to a great many nerve roots! Does that explain the many male patients with sciatica who get pain in the genitals when I do an SLR to them! It's certainly one 'biomechanical' and peripheral tissue way of reasoning the reproduction of symptoms on the front of the leg and other 'atypical' areas when doing the SLR.

Last thing on nerve elongation thoughts is on one of my favourite topics – ischaemia. Nerves love blood and the most highly metabolic are usually the first to suffer, that's the big sensory fibres – the Aβ's and the big motor fibres the Aα's. No wonder when you fall asleep with your arms overhead you lose sensation and muscle power! Next time it happens to you, test to see if your Aδ and C fibres are working by sticking a pin in your arm! The big deal clinically is that subtle weakness can be picked up by doing more than just the standard static resisted tests for the regular myotomes – you need to actually test the endurance 'to tiredness' threshold I think.

1 - Dysaesthesia means 'not normal' (dys) 'sensation' (aesthesia) and are usually described as unpleasant. Examples can be feelings of heat or burning, feelings of trickling or water, pins and needles, itching, electric shock like symptoms and so forth.

Here's an example of what I do for the calf muscle. Say the patient has sciatica affecting the left leg. I get the patient to listen to my instructions and watch my demonstration before they start:

'I want you to go up and down on tip toe, keeping your knee locked straight at all times and count every repetition you do. When you first start feeling fatigue in the muscle you can stop. I want you to remember two things, the first, is to focus on and remember the exact feeling in the muscle you had when you stopped and by that I mean in particular the intensity of the tired feeling. The second thing is remember the number of reps you did... but I'll be counting too! When you've done the good leg we'll then repeat on the painful leg and I want you to go to the exact same tiredness feeling and stop.'

Now the usual way to do calf testing is a quick test of tip-toeing – which if they can't do shows marked weakness, that's fine. If that's OK, we then get the patient to go up and down on each tip- toe five or six times and if it's pretty much the same we're happy and we leave it at that. What I do is add this extra endurance test, or to 'fatigue' test in – especially when I feel I really want to check for even the most subtle neuropathy. When this fatigue test is positive there's often a massive discrepancy between good and painful sides. For example, 20-25 reps on the good side but only 8-10 on the bad.

This test obviously isn't infallible and pain can often be inhibitory. However, it is my belief that so long as the patient understands you're interested in the pure endurance strength of the muscle, its interpretation can be reasonably valid (good research project?). If a patient stops and says, that's it, I can't do anymore, I go: 'Is that because the muscle won't let you, or is it the pain that's stopping you?'

For upper limbs I use 'elastics' to test and I arrange it so it's either general –just pull the elastic at waist height, or as localised as possible to a particular muscle group. For example, elastic under foot, do curls for biceps. For foot dorsiflexors, simply do dorsiflexion of the foot over and over again and the same for toe extension – there's no need for elaborate resistance to work those muscles to fatigue! I often do easy dips on one leg for quads, one leg bridging for hamstrings/buttocks and side lying for hip abductors. I think those L5-S1 muscles – hams and glutei are often neglected, are often weak and need assessing and addressing.

The next thing with ischaemia is to test vibration sense – a fine sensory test with a bias to Aβ fibres.

Right, I've deviated slightly from elongation tests so I'm going to finish off with the carpal tunnel as a great way to think about ischaemic testing for nerve roots and there's a bit about elongation too!

Normal hydrostatic pressure in the carpal tunnel in a neutral position is around 2.5mm Hg – (which sounds pretty low when you consider normal blood pressure to be 120/80 mm Hg). If the wrist is then flexed we know that the carpal tunnel reduces in size by 16% and the pressure increases to 30mm Hg. Apparently, it doesn't take much to stop blood flow – in the lumbar spine of a pig a pressure of 5-10mm Hg is enough to stop venous flow for example! Now, when a nerve is elongated or stretched it is known that by 8% elongation venous return starts to decline and by

15% the venous, capillary and arterial flow is completely occluded. So, what do all those figures mean to real life? Apparently, if you measure the length of the median nerve 'bed' – when the nerve is in a shortened position (think of what you do with your arm when you lie on your side in bed, it's typically flexed in the arm with a bit of scapular elevation) and then measure it again when you're arms are fully outstretched (as in 'I caught a fish this big') – there's an increase in length of around 20%. So, there's plenty of potential to stop circulation in a nerve via elongation – so do your thing with that neural mobilisation and the longer you sustain that stretch, the more ischaemic that nerve becomes! Remember, Aβ fibres in the normal can only complain by producing paraesthesia – it's OK, but it's like they're in the first few throes of slow suffocation. No wonder we all ended up with numb thumbs and fingers and prolonged paraesthesia when practicing those ULTT tests!

'How did you get on at work today love?'

'Great, I must have killed a few thousand Aβ fibres without anyone noticing, amazing what you can get away with... I'm starting to enjoy it...'

Now because AMT, ANT, neurodynamics or whatever you might want to call it, swept the world in the 1990's and beyond it left a little gap which I've been popping my head up about ever since. And that was the topic raised in the last chapter – nerve compression! I guess my failure to be heard was because it wasn't accompanied by a 'neural compression' treatment approach. Well, for the spine I guess the McKenzie extension principle got in there first! A bit like the Williams flexion exercises for back pain got in there first for neural elongation perhaps?' There's nothing new under the sun.

Let's revisit the carpal tunnel for a moment and plead for a model of reasoning that always visits the notion of neural compression alongside neural elongation, in every single movement anywhere in the body. Start with wrist flexion, as we did just now and think compression – that's compression of the median nerve in the carpal tunnel. If you sustain it, it's called 'Phalen's test' and is a test for 'carpal tunnel syndrome', which actually has dubious sensitivity[1]and specificity.[2] When it's positive, it reproduces the symptoms of carpal tunnel syndrome and usually the symptoms take quite a few seconds to come on. Now, as I said earlier, when a limb nerve is injured enough to cause a neuropathy, there's pins and needles and even numbness and it's demarcated precisely into the cutaneous innervation field of that nerve. For the median nerve, the cutaneous innervation field is precisely the lateral palm, the palmer surfaces of the thumb, the first and second fingers and half of the ring finger it only runs round onto the dorsal surface at the tips of the thumb and first two fingers.

Over the years I've seen a great many so called carpal tunnel syndromes. I can only remember a very few with this distribution, most had vague pain in the hand and vague pins and needles more akin to nerve root vagueness. Phalen's test was

1 - Sensitivity is the ability to identify true positives – that when it's positive the individual really does have the problem it's testing for.

2 - Specificity is the ability to identify true negatives – that when it's negative the individual really doesn't have the problem under test.

often asymptomatic, even after a prolonged spell of sustained flexion. Even so most patients responded well to the simple 'carpal tunnel release' surgery. (Now, here's a condition that would be so easy to do placebo surgery on, like the Mosley and O'Malley study! See chapter 7.2). However, on the Nerve Root courses[1] I taught, I often got the participants to do sustained wrist flexion (hard) for up to a minute and most times one or two would find it positive – pins and needles coming into the lateral and palmar surface of the hand. Try it!

Now, thinking nerve elongation during wrist flexion; the nerves that go over the back of the wrist will be stretched – they are the cutaneous branches of the radial nerve on the lateral dorsal side of the hand and the dorsal cutaneous branches of the ulnar nerve on the medial side. Good.

Let's now consider wrist extension and think: compression of median nerve in the carpal tunnel because the tunnel also gets smaller in extension, but also, elongation of the median nerve because the axis of flexion-extension is posterior to the course of the nerve. That's why the ULTT1 and 2a use wrist extension. The median nerve gets a double whammy in extension and because of this, should be a more sensitive test – especially if you make sure you extend the fingers to get a good elongation of the nerve. I don't know of any studies that support this. One problem I see is the real difficulty in confidently diagnosing carpal tunnel syndrome in the first place. I wouldn't mind betting that a great many median nerves, when exposed in surgery look perfectly normal, but I doubt if there's going to be a whistleblower surgeon anytime soon. Nerve conduction studies may be helpful but I believe are notoriously inaccurate, especially when the degree of neuropathy is small.

The nerves on the dorsal surface of the wrist are unlikely to be compressed by wrist extension, simply because of the limited amount of range there – just look at the slack folds of skin!

OK. Two ways of putting your arms to sleep that you might like to try...

1. Get drunk, go to bed and fold you arms up under you, including your wrists... and go prone and lie on them. The main thing is elbow flexion (compresses median and radial, elongates ulnar nerves) and wrist flexion – as discussed. Getting drunk makes sure you stay in that position for longer than you otherwise would!
2. Get drunk again for the same reason as in 1. Go to sleep lying on your back with both arms above your head – straight or bent. Think neural elongation, neural compression and the same for the main blood vessels to and from the arm too.

Write up your results and look for a publisher. Don't forget to test your C and Aδ fibres with a sharp pin!

The big thing with ischaemia is increased pressure via elongation or compression and TIME. For nerve root testing, think gently hold neural tension tests for up to a minute and gently hold neural compression tests again, for up to a minute. It's just like the carpal tunnel testing. If 'ischaemo-sensitivity' is present – the symptoms

1 - Usually thirty participants on the course.

take a little while to come on. This seems to me to be far more common with cervical nerve roots than lumbar.

What's the answer to the problem? Well, carpal tunnel syndrome sufferers tend to wake in the night with their pain and dysaesthesias and shake their hands, fiddle with them and manipulate them (remember autotomy?). What they are doing is improving the circulation and increasing the blood pressure – because they're awake and a bit fed up (adrenaline?). Remember, blood pressure drops at night and if you're not moving, that means constant pressure increase in the nerve tissue... all of which make it harder for circulation to be adequate. For nerve roots, any encroachment in the intervertebral foramen (or radicular canal if lumbar) is one thing; posture is another, neck rotated or extended for example, plus the lowered blood pressure.

The solution – at its most effective and simplest:

- get the cardiovascular system working harder – get fit
- stop smoking and all the other daft things that clog up blood supply
- actively move the areas affected by the problem and where it's coming from, far more, nicely and regularly. Do it to that 'done something feeling' that you get with exercise and do it often...
- nothing fancy needed, except for belief, understanding and a bit of patience
- if the encroachment is really significant, surgery is an option,
but it needn't be at all

  (I've never seen an ischaemosensitive nerve root in the neck not recover given time).

My spin on nerve root presentations next. Brace yourself!

Section NR 4
Read what I've read

Butler D.S. (1991) Mobilisation of the nervous system. Churchill Livingstone. Edinburgh.

Ehni B. Ehni G. Patterson R.H. (1990) Extradural spinal cord and nerve root compression from benign lesions of the cervical area. In: Youmans J.R.(ed) Nerological Surgery, Saunders, Philadelphia 2878-2916

Farmer J.C. Wisneski R. J. (1994) Cervical Spine nerve root compression. An analysis of neuroforaminal pressures with varying head and arm positions. Spine 19(16): 1850-1855.

Gifford L.S. (1997) Neurodynamics. In Pitt Brooke J. (Ed) Rehabilitation of Movement. Bailliere Tindall

Hall T. Zusman M. Elvey R. (1998) Adverse Mechanical Tension in the Nervous System? Analysis of SLR. Manual Therapy 4(2)140-146.

Hall T. and Elvey R. (1999) Nerve trunk pain: physiological diagnosis and treatment. Manual Therapy 4(2)63-73.

Maher C. (ed) (1998) Adverse Neural Tension reconsiderd. Australian Journal Of Physiotherapy Monograph No. 3. Australian Journal of Physiotherapy, Melbourne.

Sato K. and Kikuchi S. (1993) An anatomic study of foraminal nerve root lesions in the lumbar spine. Spine 18(15): 2246-2251.

Yoo J.U. Zou D. Edwards T. et al., (1992) Effect of cervical spine motion on the neuroforaminal dimensions of human cervical spine. Spine 17(10): 1131.

Section NR 5

PRACTICAL ISSUES 1: NERVE AND NERVE ROOT PAIN

Chapter NR 5.1
Practical issues 1: Nerve and nerve root pain

I've been fascinated by 'nerve pain' throughout my career. I've also been hugely frustrated by it because it can be ghastly and pretty unresponsive to treatment. I think I mentioned this when I discussed the story behind the 'Toblerone' recovery graph (chapter 13.1).

What I have come to realise is that nerve root problems are generally quite easy to indentify. There is a big 'but' however because as with most things there's a 'spectrum' that runs from 'It's so obvious you can't miss it' at one end, 'Pretty straight forward' in the middle, to the 'Really awkward and difficult, just a sniff of it' at the other end. Having said that, throughout my career I've had patients who've been to other practitioners and even Dr's and consultants and the diagnosis has been miles out, even with the 'It's so obvious you can't miss it' ones.

The main culprits are usually the practitioners who are looking to fit the patient's problem into their particular model of diagnosis and treatment. For example, I can think of a recent patient who presented with; loss of sensation in their little toe and under the foot; loss of power in their calf, their evertors and hamstrings; a very poor calf reflex and pain in the buttock and back running lightly into the calf. They were told they had a piriformis syndrome, that their sacroiliac joint was 'out' and that one leg was longer than the other. Along the way I've had similar scenarios and the patient has been told they've a lumbar disc derangement problem, a lumbar muscle imbalance problem... and so forth.

When patients come to see me and tell me they've been given these sorts of diagnoses I often ask them, while I'm doing their neurological examination, whether the practitioner who saw them did the tests that I was doing. Sadly, it is very rare for patient says yes they have... 'No one's tested your reflexes like I'm doing now?'... 'No, never... ' 'Ah, OK... '

Why do I put so much emphasis on this 'nerve root' diagnosis? Here we are:

1. It's biomedically important – losing nerve function isn't funny; a nerve root problem with neuropathy can lead to loss of sensation and muscle strength – a situation that can usefully be termed a 'minor paralysis' with variable functional consequences.

2. It's biomedically important – because a nerve root problem with a minor conduction deficit or no obvious deficit has the potential to worsen. And, we know enough about the movements and postures that physically threaten nerve roots to give appropriate advice about them. That is, movements that compress the nerve roots (extension and combinations of extension with rotation and side flexion) and movements that elongate them (flexion with straight legs, SLR etc)

3. The common low lumbar and low cervical nerve root presentations have a lengthy natural history that is important for both the clinician and the patient to understand. Believing there is a quick and instant cure is verging on 'myth' and misleading to patients, who are often very anxious. Throughout my clinical career I've heard about patients with apparent nerve root pain who've been cured in one or two treatments, but I have never witnessed

it. There's a great research project in this (following the natural history of recovery of acute nerve roots – that have been diagnosed accurately to start with!).

4. It shifts the emphasis of treatment from 'fix', to 'help resolve quicker' or 'speed recovery' and, 'prevent a long term problem from occurring'.

5. It helps the practitioner craft a balanced approach to 'advice giving'.

6. It directs you to the main 'needs' of treatment and management.

7. It engenders the need for patience and time – both from the clinician and the patient.

What follows is a clinicians' analysis of nerve root presentations. Here I am thinking of presentations whose histories are generally days, weeks or a few months and may be up to one year. Why not longer? Because, the vast majority of nerve root problems resolve reasonably well within the first eight to twelve weeks, but can carry on for up to a year. Even after that residual pains coming and going aren't uncommon. The key thing is not to confuse nerve root problems with 'chronic' maladaptive type pains that clinicians often confuse with nerve roots and here I'm thinking of whiplash and RSI in particular. I have never seen either of these conditions present with a typical nerve root problem. I would have to rack my brains to think of any that have had significant neurological deficit, as in loss of reflexes or clear-cut loss of sensation[1]. The testing of muscle power in these conditions, often suffers from difficulties of interpretation due to the common 'cog-wheel' presentation, that jerky on-off response to static testing. However, testing vibration sensitivity does reveal deficits quite commonly in these conditions, suggesting minor peripheral neuropathy is likely to be present. My point is, that while both nerve root and RSI/whiplash presentations may have 'peripheral nerve' and 'peripheral neurogenic' pain mechanisms in common the two are, for the most part, distinctly different I believe.

Recommended reading

Gifford L S (1998) Acute low cervical nerve root conditions: Symptoms, symptom behaviour and physical screening. In Touch The Journal of the Organisation of Chartered Physiotherapists in Private Practice Winter issue No. 85: 4-19

Gifford L S (2001) Acute low cervical nerve root conditions - symptom presentations and pathobiological reasoning. Manual Therapy 6 (2) 106-115

(Download both articles from: http://giffordsachesandpains.com/download-material/neurodynamics-nerve-root-and-nerve-pinch/)

I am now going to overview some important clinical aspects of low cervical (C6-C8) and low lumbar L4/5-S1) nerve root presentations.

1 - Nice research project!

Symptom distribution

Take a few moments to review the two body charts, which I would consider to be quite common symptom distribution patterns for low lumbar and low cervical nerve root presentations (figures NR 5.1 and NR 5.2)

Some points:

1. It would be very easy to say dump dermatomes, because they're so detached from clinical reality, but my recommendation is for the clinician to see them as useful guides but detached from reality. Dermatomes when first described were all about hypoalgesia the loss of sensation and not about pain distribution. So, dermatomal distribution works a little bit when considering symptoms that effect skin – meaning numbness and paraesthesia. The classic numb little toe and lateral border of the foot for S1 dermatome and S1 nerve root, is quite helpful in identifying the likely root at fault. Likewise a numb

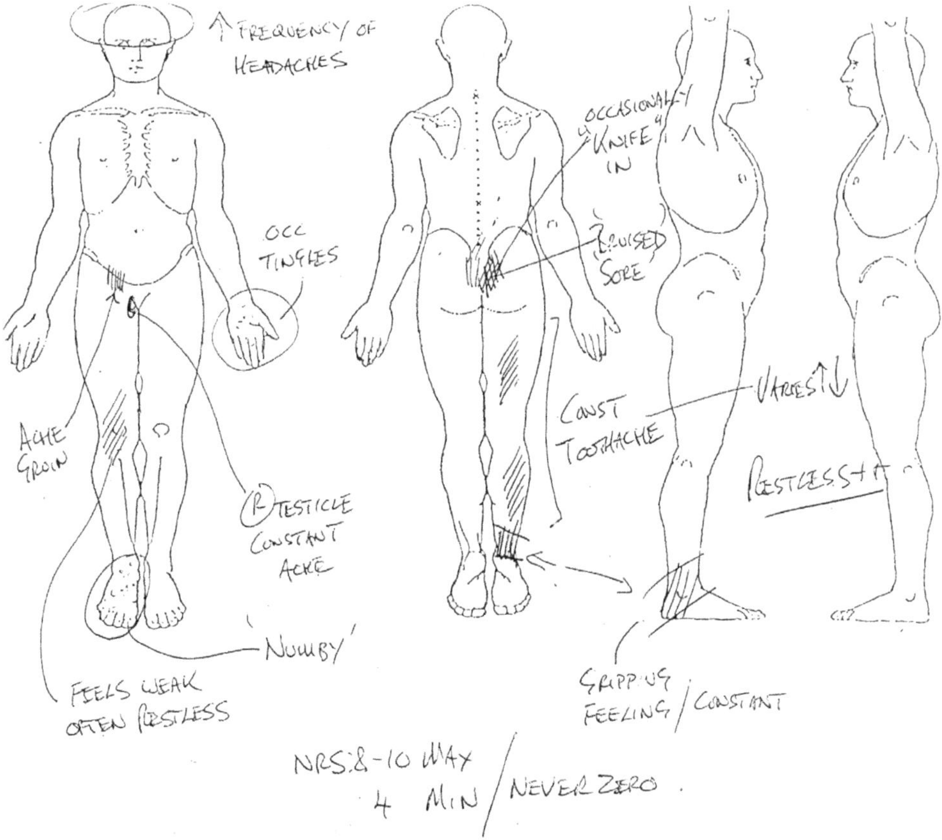

Figure NR 5.1 Common symptom distribution pattern for low lumbar nerve root presentations

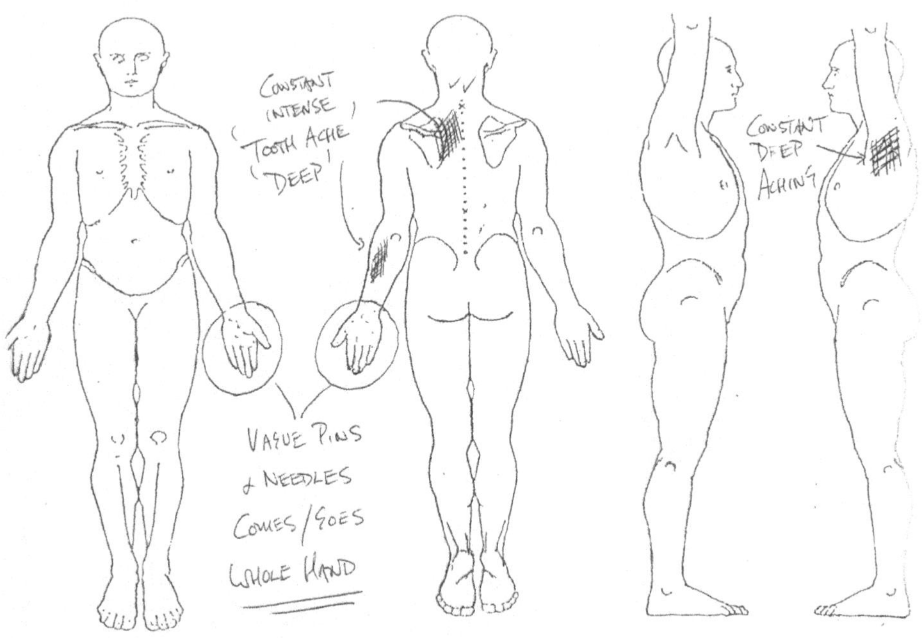

Figure NR 5.2 Common symptom distribution pattern for low cervical nerve root presentations

top of the foot for L5; a numb thumb for C6; middle fingers for C7 and little finger for C8. What they all have in common is that they occupy the most 'distal' zone of the dermatome. They're still usually very vague, so if you get very precise areas of numbness – it's best to start thinking in terms of cutaneous nerve injury. For example, a patient with a clearly defined numb area between the big and second toes on the dorsum of the foot ... Quiz question... What cutaneous nerve is that[1]?

2. As I've said, the distribution of paraesthesia sometimes fits into the rough distal dermatome and this can give useful hints in terms of identifying the level of root with the problem. However, it is not uncommon for a patient with nasty acute sciatica or low cervical 'brachialgia' to report pins and needles in the whole arm or leg or the whole hand or foot and many variations in between! Therapists must always be on the look-out for symptoms and indicators of central nervous system pathology.

3. Pain and dermatomal distribution are more of a joke and shouldn't be considered except in a very gross and vague sense. For example, figure NR 5.1 illustrates the pain distribution of a patient who'd lost calf and hamstring muscle power and whose calf reflex was zero. While there's a 'sniff' of S1 dermatome here – there's pain down the back of the leg, a great many

1 - Medial terminal branch of the deep peroneal nerve!

symptoms are way out of the S1 dermatome. Note the weird groin ache, the constant gripping round the ankle, the constant pain in the testicle and the odd knee symptoms.

4. Many years ago I came across a clever and very reaffirming bit of clinical research done by Curtis Slipman and colleagues, who introduced the notion of 'dynatomal' or pain referral maps relating to cervical nerve roots. They ended up criticising the wide reliance of clinicians on dermatomes for diagnosis of nerve root pain. Cool!

Their research protocol was very simple. While performing nerve root blocks on patients with referred or 'radicular' symptoms, Curtis and colleagues simply physically manipulated (they poked!) the nerve root they were about to block, with a 22 gauge 3 cm needle. At the same time, they asked the patient to remember the symptoms (pain and paraesthesia) produced and exactly where they were. After the block was done an 'independent observer' interviewed each patient and recorded the location of the provoked symptoms on a pain chart. They did a total of 134 nerve root stimulations on 87 subjects.

Four of the dynatome maps they made are reproduced in figure NR 5.3. 'A' in the top left relates to C4 root, 'B' to C5, 'C' to C6 and D to C7 nerve root. As you can see each body chart is divided vertically into the front of the body on the left and the back on the right. The darker the region the more commonly the pain was felt there. Let's take a closer look at 'D', which from my clinical experience is the commonest root to be affected and then C6. What I want to highlight is the extent of the symptoms on the body. Anteriorly, the left side of map 'D' shows that C7 root is capable of referring pain over the whole of the anterior aspect of the arm, the shoulder, the pectoral region, the anterior clavicular region, even the anterior neck. Posteriorly, the right half of the map shows the spread of symptoms over the whole of the scapular and on down as far as the mid to lower lateral rib area and again, the whole arm and hand. Now overlay the C7 dermatome on that map and have a laugh!

What was brilliant, when I first saw this article and the maps was that it made me feel much happier with my clinical observations – that they weren't some figment of my imagination or the patients! So often low cervical nerve root problems were coming in reporting pain, not only vaguely down their arm, but also all over their back, in the armpit (see figure NR 5.2), down the medial border of their scapula, all over their scapular, not uncommonly in the anterior pectoral area and so on. Thanks to the 'dynatome' my distress and confusion over what I was seeing was greatly helped; but it was also helped by knowing of the potential of central nervous system neurons to change and expand their receptive fields, as I have already discussed. These patients of mine weren't mad; it was just that their pain distribution seemed to be mad relative to those of the dermatomes I'd been taught. As far as I was concerned, this was yet another nail in the coffin for a great many of those who write about clinical pain. Yes, they bullshit and the clinicians who naively read their books and articles need to know this. It's also noteworthy that it may be those who write about referred pain and nerve root pain don't actually listen to the patient, or even bother with finding out about the pain distribution.

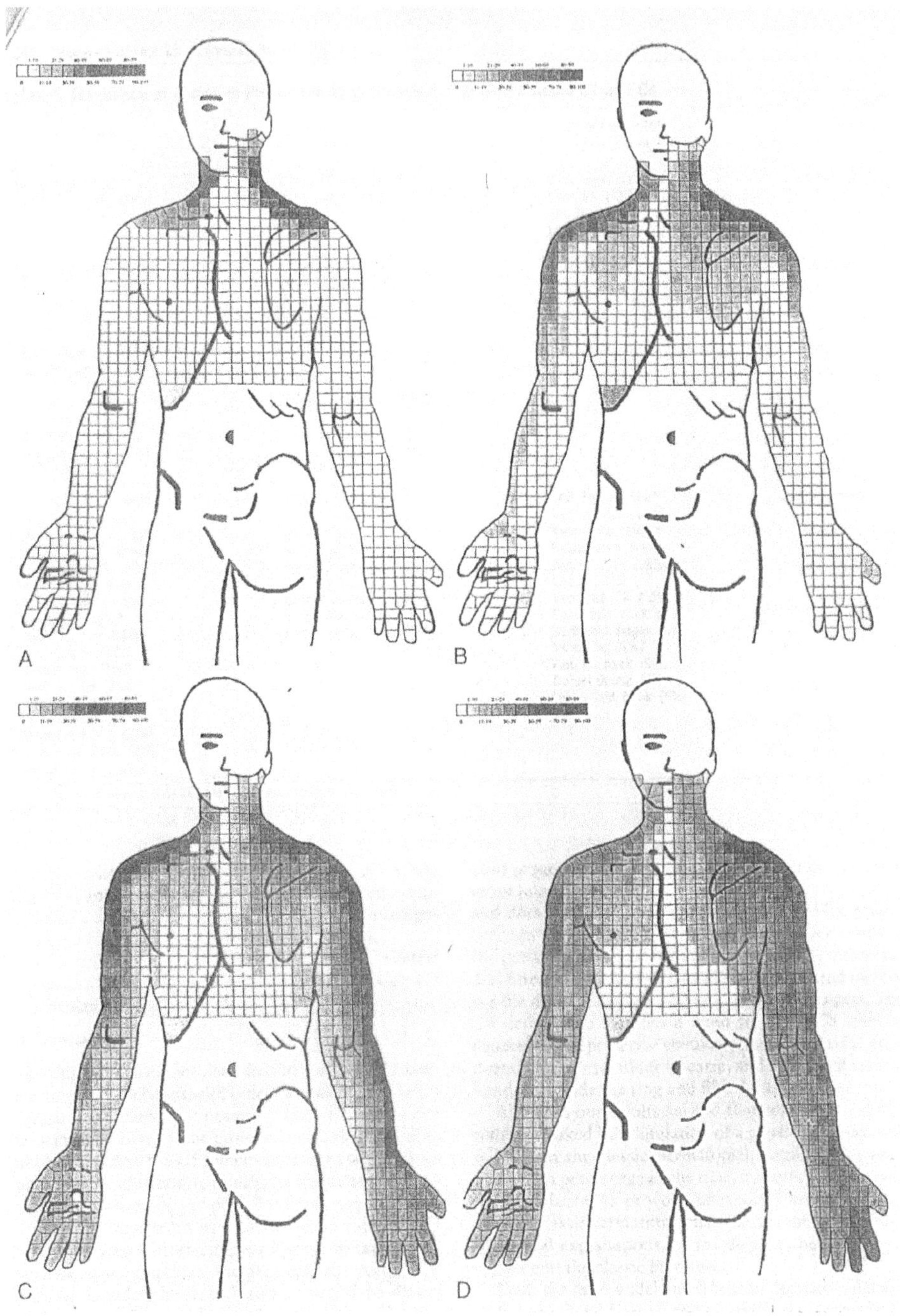

Figure NR 5.3 Dynatome maps: 'A' in the top left relates to C4 root, 'B' to C5, 'C' to C6 and D to C7 nerve root

You may recall my patient 'Karen' in chapter 1 of these books. Although her pain wasn't cervical, the apparent 'madness' of her pain distribution is given a great deal of credibility thanks to this sort of research. Lumbar and sacral 'dynatomes' are bound to be similarly 'miles out of the dermatome'. I would bet my life on it!

It would be very interesting if this research could be repeated on subjects without pain and see what the pain distribution there was in the 'normal' state!

Back to the patient and a few more points about symptom distribution:

5. Nerve root pain can be patchy (see body charts!).

6. The pain often moves from one area to another.

7. Some pains are intermittent and may or may not relate to posture and movement.

8. Sometimes nerve root pain can be quite localised, even precise. For example, just the shoulder; just the elbow to the forearm; just the buttocks or hamstrings; just the back of the knee or back of calf... and so on. The danger here is in assuming the problem stems from the joint or tissues where the pain is.

9. Symptoms are very often imprecise, the patient finds it difficult to accurately localise and can get frustrated or even embarrassed in trying to give details of the pain and its location. 'Vague' is a great term. I don't know if you had the same experiences as me when you were doing your manual therapy/clinical training, but one of the main things the tutors used to insist on was getting the exact location of all the various pains. I can remember so many occasions of almost forcing the patient to give me the exact limits of their very vague pain and getting very frustrated when they couldn't! However, the more patients I heard it from the more sceptical I became of the approach and the physiotherapists teaching me.

Symptom quality and behaviour...

This is another area where I don't think the writers about neuralgic and nerve root pain listen to the patient. In the textbooks I read about sciatica, the pain was always described as one, or all of these: shooting, stabbing, like lightening, sharp and burning. Burning and shooting are the most common.

However, in my non-textbook, 'reality' experience, which has been acquired by listening to patients for many years – sciatica is most commonly described as a DEEP ACHING, or a HORRID TOOTHACHE- LIKE pain. But, as can be seen on the figures of the body charts, many other descriptors are used too and these include those commonly found in the textbooks. Notice on the charts things like 'constant gripping feeling', 'knife', 'bruised and sore'. The key thing about nerve pain is that it's often weird and unfamiliar, when compared to ordinary aches and pains most of us get. As far as I am concerned weird pain and weird pain behaviour and distribution is very important in diagnosis of a nerve related pain problem.

Let me make a list of a few more pain qualities: deep grinding; prickling; cramping; feels like hot water; a deep compressing feeling; gripping; a cutting sensation; pulling; itchy on the skin; running water down the limb feeling... The list could go on and on but the description of the symptoms must be reasoned in parallel with their behaviour.

Let's take a brief look at symptom behaviour. Symptoms can be any one or a combination of the following...

1. Constant unrelenting, often deep in the limb or trunk.

2. Fleeting, coming and going for no apparent reason.

3. Coming for a period, often very nasty at first and staying until gradually subsiding.

4. Pain gets so intense when it comes that the patient becomes extremely restless, moving about almost writhing in agony – with no benefit whatsoever. Sometimes some patients force themselves to stay still and relax and the pain can gradually go. The patient then remains still and fearful of moving in case the pain returns.

5. Patients can report the whole limb 'cramping' for long periods, here efforts to stretch and rub the muscles and tendons make little difference. Again the patient can become very restless.

6. Some patients find that they are unable to sit at all; some cannot lie and end up sleeping in the chair. I remember one fellow whose only relief was his car seat and he spent over a month sleeping nightly in his car!

7. Some nerve roots find that resting and not moving are far better... others, that being on the move and being active are much better. Thus some stay at work, their only problem being sitting. I have helped many patients adapt their computers, so that they can operate them standing.

8. Many 'movers' dread the night and I spend a great deal of time finding a comfortable sleeping position for them. There are absolutely no rules here – especially rules like those that insist on maintaining a lordosis at all times. That's crap. The great majority of my restless lumbar patients have found the most comfortable sleeping position in flexion. For example, mattress on the floor next to a lounge chair, patient lies with feet up on the lounge chair on their back. Their backs are then supported by a very large cushion-pillow that flexes their back, so their head is in an almost upright position – think of the fetal position but on the back! For necks, neck flexion with up to three sometimes four pillows, lying on the back with pillows under the knees can be most helpful. Good old-fashioned collars – though frowned upon, can be very helpful for sleeping. The key is lots of support for the neck to keep it in the nerve roots happiest position!

Finally in this section it's worth noting '24 hour' behaviour of nerve root symptoms.

1. A great many like 'Taffy's' (see chapter NR1.1) are constant and unrelenting day and night. Ghastly!

2. Some can be terrible at night and relatively good during the day. This behaviour of pain is important to note, as it is commonly stated that 'night pain' is a significant 'red flag' for serious pathology. All I can say is that the clinician needs to weigh-up the full clinical details of any given presentation in making a diagnosis. The fact is though, that many nerve root problems with really nasty night pain are often screened with scans and x-rays for more serious pathology by anxious Drs. It is a good thing, but I always get a bit frustrated that they miss some obvious indicators that the problem in front of them is a straight forward nerve root. For example, clear impairment of conduction and if it's upper limb pain – the arm symptoms being easily reproduced by neck movements, if examined carefully. Note that night symptoms with nerve related problems is fairly common, think carpal tunnel syndrome for example. Sufferers often wake in the night shaking their arms to try and get relief.

3. Other patterns over 24 hours are: terrible on rising, then gradually better through the day; good early and worse at the end of the day; and finally – all over the place! Tobleroning as I've already noted many times! Some nerve roots have periods of total freedom followed by hours of ghastly unremitting pain.

The following points, in italics, are taken directly from Louis' Nerve Root course workbook. I don't think he was able to finish this chapter completely so I have copied these few additional notes for the reader. Philippa.

***Clinical Point**. Explaining the variable nature of the symptoms over time helps the patient deal with flare ups, rather than thinking 'It's all gone out again' when it's worse. The patient thinks 'This is normal and will settle back down.' It also helps the patient from getting despondent with treatment not working. Remember the Toblerone recovery graph.*

Let's now look at behaviour of pain related to **posture and movements**.

- *most nerve root problems seem to adopt relieving postures that tend to enlarge the spinal canal, the radicular canal and the intervertebral foramen i.e. flexion and deviation away from the side of symptoms*

  Thus the lumbar nerve root prefers to stoop in flexion when standing, may even have found crutches helpful.

- *relief is short lived, key =restless*

- *have been told to adopt good postures, or sleep on hard mattresses etc. patients usually find this impossible to maintain*

- *we need to think of adaptive and maladaptive pain and relate to postures as well*
- *being restless and constantly shifting may be as adaptive as being flexed and shifted*
- *many 'low end of the spectrum' nerve roots and/or low sensitivity ones may have great difficulty in identifying postures and movements that provoke their symptoms*

  (this is especially so with those that have a degree of 'latent' provocation)
- *many nerve root conditions with dominant distal symptoms have pretty good spinal movements and do not complain of symptoms here.*

Cervical – short term relief:

- *arm overhead, 'shoulder abduction relief' sign*
- *scapular support in elevation, not always helpful*
- *neck flexion and flexion plus deviation away from the side of pain*
- *night time – pillows and flexion*
- *deviation towards the side of pain, small percentage, often like scapula elevation and arm tucked into side*
- *protective postures of parts that hurt e.g. grip arm*

Lumbar – short term relief:

- *curled up on side*
- *supine-twisted – class manip position, painful side uppermost and rotated towards flexion – may be elements of foraminal enlargement combined with root 'slackening'?*
- *crook lying, legs up on pillows*
- *flexed standing, flexed and deviated away*
- *foot up on stool or chair while standing – to flex*
- *restless and being on move all the time*
- *taking weight off the affected leg*
- *taking weight off the affected side buttock or thigh while sitting*
- *small percentage sit bolt upright and in extension*
- *rubbing, massaging and wriggling all the time*

Symptom provocation:

- *being in one position or doing repetitive movements for a long time*
- *movements and postures that compress the root, extension reduces the*

diameter of the spinal canal, radicular canal in the lumbar spine and intervertebral foramen.

More so in the older and degenerate neck, or in the presence of oedema, disc protrusion, facet enlargement, osteophytes etc.

Cervical 'closing' – extending the neck, sustained neck extension, repeated cervical retraction exercises, movements towards the painful side. Activities like: shaving, lying supine with one pillow, looking up, washing hair under shower, swimming breaststroke and lying prone.

Lumbar 'closing' or compression – prolonged standing, lying supine or prone, walking, sitting upright, activities which involve reaching overhead.

Many patients may not find extension a problem. Ask yourself the question, 'Do they have very limited extension already due to age related changes and degeneration?' The elderly spine may adopt fixed flexion as a very adaptive 'nerve-saving' process!

- *movements and postures that tend to elongate the root*

Cervical 'elongation' – flexed postures away from side of pain. Postures and movements that depress the scapular and stretch the arm e.g. carrying shopping or just sitting with arms relaxed.

Lumbar 'elongation' – as cervical. Many lumbar 'roots' can bend with bent knees – tying shoelaces, but can't bend to floor when standing. Head flexion may come into picture – remember slump test!

Some points:

- *Remember that all movements of the limbs provide an increased sensory barrage into the afftected segments of the spinal cord. From a central pain physiology perspective it is quite possible for any movement to facilitate or inhibit symptoms – beware false positives.*

- *Other tissues are often sensitive in addition to nerve roots – nociceptive barrages can come from the surrounding segments and related tissues. These barrages may facilitate nerve root derived barrages too.*

Section NR 5
Read what I've read

Slipman C.W. (1997) Symptom provocation of fluoroscopically guided cervical nerve root stimulation. Are dynatomal maps indentical to dermatomal maps? Spine 23(20):2235-2242.

www.ingramcontent.com/pod-product-compliance
Ingram Content Group UK Ltd.
Pitfield, Milton Keynes, MK11 3LW, UK
UKHW020425250726
13967UKWH00007B/2826

9 781739 948610